The Physician Assistant's Business Practice and Legal Guide

Michele Roth-Kauffman, JD, PA-C

Associate Dean, College of Sciences,
Engineering, and Health Sciences
Chair, Physician Assistant Program
Gannon University, Erie, PA

JONES AND BARTLETT PUBLISHERS

Sudbury, Massachusetts

BOSTON   TORONTO   LONDON   SINGAPORE

World Headquarters
Jones and Bartlett Publishers
40 Tall Pine Drive
Sudbury, MA 01776
978-443-5000
info@jbpub.com
www.jbpub.com

Jones and Bartlett Publishers Canada
6339 Ormindale Way
Mississauga, ON L5V 1J2
CANADA

Jones and Bartlett Publishers International
Barb House, Barb Mews
London W6 7PA
UK

Jones and Bartlett's books and products are available through most bookstores and online booksellers. To contact Jones and Bartlett Publishers directly, call 800-832-0034, fax 978-443-8000, or visit our website www.jbpub.com. Substantial discounts on bulk quantities of Jones and Bartlett's publications are available to corporations, professional associations, and other qualified organizations. For details and specific discount information, contact the special sales department at Jones and Bartlett via the above contact information or send an email to specialsales@jbpub.com.

Production Credits
Acquisitions Editor: Jack Bruggeman
Production Director: Amy Rose
Associate Production Editor: Daniel Stone
Editorial Assistant: Kylah McNeill/Katilyn Crowley
Marketing Manager: Emily Ekle
Associate Marketing Manager: Laura Kavigian
Manufacturing Buyer: Therese Connell
Composition: Shawn Girsberger
Cover Design: Kristin Ohlin
Printing and Binding: Malloy Incorporated
Cover Printing: Malloy Incorporated

Library of Congress Cataloging-in-Publication Data
Roth-Kauffman, Michele.
   The physician assistant's business practice and legal guide / Michele Roth-Kauffman ; contributors, Mark Kauffman ... [et al.].
     p. ; cm.
   Includes index.
   ISBN: 0-7637-2674-5 (hardcover : alk. paper)
     1. Physicians' assistants—United States. 2. Physicians' assistants—Licenses—United States. 3. Physicians' assistants—Legal status, laws, etc.—United States. I. Title.
[DNLM: 1. Physician Assistants--United States. 2. Licensure—United States. 3. Professional Practice—legislation & jurisprudence—United States.]
R697.P45R686 2006
   610.73'72--dc22

                                                                                        2005004504

Printed in the United States of America
09 08 07 06 05   10 9 8 7 6 5 4 3 2 1

To my family for their love, support, and belief that I can do anything—

especially Rita (Mom), Jack (Dad), Mark, Adam, and Kevin

*To all PAs for their dedication to improving patient care and
promoting the Physician Assistant Profession*

And

*In memory of Mrs. Jisa,
former Holy Name High School Guidance Counselor (Parma Heights, Ohio)
for introducing me to the Physician Assistant Profession*

Table of Contents

Contributors

Mark Kauffman, DO, PA
Chapter 9
1) Primary Care Physician
   Medical Student/Residency Program Coordinator
   Erie Pennsylvania Veteran's Administration
2) Director of Physical Diagnosis for the Problem Based Pathway Program
   Clinical Assistant Professor of Family Medicine
   Lake Erie College of Osteopathic Medicine
3) Medical Director
   Physician Assistant Department
   Gannon University
   Erie, PA

Holly Jodon, MPAS, PA-C
Chapter 10
Faculty
Physician Assistant Department
Gannon University
Erie, PA

William Duryea, PhD, PA-C
Chapter 11
Department of Physician Assistant Studies
St. Francis University
Loretto, PA

Catherine Gillespie, DHSc, PA-C
Chapter 12
Associate Director
Physician Assistant Department
Gannon University
Erie, PA

Preface

This reference text is offered as a medical and legal resource for the physician assistant profession. It is intended for use through all phases of the professional development of the physician assistant; from the high school student sorting through career options to physician assistant students, practicing physician assistants and supervisory physicians, and those who are considering practicing with a physician assistant.

The book reviews the history and development of the profession, allowing an understanding of the role the physician assistant plays in the health care team approach to patient care. It defines the scope of practice, along with the key collaboration between the physician assistant and the supervising physician. Regulatory requirements are delineated by state, including basic requirements and maintenance of licensure and certification.

The practicing physician assistant is an asset to the community, providing quality care and continuity within the health care team. Prescriptive practices allow these providers to fluently deliver care under the auspices of their supervisory physicians. Physician assistants practice under the scope of their supervisory physician, spanning the diversity of medical practice from primary care to specialty medicine.

As a business team member, a physician assistant can generate substantial income for practices, meeting demands of increased patient volumes under a history of shrinking reimbursements. Understanding income generation allows for more compelling contract negotiations. Inappropriate coding and billing of office visits can lead to substantial loss of revenue. This text reviews the components of the history and physical examination and the development of an assessment and plan that will allow for an appropriate level of billing and reimbursement commensurate with level of service provided, optimizing the financial return and avoiding unnecessary loss of revenue.

Issues of risk management, confidentiality, and ethics are reviewed, allowing the physician assistant to practice in a safe environment, protecting both patients and providers as health care is delivered.

In summary, I hope this text serves to answer many of the questions faced by our profession on a daily basis and to further promote the profession as a growing, dynamic member of a quality health care team.

CHAPTER 1

The Physician Assistant Profession

History of the Profession • Definition of Physician Assistant • Services Provided by PAs • PA Education • Applicants to PA Programs • Initials • Regulatory Terms • Areas of Practice • PA Organizations • Demographics • Income • Outlook •Work Settings • National PA Week • PAs Compared to Physicians • PAs Compared to Nurse Practitioners • The American College of Clinicians (ACC) • Registered Nurses • Medical Assistants (MAs) • **Appendix 1** State-byState Definition of Physician Assistant

HISTORY OF THE PROFESSION

In response to a shortage and uneven distribution of primary care physicians in the mid-1960s, Dr. Eugene Stead of the Duke University Medical Center in North Carolina put together the first class of physician assistants (PAs) in 1965. The first class of PAs consisted of Navy corpsmen who had gained considerable medical training during their military service in the Vietnam War. The curriculum was based upon the medical model and the fast-track training of doctors during World War II.

The PA profession was developed in order to expand the delivery of quality medical care. It was thought that physicians could treat more patients, utilize their time more wisely, and provide better care to patients with a PA under their supervision.[1]

DEFINITION OF PHYSICIAN ASSISTANT

A physician assistant is a health care professional who has graduated from an accredited PA educational program and is authorized by the state to practice medicine under the supervision of a licensed physician. A PA who is employed by the federal government is credentialed to practice and subject to federal guidelines, which are not necessarily the same as state regulations.

The duties of a physician assistant are delegated by the supervising physician and must be within the scope of practice of the supervising physician, within the PA's training and experience, and allowed by law.[2]

Physician assistants take patient histories and perform physical examinations, develop a differential diagnosis for each of their patients' medical disorders, order and interpret laboratory tests, asses patients, tailor treatment plans to individual patient needs, prescribe medications, suture wounds, assist in surgery, provide patient education and counseling, provide treatments in emergency situations, provide rehabilitative services, and make rounds in nursing homes and hospitals.

Forty-eight states, the District of Columbia, and Guam have enacted laws that allow physicians to delegate prescriptive authority to PAs; Indiana and Ohio are the only states that have not.

Physician assistants are also referred to as *physician extenders* and *mid-level practitioners*.

Physician Extenders

The term *physician extender* refers to either a physician assistant or a nurse practitioner. Physicians' associations usually use the term.[3]

Mid-Level Practitioners

States, the federal government, and physician associations use the term *mid-level practitioner*.

> Pursuant to Title 21, Code of Federal Regulations, Section 1300.01(b28), the term *mid-level practitioner* means an individual practitioner other than a physician, dentist, veterinarian, or podiatrist, who is licensed, registered, or otherwise permitted by the United States or the jurisdiction in which he/she practices, to dispense a controlled substance in the course of professional practice. Examples of mid-level practitioners include, but are not limited to, health care providers such as nurse practitioners, nurse midwives, nurse anesthetists, clinical nurse specialists, and physician assistants who are authorized to dispense controlled substances by the state in which they practice.[4]

SERVICES PROVIDED BY PAs

PAs may perform any service delegated to them by their supervising physician that is in the scope of the practice of the supervising physician, as long as the PA is trained to provide that service and it is authorized by the laws and the regulatory body of the state in which the PA is practicing.

PAs' responsibilities include:

- Compiling complete patient histories that detail the patient's chief complaint, history of present illness, past medical history, social history, immunizations, past surgical history, past hospitalizations, and the review of systems on healthy and acutely ill patients

- Performing comprehensive or problem-specific physical exams, including drivers physicals, school and sports physicals, obstetrical exams, and yearly gynecological examinations
- Ordering and interpreting diagnostic tests for screening and diagnosis, such as basic metabolic panels, urinalysis, complete blood counts, and electrocardiograms
- Ordering and interpreting X-rays
- Performing therapeutic procedures and corrective measures, including joint injections, arthrocentesis, minor surgical procedures, suturing, biopsies of the skin, cryotherapy, and cast removal
- Making referrals of individuals to the appropriate specialists, including physicians, physical therapists, or other health care providers
- Developing and monitoring treatment plans based on patient diagnosis and response to therapy
- Prescribing and ordering the appropriate diet for individual health needs
- Educating patients on disease prevention, general health, compliance, and risk management
- Informing patients of treatment options and encouraging patients to take an active role in their health care
- Providing crisis intervention and referrals for psychiatric evaluation
- Prescribing medications and other treatments as well as educating patients on side effects and benefits of the treatment
- Obtaining informed consent for treatment
- Providing family planning services and prenatal care
- Immunizing children and adults and providing well-child care
- Assisting in surgery and providing preoperative and postoperative care
- Providing care in emergency or urgent care centers
- Participating in research activities and projects
- Providing educational services in the community
- Precepting physician assistant, medical, and other health-science students
- Participating in on-call activities
- Developing educational materials and practice guidelines
- Serving as a safety-compliance officer for the practice
- Initiating and maintaining follow-up on abnormal lab results and noncompliant patients
- Making rounds in nursing homes and hospitals
- Providing consultation services for patients who have been admitted to the hospital, nursing home, or rehabilitation center
- Corresponding with government agencies, employers, and other health care professionals regarding patients as necessary while complying with federal privacy regulations
- Being aware of socioeconomic and cultural issues that affect the availability of and compliance with health care

- Linking patients with the appropriate community services and resources
- Supervising and providing educational opportunities for other PAs, nurses, medical assistants, and nonlicensed health care workers
- Providing education on the PA profession at health fairs and school programs
- Volunteering at community and workplace programs
- Representing the PA profession and providing education on the profession before legislative bodies, agencies, and private business

The responsibilities delegated to a PA depend upon the specialty of the supervising physician, the practice setting, the education and experience of the PA, and the laws and regulations of the state in which the PA is practicing. All states require a PA to be licensed, registered, or to hold a certificate.

PA EDUCATION

Physician assistant education follows the medical model, which complements physician training, and is competency based. A physician assistant student is required to demonstrate proficiency in medical knowledge and meet behavioral and clinical objectives. Medical doctor (MD), doctor of osteopathy (DO), doctor of dental science (DDS), and juris doctor (JD) degrees are also competency based.

There are 135 PA educational programs in the United States, which are accredited by the Accreditation Review Commission on Education for the Physician Assistant Inc. (ARC-PA). All programs are required to meet ARC-PA standards. Site visits are made periodically to each program in order to assure compliance with the standards.

Classroom and laboratory instruction in the basic medical sciences including anatomy, physiology, pathophysiology, pathology, biochemistry, microbiology, pharmacology, physical diagnosis, clinical laboratory science, behavioral medicine, medical ethics, and clinical medicine occur prior to the clinical phase of the program. The clinical curriculum must include rotations in internal medicine including exposure to geriatrics and nursing home care; family medicine including exposure to pediatrics; behavioral medicine; pre- and postnatal care; and gynecology, surgery, and emergency medicine.[5]

Physician assistants are trained in primary care programs and receive a broad education in medicine. This allows PAs to practice in the areas of primary care medicine, internal medicine, family medicine, pediatrics, and obstetrics and gynecology, as well as surgery and surgical subspecialties. There are also several postgraduate programs, which offer PAs additional training in medical specialties such as neonatology, orthopedics, oncology, and cardiovascular surgery.

The typical PA program is 22 to 27 months in length.[6] The majority of the first half of the program is spent in the classroom and is considered the didactic phase. The PA student spends the last half of the program in doctors' offices, clinics, and hospitals where he or she is exposed to intensive hands-on clinical experiences in multiple medical disciplines. Physician assistant students complete over 2000 hours of supervised clinical practice prior to graduation. Each program has its own set of prerequisites, which usually include courses in chemistry, biology, psychology, and medical terminology. Many programs require or give preference to candidates with prior medical experience.

There are courses of study available that allow students to enter into 4- or 5-year programs. The student typically completes the prerequisites for entry into the professional phase of the program in the first 2 or 3 years and then enters the professional phase of the program, which runs the last 22 to 27 months. These programs offer entry to the profession to students straight out of high school and to nontraditional students who do not have a bachelor's degree.

The profession has not adopted a minimum degree, preferring to use competency as a way of measuring skill. The American Academy of Physician Assistants (AAPA) endorses the baccalaureate degree as the minimum degree for PAs.[7] Whether or not the master's degree should become the minimum degree required for entry into the profession continues to be debated. Proponents of the master's degree requirement believe that it would bring greater acceptance to the profession by both patients and other health care professionals. Opponents believe that one of the disadvantages of requiring a master's degree is that it could make it more difficult for minorities to gain entry into the profession. Currently, 90 of the 137 accredited programs confer a master's degree upon completion of their program of study.[8]

After graduation, PAs are required to log 100 hours of continuing medical education every 2 years in order to maintain certification.

Information obtained in the 2004 AAPA Physician Assistant Census revealed that 50% of the respondents received a bachelor's degree from PA school and 22% received a master's-level PA degree. Overall, 35% of respondents hold a master's degree and 2% a doctoral degree. Of the 58,826 individuals eligible to practice as PAs, 23,494 completed surveys; this represents 38% of all individuals eligible to practice as PAs.[9]

Since the beginning of 2005, Mississippi has required PAs to have a master's degree in a science- or health-related field in order to practice in the state.

APPLICANTS TO PA PROGRAMS

The average age of a student applying to a PA program is 27.5. In 2003, 81% of all students enrolled in PA programs had earned at least a bachelor's degree and had a mean 32.4 months of prior medical experience.[10] It is common for emergency medical technicians (EMTs), paramedics, and nurses to apply to PA programs.

Applicants to PA programs are required to meet the following technical standards:

A candidate for admission to the PA program must have the use of certain sensory and motor functions to permit him or her to carry out the activities described in the sections that follow. Graduation from the program signifies that the individual is prepared for entry into clinical practice or into postgraduate training programs. Therefore, it follows that graduates must have the knowledge and skills needed to function in a broad variety of clinical situations and to render a wide spectrum of diagnostic and therapeutic care. The candidate and student must be able to consistently, quickly, and accurately integrate all information received by whatever senses are employed. Also, they must have the intellectual ability to learn, integrate, analyze, and synthesize data.

A candidate for a PA program ordinarily must have abilities and skills of five varieties, including observation; communication; motor; intellectual; conceptual, integrative, and quantitative; and behavioral and social. Where technological assistance is available in the program, it may be permitted for disabilities in certain areas. Under all circumstances, a candidate should possess certain qualities that allow him/her to perform in a reasonably independent manner:

1. *Observation*—Candidates and students ordinarily must have sufficient vision to be able to observe demonstrations, experiments, and laboratory exercises. They must be able to observe a patient accurately at a distance and close at hand.

2. *Communication*—Candidates and students ordinarily must be able to communicate with patients and colleagues. They should be able to hear, but if technological compensation is available, it may be permitted for some handicaps in this area. Candidates and students must be able to read, write, and speak English.

3. *Motor*—Candidates and students ordinarily should have sufficient motor function such that they are able to execute movements reasonably required to provide general care and emergency treatment to patients. Examples of emergency treatment reasonably required of physician assistants are cardiopulmonary resuscitation, administration of intravenous medication, the application of pressure to stop bleeding, the opening of obstructed airways, the suturing of simple wounds, and the performance of simple obstetrical maneuvers. These actions require coordination of both gross and fine muscular movements, equilibrium, and functional use of the senses of touch and vision.

4. *Intellectual, conceptual, integrative, and quantitative abilities*—These abilities include measurement, calculation, reasoning, analysis, and synthesis. Problem solving, the critical intellectual skill demanded of a physician assistant, requires all of these intellectual abilities. In addition, candidates and students should be able to comprehend three-dimensional relationships and understand the spatial relationships of structures.

5. *Behavioral and social abilities*—Candidates and students must possess the emotional health required for full utilization of the intellectual abilities, the the exercise of good judgment, the prompt completion of all responsibilities attendant to the assessment and care of patients, and the development

of mature, sensitive, and effective relationships with patients. Candidates and students must be able to tolerate physically taxing workloads, adapt to changing environments, display flexibility, and learn to function in the face of uncertainties inherent in the clinical problems of many patients. Compassion, integrity, concern for others, interpersonal skills, interest, and motivation are all personal qualities to be assessed during the admissions and educational processes.

PA programs are committed to provide reasonable accommodations to students with an identifiable disability as defined by the Americans with Disabilities Act. In doing so, however, PA programs must maintain the integrity of their curriculum and preserve those elements deemed essential to educating candidates to become effective physician assistants.

INITIALS

Physician Assistant-Certified (PA-C) designates a person who has completed the designated course of study, graduated from an accredited physician assistant program, and passed the Physician Assistant National Certifying Exam (PANCE) developed by the National Board of Medical Examiners and administered by the National Commission on Certification of Physician Assistants (NCCPA). The NCCPA is an independent organization responsible for administering the national exam and certifying physician assistants. Commissioners of the NCCPA represent a number of different medical professions including physicians and physician assistants. In order to maintain certification and continue to use the *C* after *PA* a physician assistant must log 100 hours of continuing medical education (CME) every 2 years and pass a recertification exam every 6 years. A physician assistant is required to log his or her CME credits with the NCCPA. The NCCPA has a system for auditing physician assistants' CME credits in order to ensure that the credits logged meet the required standards.

REGULATORY TERMS

Licensure, certification, and *registration* are the three terms used in state laws for the credentialing of physician assistants. Physician assistants who are currently working in states that certify or register PAs should begin to work through the legislative process in order to change those state laws. It is important for the profession to work toward licensure as the credential for all PAs.

The Pew Health Professions Commission Task Force on Health Care Workforce Regulation recommends that states "license" health professions. "Certification" should be used by organizations that attest to the competency of individual health professionals.[11] In order for a physician assistant to be certified by the National Commission on Certification of Physician Assistants, a candidate must have graduated from an accredited physician assistant program and must pass the national certification exam. "Licensure" of physician assistants by the states will promote clarity and acceptance by the public and other health care professions.

In order for a physician assistant to practice in a state he or she must be granted permission. The state will contact the program the PA graduated from for verification that the prescribed course of study was completed. The PA must have the NCCPA send his or her passing board results directly to the state, or provide a letter verifying that the PA passed the exam. PA practice is regulated by each state; however, there are several states that do not refer to this practice as *licensure*. "Licensure is the most rigorous method of regulation.... Licensing physician assistants holds the profession to rigorous standards and creates credential parity."[12]

Many laws and insurance provisions refer to *licensed providers*. In states where physician assistants are not licensed, PAs have been denied permission to provide services to patients and/or have not been eligible for reimbursement for certain services provided. By obtaining licensure, PAs increase their marketability because they are allowed to perform more duties and be reimbursed for them. Obtaining licensure also makes it less likely that PAs will be confused with "unlicensed assistive personnel."[13]

One of the requirements for physician assistants to obtain permission to practice in a state is that they have a supervising physician. Licensure will not allow a physician assistant to practice independently or collect payment for reimbursable services. All reimbursements for PA services are made directly to the supervising physician, practice, clinic, or hospital that employs the PA.[14]

> The American Academy of Physician Assistants recommends licensure for physician assistants. Currently in the 50 states and DC, PAs are licensed in 44 jurisdictions, certified in four, and registered in three.[15]

AREAS OF PRACTICE

PAs are found in all areas of medicine and practice in over 61 specialty fields, including family/general practice, general internal medicine, obstetrics and gynecology, pediatrics, general surgery and surgical subspecialties, emergency medicine, and subspecialties of internal medicine.[16] PAs assist in surgery, perform invasive procedures, supervise other PAs and other clinical staff, and precept PA students and students of other health professions. PAs serve patient populations that range from newborns to the elderly.

PA ORGANIZATIONS

American Academy of Physician Assistants (AAPA)

The AAPA is the only national organization representing PAs in all medical specialties. AAPA was founded in 1968 and currently has 57 constituent chapters representing PAs in all 50 states, the District of Columbia, Guam, and the federal services.

AAPA's mission is to "promote quality, cost effective, accessible health care and to promote the professional and personal development of physician assistants."[17]

The AAPA is active in educational efforts geared toward the general public in order to increase knowledge of the PA profession, provides continuing medical education opportunities for PAs, and conducts research on PAs and the PA profession.

The AAPA's vision is that "physician assistants will be worldwide leaders vital to providing and improving the medical care of all people."[18]

Association of Physician Assistant Programs (APAP)

APAP, the national organization representing physician assistant programs, was established in 1972. "APAP's mission is to assist PA educational programs in the instruction of highly educated physician assistants."[19]

The association offers conferences and workshops aimed at faculty and leadership development.

Accreditation Review Commission on Education for the Physician Assistant (ARC-PA)

ARC-PA defines the minimum standards for PA education and ensures program compliance by performing periodic site visits. The accrediting agency is responsible for protecting the interests of the public and the PA profession.[20]

ARC-PA standards are approved by the:

- American Academy of Family Physicians
- American Academy of Pediatrics
- American Academy of Physician Assistants
- American College of Physicians
- American Society of Internal Medicine
- American College of Surgeons
- American Medical Association
- Association of Physician Assistant Programs

National Commission on the Certification of Physician Assistants (NCCPA)

The NCCPA is an independent organization responsible for the certification of PAs. The NCCPA administers the Physician Assistant National Certifying Exam (PANCE). The exam is a 360-question multiple-choice exam administered 50 weeks out of the year. Passing the exam is a prerequisite for licensure, certification, or registration in all 50 states. Only graduates of an accredited physician assistant program are eligible to sit for the exam. Candidates cannot sit for the exam prior to graduation.[21]

DEMOGRAPHICS

The AAPA estimates that there were 61,891 individuals eligible to practice as PAs in the United States in 2004 and that there were 58,826 PAs in clinical practice at the beginning of 2004. New York (9.7%), California (8.3%), Texas (6.2%), Pennsylvania (5.7%), Florida (5.4%), and North Carolina (5.2%) had the highest number of clinically practicing PAs who responded to the 2004 census. In 2005 the AAPA projects that New York and California will be the states with the greatest number of PAs practicing, and Mississippi and Arkansas are projected to have the smallest number of practicing PAs in 2005.[22]

INCOME

The median total annual income from primary employers for PAs who are not self-employed and who work at least 32 hours per week was reported as $74,264, with a mean of $78,257 in 2004. The median total annual income reported by PAs who graduated in 2003 was $65,783, with a mean of $67,797.[23]

OUTLOOK

The number of PA jobs is expected to increase by 36% or more between 2000 and 2010 due to the expansion of the health care industry and the focus on cost containment. Job opportunities in areas that have a difficult time attracting physicians, such as rural areas and inner cities, will continue to offer employment to PAs. PAs will also be utilized in states that have imposed legal limitations on the number of hours worked by physician residents to supply some of the services previously provided by physician residents.[24]

WORK SETTINGS

The largest group of PAs (43%) who responded to the 2004 census are employed by a single or multispecialty physician group practice. Hospitals employ 22%, solo physicians employ 14%, and 10% of respondents work for some type of government agency. Just over 2% of respondents work for the Department of Veterans Affairs, making it the largest single government employer of PAs. State governments collectively employ approximately 2% of the 2004 respondents.

The most prevalent work setting for PAs is a hospital (reported by 37% of respondents). Another 29% reported working in a group practice office setting. Eight percent work in a federally qualified health center or community health center.

The majority of respondents (87%) work full time with a 44.4-hour (median 42-hour) work week. Thirty-nine percent of respondents take call. PAs were on call a mean of 99 hours per month.[25]

NATIONAL PA WEEK

National PA Week is celebrated October 6–13 and commemorates the graduation of the first class of PA students from the Duke University Medical Center's PA program. National PA Week is celebrated in a variety of ways. PAs perform community service projects such as free blood pressure screenings or blood drives, sponsor educational programs, or visit their legislative representatives in order to increase their awareness of the PA profession.

PAs COMPARED TO PHYSICIANS

Physician assistant education mirrors physician education. PA program curricula follow the "medical model." In institutions that house both PA schools and medical schools, PA students attend many of same classes as medical students.

One of the main differences between PAs and physicians is the length of time in training. Although the core content of the curriculum is similar, physicians spend an average of 42 months in formal education whereas the professional phase of PA training averages 22–27 months. Physicians are also required to do an internship year (which may be included as part of their residency). The majority of physicians also complete a residency in a specialty in order to be eligible for board certification. Residencies range from 2 to 5 years. Additional training beyond residency in the form of fellowships is required for certain areas of specialization, such as transplant surgery, or when a physician changes his or her area of specialization.

"A physician has complete responsibility for the care of the patient. PAs share that responsibility with the supervising physician."[26]

PAs COMPARED TO NURSE PRACTITIONERS

There are several differences between a nurse practitioner (NP) and a physician assistant. The most important difference is that a nurse practitioner can work independently under his or her license if state law allows it. A physician assistant always works under the supervision of a physician and does not practice independently.

Nurse practitioners are nurses with an additional 1 to 2 years of training and describe themselves as nurses with a broadened scope of practice. Physician assistants come from a variety of health care backgrounds, including nursing.

NPs have a specific area of certification such as family nurse practitioner (FNP), pediatric NP, and obstetrical/gynecological NP. Physician assistants receive primary care training and are not limited to one specialty.

NPs are not required to pass a certification exam in all states. All physician assistants are required to pass the national exam administered by the NCCPA before they are certified.

PAs and NPs operate under different state laws and regulations. Medical boards regulate PAs and nursing boards regulate NPs.

Even though there are many differences between PAs and NPs, their roles in health care can be similar. In some states the services and job descriptions of NPs and PAs are interchangeable. This is especially true if an NP is employed by a physician.

Due to these similarities the University of California, Davis, FNP/PA Program educates both groups of professionals together.[27]

THE AMERICAN COLLEGE OF CLINICIANS (ACC)

The ACC was founded in 2003 and is the first national organization aimed at uniting PAs and NPs. The organization advocates the rights of all advanced-practice clinicians. One of the organization's goals is to encourage the professions to work together in order to improve conditions for both professions. The ACC plans to educate physicians, pharmacists, and the public about NPs and PAs. Ultimately, the organization hopes that PAs and NPs will join together to work on legislative and reimbursement issues together.[28]

REGISTERED NURSES

Nursing is the largest health care occupation. Over half of all nurses are employed in hospital inpatient or outpatient settings. Nurses are also employed in clinics and physician offices, nursing homes, schools, government, residential care agencies, home health care, research, management, public relations firms, insurance agencies, and by private individuals. Nurses are trained in a nursing model that includes classroom instruction as well as supervised clinical experiences in hospitals and nursing homes, home health care, and outpatient clinics. In order to obtain a nursing license, a student must graduate from an approved nursing program and pass a national licensing examination.

Registered nurses (RNs) may hold an associate degree in nursing (ADN), Bachelor of Science degree in nursing (BSN), or a diploma from a hospital-administered program. A graduate from an ADN, BSN, or diploma program is eligible for licensure after successful completion of the licensing exam. State laws govern the scope of practice for nurses. Nurses are required to renew their license periodically, and some states require nurses to obtain some form of continuing education credits.

Clinical duties of nurses include:

- Observing and assessing patients
- Recording patients' symptoms, reactions, and progress in patient charts
- Developing and managing nursing care plans
- Preparing patients and assisting physicians, NPs, and PAs during procedures and examinations
- Administering medications and injections and starting intravenous fluids following an order given by a health care provider with prescriptive privileges

- Providing care to patients in the hospital and carrying out medical plans
- Helping patients cope with illness and promoting wellness and disease prevention
- Assisting patients in rehabilitation
- Changing dressing on wounds and incisions
- Arranging for health screenings and immunizations
- Supervising licensed practical nurses and nurses aides
- Performing routine laboratory and office work and maintaining records
- Providing nursing services to patients in their homes
- Offering health counseling and education for patients and their families
- Developing educational programs for the community[29]

MEDICAL ASSISTANTS (MAs)

Medical assistants handle administrative and clinical duties in a physician office and should not be confused with physician assistants.[30] Administrative duties handled by MAs include:

- Greeting patients and answering phones
- Updating and filing patient records
- Filling out insurance forms
- Corresponding with patients
- Scheduling appointments
- Arranging for hospital admissions and testing
- Billing and bookkeeping

State laws regulate MAs' clinical duties. Clinical duties of MAs include:

- Taking medical histories
- Recording vital signs
- Explaining procedures to patients
- Preparing patients for exams
- Assisting the provider during an exam
- Collecting and preparing laboratory specimens
- Performing basic laboratory tests in the office
- Sterilizing medical instruments
- Administering medications as directed
- Drawing blood
- Preparing patients for X-rays
- Changing dressings
- Performing electrocardiograms
- Calling in prescriptions
- Removing sutures
- Arranging examining room equipment
- Maintaining supplies and equipment

References

1. The American Academy of Physician Assistants Web site. Available at http://www.aapa.org. Accessed November 2003.

2. The American Academy of Physician Assistants Web Site. Available at http://www.aapa.org. Accessed November 2003.

3. Buppert, C. (2003). *Nurse Practitioner's Business Practice and Legal Guide* (p. 2). Gaithersburg, MD: Aspen.

4. The US Department of Justice Drug Enforcement Administration Web site. Available at http://www.deadivision.usdoj.gov/drugreg/practitioners/index.html. Accessed November 2003.

5. Accreditation Review Commission on Education for the Physician Assistant. (2001). *Accreditation Standards for Physician Assistant Education*, Marshfield, WI: ARC-PA.

6. The American Academy of Physician Assistants Web site. Available at http://www.aapa.org. Accessed December 2003.

7. The American Academy of Physician Assistants Web site. Available at http://www.aapa.org. Accessed March 2005.

8. The American Academy of Physician Assistants Web site. Available at http://www.aapa.org. Accessed December 2003.

9. The American Academy of Physician Assistants Web site. Available at http://www.aapa.org. Accessed October 2003.

10. Simon AF. (2004). *20th Annual Report on Physician Assistant Programs in the United States, 2003–2004.* (pp. 37–55). Alexandria, VA: Association of Physician Assistant Programs.

11. The American Academy of Physician Assistants Web site. Available at http://www.aapa.org. Accessed December 2003.

12. The American Academy of Physician Assistants Web site. Available at http://www.aapa.org. Accessed December 2003.

13. The American Academy of Physician Assistants Web site. Available at http://www.aapa.org. Accessed December 2003. .

14. The American Academy of Physician Assistants Web site. Available at http://www.aapa.org. Accessed December 2003.

15. The American Academy of Physician Assistants Web site. Available at http://www.aapa.org. Accessed March 2005.

16. The American Academy of Physician Assistants Web site. Available at http://www.aapa.org. Accessed December 2003.

17. The American Academy of Physician Assistants Web site. Available at http://www.aapa.org. Accessed December 2003.

18. The American Academy of Physician Assistants Web site. Available at http://www.aapa.org. Accessed December 2003.

19. The American Academy of Physician Assistants Web site. Available at http://www.aapa.org. Accessed December 2003.

20. The Accreditation Review Commission on Education for the Physician Assistant, Inc., Web site. Available at http://www.arc-pa.org. Accessed December 2003.

21. National Commission on the Certification of Physician Assistants. Available at http://www.nccpa.net. Accessed December 2003.

22. The American Academy of Physician Assistants Web site. Available at http://www.aapa.org. Accessed October 2004.

23. The American Academy of Physician Assistants Web site. Available at http://www.aapa.org. Accessed October 2004.

24. The United States Department of Labor, Bureau of Labor Statistics Web site. *Occupational Outlook Handbook, 2002–03 Edition.* Available at http://www.bls.gov. Accessed December 2003.

25. The American Academy of Physician Assistants Web site. Available at http://www.aapa.org. Accessed October 2004.

26. The American Academy of Physician Assistants Web site. Available at http://www.aapa.org. Accessed December 2003.

27. UC Davis Web site. Available at http://fnppa.ucdavis.edu. Accessed December 2003.

28. Herrick, T. (2003). The American College of Clinicians is born. *Clinicians News*, 7(9), 1.

29. The United States Department of Labor, Bureau of Labor Statistics Web site. *Occupational Outlook Handbook*, 2002–03 Edition. Availaible at http://www.bls.gov. Accessed December 2003.

30. The United States Department of Labor, Bureau of Labor Statistics Web site, *Occupational Outlook Handbook*, 2002-03 Edition. Available at http://www.bls.gov. Accessed December 2003.

State by State Definition of Physician Assistant

ALABAMA

ASSISTANT TO PHYSICIAN. A person who is a graduate of an approved program, is licensed by the Board, and is registered by the Board to perform medical services under the supervision of a physician approved by the Board to supervise the assistant.

ALABAMA ADMIN. CODE R. 540-X-7-.01(1)

ALASKA

"physician assistant" means a person specially trained to perform many of the functions and duties of the physician, including examination, diagnosis and treatment, and who is licensed under this chapter to do so;

12 ALASKA ADMIN. CODE 40.990(13)

ARIZONA

"Physician assistant" means a person who is licensed pursuant to this chapter and who performs health care tasks pursuant to a dependent relationship with a physician.

12 ARIZONA REV. STAT. ANN. SEC. 32-2501.13

ARKANSAS

"Physician assistant" means a person who has:
  (i) Graduated from a physician assistant or surgeon assistant program accredited by the American Medical Association's Committee on Allied Health Education and Accreditation or the Commission on Accreditation of Allied Health Education Programs; and
  (ii) Passed the certifying examination administered by the National Commission on Certification of Physician Assistants.

(B) The physician assistant is a dependent medical practitioner who:
    (i) Provides health care services under the supervision of a physician; and
    (ii) Works under a physician-drafted protocol approved by the Arkansas State Medical Board, which describes how the physician assistant and the physician will work together and any practice guidelines required by the supervising physician.

ARKANSAS CODE 17-105-101(2)

CALIFORNIA

"Physician assistant" means a person who meets the requirements of this chapter and is licensed by the committee.

CALIFORNIA BUS. & PROF. CODE SEC. 3051

COLORADO

A person licensed under the laws of this state to practice medicine may delegate to a physician assistant licensed by the board the authority to perform acts that constitute the practice of medicine to the extent and in the manner authorized by rules and regulations promulgated by the board, including the authority to prescribe medication, including controlled substances, and dispense only such drugs as designated by the board. Such acts shall be consistent with sound medical practice. Each prescription issued by a physician assistant licensed by the board shall have imprinted thereon the name of his or her supervising physician. Nothing in this subsection (5) shall limit the ability of otherwise licensed health personnel to perform delegated acts. The dispensing of prescription medication by a physician assistant shall be subject to the provisions of section 12-22-121 (6).

COLORADO REV. STAT. SEC. 12-36-106(5)(A)

CONNECTICUT

"Physician assistant" means an individual who: (A) Functions in a dependant relationship with a physician licensed pursuant to this chapter; and (B) is licensed pursuant to section 20-12b to provide patient services under the supervision, control, responsibility and direction of said physician.

CONNECTICUT GEN. STATUTE SEC. 20-12A (5)

DELAWARE

A "physician's assistant" is defined as an individual who has graduated from a physician's or surgeon's assistant program which has been accredited by the Committee on Allied Health Education and Accreditation (CAHEA) of the American Medical Association (AMA), or a successor agency acceptable to and approved by the Board, has passed a national certifying examination acceptable to the Physician's Assistant Advisory Council of the Board and approved by the full Board, and who is licensed under this chapter to practice as a physician's assistant. Physician's assistants who are currently registered in the State but who are not graduates of an approved program of the type outlined above may be licensed to practice as, and use the title "physician's assistant," provided the individual has successfully passed 1 of the national certifying examinations developed and administered by the National Board of Medical Examiners (NBME) or the National Commission on Certification of Physician's Assistants (NCCPA) on or prior to October 1987, and has maintained Continuing Medical Education (CME) credits as required by rules and regulations developed under this chapter.

TIT. 24 DEL. CODE SEC. 1770A-1

DISTRICT OF COLUMBIA

Physician Assistant—a person licensed to practice as a physician assistant under the Act.

TIT. 17 D.C. MUN. REGS. SEC. 4999

FLORIDA

"Physician assistant" means a person who is a graduate of an approved program or its equivalent or meets standards approved by the boards and is licensed to perform medical services delegated by the supervising physician.

FLORIDA STAT. ANN. SEC. 458.347 (2)(E)

GEORGIA

"Physician's assistant" means a skilled person qualified by academic and practical training to provide patients' services not necessarily within the physical presence but under the personal direction or supervision of the applying physician.

GEORGIA CODE ANN. SEC. 43-34-102 (5)

HAWAII

"Physician assistant" means an individual who has been certified by the board to practice medicine with physician supervision. A physician assistant may perform those duties and responsibilities delegated by the physician assistant's supervising physician.

HAWAII ADMIN. R SEC. 16-85-45.5

IDAHO

Physician Assistant. A person who is a graduate of an approved program and who is qualified by general education, training, experience and personal character, and who has been authorized by the Board, to render patient services under the direction of a supervising physician.

IDAHO ADMIN. CODE SEC. 22.01.03.05

ILLINOIS

"Physician assistant" means any person not a physician who has been certified as a physician assistant by the National Commission on the Certification of Physician Assistants or equivalent successor agency and performs procedures under the supervision of a physician as defined in this Act. A physician assistant may perform such procedures within the specialty of the supervising physician, except that such physician shall exercise such direction, supervision and control over such physician assistants as will assure that patients shall receive quality medical care. Physician assistants shall be capable of performing a variety of tasks within the specialty of medical care under the supervision of a physician. Supervision of the physician assistant shall not be construed to necessarily require the personal presence of the supervising physician at all times at the place where services are rendered, as long as there is communication available for consultation by radio, telephone or telecommunications within established guidelines as determined by the physician/physician assistant team. The supervising physician may delegate tasks and duties to the physician assistant. Delegated tasks or duties shall be consistent with physician assistant education, training, and experience. The delegated tasks or duties shall be specific to the practice setting and shall be implemented and reviewed under guidelines established by the physician or physician/physician assistant team. A physician assistant, acting as an agent of the physician, shall be permitted to transmit the supervising physician's orders as determined by the institution's by-laws, policies, procedures, or job description within which the physician/physician assistant team practices. Physician assistants shall practice only within the established guidelines.

ILLINOIS COMP. STAT. 225/95 (3)

INDIANA

"Physician assistant" means an individual who has:
(1) graduated from a physician assistant or surgeon assistant program accredited by an accrediting agency;
(2) passed the certifying examination administered by the NCCPA and maintains certification by the NCCPA; and
(3) been certified by the committee.

INDIANA REV. CODE SEC. 25-27.5-2-10

"Physician assistant" means an individual who has:
(1) graduated from an approved physician assistant or surgeon assistant program; and (2) passed the certifying examination and maintains certification by the NCCPA.

INDIANA ADMIN. CODE TIT. 844 R. 2.2-1-5

IOWA

"Physician assistant" means a person licensed as a physician assistant by the board.

IOWA ADMIN. CODE R. 645-326.1

KANSAS

"Physician assistant" means a person who is licensed in accordance with the provisions of K.S.A. 2000 Supp. 65-28a04 and amendments thereto and who provides patient services under the direction and supervision of a responsible physician.

KANSAS STAT. ANN. 65-28A02(4)

KENTUCKY

"Physician assistant" means a person who:

(a) Has graduated from a physician assistant or surgeon assistant program accredited by the Accreditation Review Commission on Education for Physician Assistants or its predecessor or successor agencies and has passed the certifying examination administered by the National Commission on Certification of Physician Assistants or its predecessor or successor agencies;

or

(b) Possesses a current physician assistant certificate issued by the board prior to July 15, 2002

KENTUCKY REV. STAT. SEC. 311.840(3)

LOUISIANA

Physician assistants are skilled members of the health care profession who work under the supervision of licensed physicians. They are qualified to take patient histories, perform physical examinations, and order and interpret certain diagnostic tests. A physician assistant may implement treatment plans as delegated by the supervising physician and explain them to patients.

LOUISIANA REV. STAT. SEC. 1360.21(B)

"Physician assistant" or "assistant" means a person who is a graduate of a program accredited by the Committee on Allied Health Education and Accreditation or its successors and who has successfully passed the national certificate examination administered by the National Commission on the Certification of Physicians' Assistants or its predecessors and who is approved and licensed by the Louisiana State Board of Medical Examiners to perform medical services under the supervision of a physician or group of physicians who are licensed by and registered with the board to supervise such assistant.

"Physician assistant-certified (PA-C)" means a physician assistant who is currently certified by the National Commission on the Certification of Physicians' Assistants or its successors.

LOUISIANA REV. STAT. SEC. 1360.22(5-6)

MAINE

Physician Assistant means a person who has graduated from a physician assistant or surgeon assistant program accredited by the American Medical Association Committee on Allied Health Education and Accreditation, or the Commission for Accreditation of the Allied Health Education Programs or its successor; and/or who has passed the certifying examination administered by the National Commission on Certification of Physician Assistants or its successor. Only physician assistants who are currently certified by the N.C.C.P.A. may use the initials PA-C.

CODE MAINE R. SEC. 02 373 (G)

MARYLAND

"Physician assistant" means an individual who is certified to perform delegated medical acts under the supervision of the supervising physician.

MARYLAND REGS. CODE TIT. 10 SEC. 32.03.02

MASSACHUSETTS

Physician assistant means a person who meets the requirements for registration as set forth in M.G.L. c. 112, § 9I and who may provide medical services appropriate to his or her training, experience and skills under the supervision of a registered physician.

CODE MASSACHUSETTS REGS. TIT. 263 SEC. 2.03

MICHIGAN

"Practice as a physician's assistant" means the practice of medicine or osteopathic medicine and surgery performed under the supervision of a physician or physicians licensed under this part or part 175.

MICHIGAN COMPLIED LAWS SEC. 333.17001

MINNESOTA

"Physician assistant" or "registered physician assistant" means a person registered pursuant to this chapter who is qualified by academic or practical training or both to provide patient services as specified in this chapter, under the supervision of a supervising physician.

MINNESOTA STAT. ANN. SEC. 147A.01(18)

MISSISSIPPI

"Physician assistant" means a person who meets the Board's criteria for licensure as a physician assistant and is licensed as a physician assistant by the Board. Nothing in this act authorizes the licensure of anesthesiologist's assistants.

MISSISSIPPI CODE ANN. SEC. 573-26-1

MISSOURI

"Physician assistant", a person who has graduated from a physician assistant program accredited by the American Medical Association's Committee on Allied Health Education and Accreditation or by its successor agency, who has passed the certifying examination administered by the National Commission on Certification of Physician Assistants and has active certification by the National Commission on Certification of Physician Assistants who provides health care services delegated by a licensed physician. A person who has been employed as a physician assistant for three years prior to August 28, 1989, who has passed the National Commission on Certification of Physician Assistants examination, and has active certification of the National Commission on Certification of Physician Assistants.

MISSOURI REV. STAT. SEC. 334.735 (6)

MONTANA

"Physician assistant-certified" means a member of a health care team, approved by the board, who provides medical services that may include examination, diagnosis, prescription of medications, and treatment, as approved by the board, under the supervision of a physician licensed by the board.

MONTANA CODE ANN. SEC. 37-20-401

NEBRASKA

Physician assistant means any person who graduates from a program approved by the Commission on Accreditation of Allied Health Education Programs or its predecessor or successor agency and the board, who satisfactorily completes a proficiency examination, and whom the board, with the concurrence of the department, approves to perform medical services under the supervision of a physician or group of physicians approved by the board to supervise such assistant.

NEBRASKA REV. STAT. SEC. 71-1.107.16 (7)

NEVADA

"Physician assistant" means a person who is a graduate of an academic program approved by the Board or who, by general education, practical training and experience determined to be satisfactory by the Board, is qualified to perform medical services under the supervision of a supervising physician and who has been issued a license by the Board.

NEVADA REV. STAT. SEC. 630.015

NEW HAMPSHIRE

"Physician assistant" or "P.A." means a person qualified both by academic and practical training in a program approved by the board to provide patient services under the supervision and direction of a licensed physician in a variety of medical care settings.

NEW HAMPSHIRRE REV. STAT. ANN. SEC. 326-D:1

NEW JERSEY

"Physician assistant" means a person who holds a current, valid license issued pursuant to section 4 of this act.

NEW JERSEY STAT. ANN. SEC. 45: 9-27.11

NEW MEXICO

"Physician assistant" means a health professional who is licensed by the board to practice as a physician assistant and who provides services to patients under the supervision and direction of a licensed physician....

NEW MEXICO STAT. ANN. SEC. 61-6-6

NEW YORK

The term "physician assistant" means a person who is registered as a physician assistant pursuant to this article.

NEW YORK STAT. C. L. SEC. 6540

NORTH CAROLINA

Any person who is licensed under the provisions of G.S. 90-11 to perform medical acts, tasks, and functions as an assistant to a physician may use the title "physician assistant".

NORTH CAROLINA GEN. STAT. SEC. 90-18.1(A)

"Physician Assistant" means a person licensed by and registered with the Board to perform medical acts, tasks, or functions under the supervision of a physician licensed by the Board, who performs tasks traditionally performed by the physician, and who has graduated from a physician assistant or surgeon assistant program accredited by the Commission on Accreditation of Allied Health Education Programs, or its predecessor or successor agencies.

21 NORTH CAROLINA ANN. CODE 32 SEC. .0101

NORTH DAKOTA

The terms "physician assistant" and "certified physician assistant" and the initials "PA-C" may only be used to identify a person who has been issued a certificate of qualification by the board of medical examiners. A person who uses those terms or initials as identification without having received a certificate of qualification is engaging in the practice of medicine without a license.

NORTH DAKOTA MED. PRAC. ACT SEC. 43-17-02.2

The physician assistant is a skilled person, qualified by academic and clinical training to provide patient services under the supervision and responsibility of a licensed doctor of medicine or osteopathy who is responsible for the performance of that assistant. The assistant may be involved with the patients of the physician in any medical setting for which the physician is responsible.

NORTH DAKOTA ADMIN. CODE SEC. 50-03-01-01

OHIO

"Physician assistant" means a skilled person qualified by academic and clinical training to provide services to patients as a physician assistant under the supervision and direction of one or more physicians who are responsible for the physician assistant's performance.

OHIO REV. CODE SEC. 4730.01

OKLAHOMA

"Physician assistant" means a health care professional, qualified by academic and clinical education and licensed by the State Board of Medical Licensure and Supervision, to provide health care services in any patient care setting at the direction and under the supervision of a physician or group of physicians.

OKLAHOMA STAT. ANN. TIT. 59 SEC. 519.2

OREGON

A physician assistant is a person qualified by education, training, experience, and personal character to provide medical services under the direction and supervision of a physician licensed under ORS Chapter 677, in active practice and in good standing with the Board. The purpose of the physician assistant program is to enable physicians licensed under ORS 677 to extend high quality medical care to more people throughout the state.

OREGON ADMIN. RULES SEC. 847-050-0005

"Physician assistant" means a person who is licensed as such in accordance with ORS 677.265, 677.495, 677.0505, 677.510, 677.515, 677.520, and 677.525.

OREGON ADMIN. RULES SEC. 847-050-0010

PENNSYLVANIA

Physician assistant—An individual who is certified as a physician assistant by the Board.

PENNSYLVANIA ADMIN. CODE SEC. 18.122

RHODE ISLAND

"Physician assistant" means a person, not a physician nor holding a medical doctor or equivalent degree, who is qualified by academic and practical training to provide those certain patient services in which he/she is trained under the supervision, control, responsibility and direction of a licensed physician.

RHODE ISLAND R5-54-PA-1.11

SOUTH CAROLINA

'Physician assistant' means a health care professional licensed to assist in the practice of medicine with a physician supervisor.

SOUTH CAROLINA PA PRAC. ACT SEC. 40-47-905(5)

SOUTH DAKOTA

"Assistant to the primary care physician," a person who is a graduate of an approved program of instruction in primary health care, who has passed a licensure examination administered by the board, and is approved by the board to perform direct patient care services under the supervision of a primary care physician or physicians approved by the board to supervise such an assistant;

"Assistant to the specialist physician," a person who is a graduate of an approved program for instruction in a recognized clinical specialty, who has passed a licensure examination administered by the board and is approved by the board to perform direct patient care services in said specialty under the supervision of a specialist physician or physicians approved by the board to supervise such assistant;

"Physician assistant," a person who is either an assistant to the primary care physician or an assistant to the specialist physician.

SOUTH DAKOTA CODIFIED LAWS 36-4A-1

TENNESSEE

A physician assistant who holds state license in accordance with T.C.A. § 63-19-105.

RRT SEC.0880-3-02

TEXAS

Physician assistant - A person licensed as a physician assistant by the Texas State Board of Physician Assistant Examiners.

TEXAS CODE ANN. SEC. 185.2

UTAH

"Practice as a physician assistant" means:
(a) the professional activities and conduct of a physician assistant in diagnosing, treating, advising, or prescribing for any human disease, ailment, injury, infirmity, deformity, pain, or other condition, dependent upon and under the supervision of a supervising physician or substitute supervising physician in accordance with a delegation of services agreement; and
(b) the physician assistant acts as the agent of the supervising physician or substitute supervising physician when acting in accordance with a delegation of services agreement.

UTAH CODE ANN. SEC. 58-70A-102

VERMONT

Physician assistants practice medicine with physician supervision. Physician assistants may perform those duties and responsibilities, including the prescribing and dispensing of drugs and medical devices that are delegated by their supervision physician.

VERMONT RULES OF THE BD. OF MED. SEC. II.5.1

VIRGINIA

"Physician assistant" means an individual who has met the requirements of the Board for licensure and who works under the supervision of a licensed doctor of medicine, osteopathy, or podiatry.

CODE OF VIRGINIA SEC. 54.1-2900

WASHINGTON

"Physician assistant" means a person who is licensed by the commission to practice medicine to a limited extent only under the supervision of a physician as defined in chapter 18.71 RCW and who is academically and clinically prepared to provide health care services and perform diagnostic, therapeutic, preventative, and health maintenance services.

REV. CODE WASHINGTON SEC. 18.71A.010

"Physician assistant" means an individual who either:
(a) Successfully completed an accredited and commission approved physician assistant program, is eligible for the NCCPA examination and was licensed in Washington state prior to July 1, 1999;
(b) Qualified based on work experience and education and was licensed prior to July 1, 1989;
(c) Graduated from an international medical school and was licensed prior to July 1, 1989; or
(d) Holds an interim permit issued pursuant to RCW.

WASHINGTON ANN. CODE SEC. 246-918-005

WEST VIRGINIA

"Physician assistant" means an assistant to a physician who is a graduate of an approved program of instruction in primary health care or surgery, has attained a baccalaureate or master's degree, has passed the national certification examination and is qualified to perform direct patient care services under the supervision of a physician.

WEST VIRGINIA CODE SEC. 30-3-16

WISCONSIN

"Physician assistant" means an individual licensed by the medical examining board to provide medical care with physician supervision and direction.

WISCONSIN STAT. SEC. 448.01(6)

WYOMING

"Physician assistant" means any person who:
(A) Graduates from a physician assistant education program approved by CAAHEP or its predecessor or successor agency;
(B) Satisfactorily completes a certification examination administered by NCCPA or other national physician assistant certifying agency established for such purposes which has been reviewed and approved by the board, and is currently certified;
(C) The board approves to assist in the practice of medicine under the supervision of a physician or group of physicians approved by the board to supervise such assistant.

WYOMING STAT. ANN. SEC. 33-26-501

CHAPTER 2

Scope of Practice

PA Education and Experience • State Laws and Regulations • Institutional Policy • Delegatory Decisions Made by the Supervising Physician • Physician Assistants in the Emergency Room • Natural Disasters • Letters of Agreement/Written Agreements • Relationships with Pharmaceutical Companies • Addtional Resources • **Appendix 2-A** Scope of Practice State-by-State • **Appendix 2-B** Supervision Requirements State-by-State • **Appendix 2-C** Sample Written Agreements

PA EDUCATION AND EXPERIENCE

A physician assistant's scope of practice should be limited to those duties and responsibilities that the PA is adequately trained for. A PA's education and experience may be gained:

- During training in an accredited PA program.
- Through clinical practice and training provided by the supervising physician.
- Through continuing medical education courses.

STATE LAWS AND REGULATIONS

There are variations in the state laws that regulate PAs. However, state laws regulating physician assistant practice have evolved from checklists, which delineated every procedure and task a PA was allowed to perform, to broader regulations that allow for physicians to make determinations on the skill level of the PAs they supervise. States may define PAs' scope of practice through statutes enacted by the legislature or through a regulatory board, usually the state Board of Medicine. In this instance the rules and regulations developed by the board will define PA scope of practice. Rules and regulations carry the same force as statutes. Violation of a statute or regulation may result in a fine and/or a licensure action, which may include loss of licensure permanently or for a prescribed period of time.

It is vital that a PA obtain both the state statutes and the regulatory board's rules pertaining to PAs in order to be sure he or she is in compliance with both prior to beginning practice.

INSTITUTIONAL POLICY

Beyond the regulation by state laws, physician assistants are also governed by institutional regulations and policies. Various health care facilities such as nursing homes, hospitals, and acute care centers grant privileges based on physician assistants' qualifications and responsibilities deemed appropriate by their supervising physicians. This process mimics the credentialing process for the physician providers. Institutional regulations and policies cannot exceed regulations set forth by state boards of medicine. Institutions have the right to limit the responsibilities assigned to PAs whom they employ or grant privileges to.

DELEGATORY DECISIONS MADE BY THE SUPERVISING PHYSICIAN

A PA's supervising physician determines which services the PA will provide and the responsibilities the PA will have, after the physician determines the PA's skill level and competency through direct observation. A PA must have a supervising physician who has been approved by the medical board of the state prior to beginning to practice; some states also require a PA to have substitute supervising physicians approved as well. Many states require a collaborative or written agreement or a job description to be approved by the board before the board will issue a PA a license. This agreement will outline the PA's responsibilities and duties, prescriptive practice, and the level of physician supervision.

The American Medical Association (AMA) recognized these concepts when its 1995 House of Delegates adopted the following guidelines for physician–physician assistant practice:

- The physician is responsible for managing the health care of patients in all practice settings.
- Health care services delivered by physicians and physician assistants must be within the scope of each practitioner's authorized practice as defined by law.
- The physician is ultimately responsible for coordinating and managing the care of patients and, with the appropriate input from the physician assistant, insuring the quality of health care provided to the patients.
- The physician is responsible for supervision of the physician assistant in all settings.
- The role of the physician assistant in the delivery of care should be defined through mutually agreed-upon guidelines that are developed by the physician and the physician assistant and based on the physician's delegatory style.
- The physician must be available for consultation with the physician assistant at all times either in person or through telecommunications systems or other means.

- The extent of involvement by the physician assistant in the assessment and implementation of treatment will depend upon the complexity and acuity of the patient's condition and the training and experience and preparation of the physician assistant as adjudged by the physician.
- Patients should be made clearly aware at all times whether they are being cared for by a physician or a physician assistant.
- The physician and physician assistant together should review all delegated patient services on a regular basis, as well as the mutually agreed-upon guidelines for the practice.The physician is responsible for clarifying and familiarizing the physician assistant with his or her supervising method and style of delegating patient care.[1]

"PAs have great respect for the depth of training received by physicians, and acknowledge physicians as the best educated and most comprehensive providers on the health care team."[2]

Supervising physicians must also comply with statutes and regulations governing physician assistants. Many states have statutes that outline the duties and responsibilities of supervising physicians. For example, Kentucky's statute states:

A supervising physician shall:
(1) Restrict the services of a physician assistant to services within the physician assistant's scope of practice and to the provisions of KRS 311.840 to 311.862;
(2) Prohibit a physician assistant from prescribing or dispensing controlled substances;
(3) Inform all patients in contact with a physician assistant of the status of the physician assistant;
(4) Post a notice stating that a physician assistant practices medicine or osteopathy in all locations where the physician assistant may practice;
(5) Require a physician assistant to wear identification that clearly states that he or she is a physician assistant;
(6) Prohibit a physician assistant from independently billing any patient or other payor for services rendered by the physician assistant;
(7) If necessary, participate with the governing body of any hospital or other licensed health care facility in a credentialing process established by the facility;
(8) Not require a physician assistant to perform services or other acts that the physician assistant feels incapable of carrying out safely and properly;
(9) Maintain adequate, active, and continuous supervision of a physician assistant's activities to assure that the physician assistant is

performing as directed and complying with the requirements of KRS 311.840 to 311.862 and all related administrative regulations;

(10) Sign all records of service rendered by a physician assistant in a timely manner as certification that the physician assistant performed the services as delegated;

(11) (a) Reevaluate the reliability, accountability, and professional knowledge of a physician assistant two (2) years after the physician assistant's original certification in this Commonwealth and every two (2) years thereafter; and (b) based on the reevaluation, recommend approval or disapproval of certification or recertification to the board; and

(12) Notify the board within three (3) business days if the supervising physician:

(a) Ceases to supervise or employ the physician assistant; or

(b) Believes in good faith that a physician assistant violated any disciplinary rule of the medical board.

KRS 311.856

PHYSICIAN ASSISTANTS IN THE EMERGENCY ROOM

The Emergency Medical Treatment and Labor Act (42 USC sec. 1864, Ch. 7) took effect in 1986 in order to ensure all individuals access to emergency care and prevent inappropriate transfers to other facilities. A hospital must provide appropriate medical screening to any individual requesting emergency medical care. If an emergent medical condition exists, the patient must receive the appropriate medical treatment in order to stabilize the patient. A patient can be transferred if the hospital cannot provide the medical care necessary to stabilize the patient and the specific criteria in the law regarding transfers are met.

Physician assistants can perform the screening exams required by the Emergency Medical Treatment and Labor Act (EMTLA) as long as the hospital grants the authority to PAs through privileges or a similar mechanism.[1]

> In the case of a hospital that has an emergency department, if an individual (whether or not eligible for Medicare benefits and regardless of the ability to pay) comes by him or herself or with another person to the emergency department and a request is made on the individual's behalf for an examination or treatment of a medical condition by qualified medical personnel (as determined by the hospital in its rules and regulations), the hospital must provide an appropriate medical screening examination within the capabilities of the hospital's emergency department, to determine whether or not an emergency medical condition exists. *The examination must be conducted by individuals determined qualified by hospital bylaws or rules and regulations.* (Emphasis added) [42 CFR sec. 489.24 (a)]

The Centers for Medicare and Medicaid Services 2004 Interpretive Guidelines state:

> A hospital must formally determine who is qualified to perform the initial medical screening examination, i.e., qualified medical person (QMP). While it is permissible for hospitals to designate a nonphysician practitioner as the qualified medical person, the designated nonphysician practitioners must be set forth in a document that is approved by the governing body of the hospital. Those health practitioners designated to perform medical screening examinations are to be identified in the hospital bylaws or in the rules and regulations governing the medical staff following governing body approval. It is not acceptable for the hospital to allow the medical director of the emergency department to make what may be informal personnel appointments that could frequently change.[2]

A physician assistant, after consultation with a physician, may decide that a patient transfer is appropriate. A physician assistant may sign the transfer order, which must be countersigned by a physician within a reasonable amount of time:

> If a physician is not physically present in the emergency room at the time an individual is transferred, a qualified medical person (as determined by the hospital in its bylaws or rules and regulations) has signed a certificate described in paragraph (d)(1)(ii)(B) of this section after a physician (as defined by section 1861(r)(1) of the Act) in consultation with the qualified medical person, agrees with the certification and subsequently countersigns the certification. [42CFR sec. 489.24(d)(ii)(C)]

The Centers for Medicare and Medicaid Services 2004 Interpretive Guidelines state:

> A QMP may sign the certification of benefits versus risks of transfer only after consultation with the physician who authorizes the transfer. If a QMP determines that the transfer to another facility is in the best interest of the individual and signs the certification of benefits versus risks, a physician's countersignature must be obtained within the established timeframe according to hospital policies and procedures.[3]

Physicians in the emergency department may delegate on-call services to PAs. The Centers for Medicare and Medicaid Services 2004 Interpretive Guidelines state:

> The decision as to whether the on-call physician responds in person or directs a nonphysician practitioner (physician assistant, nurse prac-

titioner, orthopedic tech) as his or her representative to present to the dedicated ED is made by the responsible on-call physician, based on the individual's medical need and the capabilities of the hospital and applicable state scope of practice laws, hospital bylaws, and rules and regulations. The on-call physician is ultimately responsible for the individual regardless of who responds to the call.[4]

NATURAL DISASTERS

PAs may provide medical assistance during disasters and emergencies without a supervising physician available under the state laws of Arizona, California, Delaware, Iowa, Kentucky, Louisiana, Maryland, Minnesota, North Carolina, and Wyoming. PAs in the remainder of the states can volunteer at the hospital or Red Cross in a nonmedical capacity but cannot volunteer as a PA unless there is direct communication with their supervising physician or the PA is working as part of a Disaster Medical Assistance Team (DMAT).

For the most part Good Samaritan acts will not cover PAs assisting in disaster or emergency situations. Good Samaritan acts provide immunity for medical professionals who stop to assist a person in an emergency situation. There have been a few amendments to Good Samaritan acts allowing PAs to assist in natural disasters. Generally, the authority for PAs to provide medical assistance in disaster and emergency situations is granted by separate law.[5]

The AAPA has adopted model language for legislation to address this issue. The legislative language can be found at the AAPA's Web site at www.aapa.org/gandp/modelaw.html, Participation in Disaster and Emergency Care.

LETTERS OF AGREEMENT/WRITTEN AGREEMENTS

Letters of agreement and written agreements are documents that define a PA's scope of practice and duties, including the medications to be prescribed, the relationship with the supervising physician, and the locations at which the PA will be utilized. There are states (for example, Pennsylvania) that require a letter of agreement to be approved by the state Board of Medicine prior to issuing a license to the physician assistant. There are also states that tie PAs' prescriptive privileges to formularies. (See Table 2-1.)

Table 2-1 States That Restrict PA Prescriptive Practice Through Formularies

Alabama	Oklahoma
Florida	Pennsylvania
Georgia	South Carolina
Minnesota	Vermont
New Mexico	West Virginia

If a particular state requires a letter of agreement, the format may be clearly delineated in the statute or regulation that makes the requirement, or the state Board of Medicine may include a sample in the licensure application. Another option is to contact the state society of physician assistants to see if it has a sample format or can provide samples of letters of agreement from PAs practicing within that state. (See Appendix 2-C for sample letters of agreement/written agreements.)

RELATIONSHIPS WITH PHARMACEUTICAL COMPANIES

If meeting with pharmaceutical sales representatives will be part of the duties a supervising physician assigns to a PA, it is important that the PA is familiar with Pharmaceutical Research and Manufacturers of America (PhRMA) Code on Interactions with Healthcare Professionals found at www.phrma.org/publications/policy/2004-01-19.391.pdf and the American Medical Association's Ethical Guidelines on Gifts to Physicians from the Industry found at www.ama-assn.org/ama/pub/article/4001-7922.html and www.ama-assn.org/ama1/pub/upload/mm/473/ama_m4_ph.pdf. The guidelines indicate that acceptance of items that contribute to the medical aspect of practice such as medical books, pens, note pads, and stethoscopes are allowable. Personal items including dinners, vacations, cash payments, golf balls, golf clubs, or sports bags are unacceptable. If you are uncertain as to whether to accept an item from a pharmaceutical sales representative or other vendor, determine if the item would be considered a benefit to patient care and only accept items that can clearly benefit the patient or the practice. Acceptance of items of personal benefit or travel or other expenses of providers to attend educational seminars that are provided by pharmaceutical companies or other vendors may lead to governmental investigations.

ADDITIONAL RESOURCES

Office of the Inspector General, U.S. Department of Health and Human Services, Compliance Program Guidelines for Pharmaceutical Manufacturers found at http://oig.hhs.gov/authorities/docs/03/050503FRCPGPharmac.pdf

Advanced Medical Technology Association, Code of Ethics on Interactions with Health Care Professionals found at www.advamed.org/publicdocs/code_of_ethics.pdf

American Council for Continuing Education, Standards for Commercial Support found at www.accme.org?incoming/174_Standards%20for%20Commercial%20Support_April%202004.pdf

REFERENCES

1. The American Academy of Physician Assistants Web site. FAQs: EMTALA and PAs. Available at http://www.aapa.org. Accessed March 2005.

2. Missouri Hospital Association Web site. State Operations Manual Appendix V—Interpretative Guidelines—Responsibilities of Medicare Participating Hospitals in Emergency Cases. Available at http://web.mhanet.com/asp/Regulations/pdf/2004_emtala_interpretive_guidelines.pdf (p. 4). Accessed March 2005.

3. Missouri Hospital Association Web site. State Operations Manual Appendix V—Interpretative Guidelines—Responsibilities of Medicare Participating Hospitals in Emergency Cases. Available at http://web.mhanet.com/asp/Regulations/pdf/2004_emtala_interpretive_guidelines.pdf (p. 45). Accessed March 2005.

4. Missouri Hospital Association Web site. State Operations Manual Appendix V—Interpretative Guidelines—Responsibilities of Medicare Participating Hospitals in Emergency Cases. Available at http://web.mhanet.com/asp/Regulations/pdf/2004_emtala_interpretive_guidelines.pdf (p. 22). Accessed March 2005.

5. Good Samaritan act not enough to allow PAs to assist in natural disasters. (2004, October 15). *AAPA News*, 5.

Scope of Practice
State-by-State

ALABAMA

(1) There shall be at all times a direct continuing and close supervisory relationship between the physician assistant and the physician to whom that assistant is registered. The supervising physician shall at all times be responsible for the activities of the physician assistant.

(2) The physician assistant shall provide medical services within the education, training, and experience of the physician assistant that are delegated by the supervising physician. These services include, but are not limited to:
   (a) Obtaining patient histories and performing physical examinations;
   (b) Ordering and/or performing diagnostic and therapeutic procedures;
   (c) Formulating a working diagnosis;
   (d) Developing and implementing a treatment plan;
   (e) Monitoring the effectiveness of therapeutic interventions;
   (f) Assisting at surgery;
   (g) Offering counseling and education to meet patient needs; and
   (h) Making appropriate referrals.

(3) The job description in the form specified in Appendix B to Chapter 7 is approved by the Board as a model job description which shall be acceptable to the Board if submitted by a qualified applicant for registration in compliance with these Rules.

(4) A physician assistant is prohibited from performing any medical service, procedure, function, or activity which is not specifically listed, in detail, in the job description approved by the Board.

(5) Requests for changes in the job description of the assistant, including addition of specialized duties and tasks, shall be submitted,

in writing, by the supervising physician to the Board for prior approval.

(6) Should the supervising physician contemplate a request for additional duties for the assistant for addition to the assistant's Job Description, a written request shall be submitted to and approved by the Board prior to any additional duty or procedure being performed by the assistant.

(7) When any addition of a duty or procedure to the assistant's Job Description is contemplated, a written request for training of the assistant in the duty or procedure shall be submitted to and approved by the Board prior to the assistant actually receiving any training in the duty or procedure.

ALABAMA ADMIN. CODE R. 540-X-7-.25

Limitations upon utilization of physician assistants (P.A.).

(1) A physician who practices in a surgical specialty may have registered to him or her not more than two physician assistants. A supervising physician must be present in the operating room or be immediately available to that operating room whenever a physician assistant is involved in the care of a patient in the operating room. Whenever a physician assistant performs or assists in performing invasive procedures with involvement deeper than the complete dermis, the supervising physician must be present in the operating room, unless otherwise specifically approved by the Board.

(2) Except for a physician subject to paragraph (1) of this rule, a physician may have registered to him or her not more than three physician assistants. The cumulative work times for all physician assistants being supervised by an individual primary supervising physician pursuant to paragraph (2) shall not exceed 80 hours per week.

(3) A physician assistant may be registered to more than one supervising physician at any one time. The number of supervising physicians to whom a physician assistant may be registered shall be restricted by the Board if the Board, in its discretion, determines that such restriction is appropriate to maintain the quality of medical services being provided or to otherwise protect the public health, safety and welfare.

(4) Employees of the State Health Department or of a county board of health are specifically exempt from the requirements of paragraph (2) of this rule. The Board of Medical Examiners, in its discretion, may determine how many physician assistants may be registered

to and/or supervised by a physician employed by the State Health Department or by a county board of health.

ALABAAMA ADMIN. CODE R. 540-X-7-.26

Prohibited activities and functions—physician assistants (P.A.).

(1) Notwithstanding any other provision of law, a physician assistant may perform medical service when such services are rendered under the supervision of a licensed physician or physicians approved by the Board; except, that no medical services may be performed except under the supervision of an ophthalmologist in the office in which such physician normally actually practices his profession and nowhere else in any of the following areas:

    (a) The measurement of the powers or range of human vision or the determination of the accommodation and refractive state of the human eye or the scope of its functions in general or the fitting or adaptation of lenses or frames for the aid thereof.

    (b) The prescribing or directing the use of or using any optical device in connection with ocular exercises, visual training or orthoptics.

    (c) The prescribing of contact lenses for or the fitting or adaptation of contact lenses to the human eye. Nothing in this section shall preclude the performance of routine visual screening.

(2) Any medical service, procedure, activity or function not specifically enumerated in the job description approved by the Board is prohibited.

(3) There shall be no practice by a physician assistant who is not licensed and registered by the Board.

(4) There shall be no independent practice by a physician assistant who is licensed and/or registered by the Board.

ALABAMA ADMIN. CODE R. 540-X-7-.27

ALASKA

PERFORMANCE AND ASSESSMENT OF PRACTICE. (a) A person may perform medical diagnosis and treatment as a physician assistant only if licensed by the board and authorized to practice under 12 AAC 40.408 and only within the scope of practice of the collaborating physician.

(b) A periodic method of assessment of the quality of practice must be established by the collaborating physician before an applicant is granted authorization to practice. In this subsection, "periodic method of assessment" means evaluation of medical care and clinic management.

12 ALASKA ADMIN. CODE 40.430

ARIZONA

Health care tasks; scope of practice; restrictions; civil penalty

(A) After a supervising physician receives board approval of a notice of supervision, that physician may delegate health care tasks to the physician assistant. The physician assistant may perform these tasks in any setting authorized by the approved supervising physician and the board, pursuant to subsections E and F of this section, including clinics, hospitals, ambulatory surgical centers, patient homes, nursing homes and other health care institutions. These tasks may include:

(1) Obtaining patient histories.

2. Performing physical examinations.

3. Ordering and performing diagnostic and therapeutic procedures.

4. Formulating a diagnostic impression.

5. Developing and implementing a treatment plan.

6. Monitoring the effectiveness of therapeutic interventions.

7. Assisting in surgery.

8. Offering counseling and education to meet patient needs.

9. Making appropriate referrals.

10. Prescribing schedule IV or V controlled substances as defined in the federal controlled substances act of 1970 (P.L. 91-513; 84 Stat. 1242; 21 United States code section 802) and prescription-only medications.

11. Prescribing schedule II and III controlled substances as defined in the federal controlled substances act of 1970.

12. Performing minor surgery as defined in section 32-2501.

13. Performing other nonsurgical health care tasks that are normally taught in courses of training approved by the board, that are consistent with the training and experience of the physician assistant and that have been properly delegated by the approved supervising physician.

(B) The approved supervising physician shall:

1. Meet the requirements established by the board for supervising a physician assistant and receive written board notification of this compliance.

2. Accept responsibility for all tasks and duties the physician delegates to a physician assistant.

3. Notify the board and the physician assistant in writing if the physician assistant exceeds the scope of the delegated health care tasks.

4. Notify the board if the physician has delegated authority to the

physician assistant to prescribe medication. The physician shall also notify the board if the physician makes any changes to this authority.

C. Supervision does not require the personal presence of the physician at the place where health care tasks are performed. The board by order may require the personal presence of a physician when designated health care tasks are performed.

D. A physician assistant shall meet in person with the supervising physician at least once each week to discuss patient management. If the supervising physician is unavailable due to vacation, illness or continuing education programs, a physician assistant may meet with the supervising physician's agent. If the supervising physician is unavailable for any other reason, the fulfillment of this responsibility by the supervising physician's agent is subject to board approval.

E. A physician assistant shall not perform health care tasks in a place which is geographically separated from the supervising physician's primary place for meeting patients without the authorization of the supervising physician and the board.

F. The board may approve the performance of health care tasks by a physician assistant in a place which is geographically separated from the supervising physician's primary place for meeting patients if:
1. Adequate provision for immediate communication between the supervising physician or supervising physician's agent and the physician assistant exists.
2. The physician assistant's performance of health care tasks is adequately supervised and reviewed.
3. A printed announcement which contains the names of the physician assistant and supervising physician and states that the facility employs a physician assistant who is performing health care tasks under the supervision of a licensed physician is posted in the waiting room of the geographically separated site.

G. At all times while a physician assistant is on duty, he shall wear a name tag with the designation "physician assistant" on it.

H. The board by rule may prescribe a civil penalty for a violation of this article relating to charting, wearing tags, identifying prescriptions and posting signs in geographically separated locations. The penalty shall not exceed fifty dollars for each violation. The board shall deposit, pursuant to sections 35-146 and 35-147, all monies it receives from this penalty in the state general fund. A physician assistant and the supervising physician may contest the imposition of this penalty pursuant to board rule. The imposition of a civil penalty is public information, and the board may use this information in any future disciplinary actions.

ARIZONA REV. STAT. ANN. SEC. 32-2531

ARKANSAS

Physician assistants provide health care services with physician supervision. The supervising physician shall be identified on all prescriptions and orders. Physician assistants may perform those duties and responsibilities, including the prescribing, ordering, and administering drugs and medical devices, that are delegated by their supervising physicians.

(a) Physician assistants shall be considered the agents of their supervising physicians in the performance of all practice related activities, including but not limited to, the ordering of diagnostic, therapeutic, and other medical services.

(b) Physician assistants may perform health care services in any setting authorized by the supervising physician in accordance with any applicable facility policy.

(c) Nothing in this chapter shall be construed to authorize a physician assistant to:

(1) Examine the human eye or visual system for the purpose of prescribing glasses or contact lenses or the determination of the refractive power for surgical procedures;

(2) Adapt, fill, duplicate, modify, supply, or sell contact lenses or prescription eye glasses; or

(3) Prescribe, direct the use of, or use any optical device in connection with ocular exercises, vision training, or orthoptics.

ARKANSAS CODE 17-105-107

CALIFORNIA

A physician assistant may perform those medical services as set forth by the regulations of the board when the services are rendered under the supervision of a licensed physician and surgeon or of physicians and surgeons approved by the board, except as provided in Section 3502.5.

(b) Notwithstanding any other provision of law, a physician assistant performing medical services under the supervision of a physician and surgeon may assist a doctor of podiatric medicine who is a partner, shareholder, or employee in the same medical group as the supervising physician. A physician assistant who assists a doctor of podiatric medicine pursuant to this subdivision shall do so only according to patient-specific orders from the supervising physician and surgeon. The supervising physician and surgeon shall be physically available to the physician assistant for consultation when such assistance is rendered. A physician assistant assisting a doctor of podiatric medicine shall be limited to performing those duties included within the scope of practice of a doctor of podiatric medicine.

(c) No medical services may be performed under this chapter in any of the following areas:

    (1) The determination of the refractive states of the human eye, or the fitting or adaptation of lenses or frames for the aid thereof.

    (2) The prescribing or directing the use of, or using, any optical device in connection with ocular exercises, visual training or orthoptics.

    (3) The prescribing of contact lenses for, or the fitting or adaptation of contact lenses to, the human eye.

    (4) The practice of dentistry or dental hygiene or the work of a dental auxiliary.

(d) This section shall not be construed in a manner that shall preclude the performance of routine visual screening.

CALIFORNIA BUS. & PROF. CODE SEC. 3502

A physician assistant may only provide those medical services which he or she is competent to perform and which are consistent with the physician assistant's education, training, and experience, and which are delegated in writing by a supervising physician who is responsible for the patients cared for by that physician assistant. The committee or division or their representative may require proof or demonstration of competence from any physician assistant for any tasks, procedures or management he or she is performing. A physician assistant shall consult with a physician regarding any task, procedure or diagnostic problem which the physician assistant determines exceeds his or her level of competence or shall refer such cases to a physician.

CALIFORNIA CODE REGS. SEC. 1399.540

Because physician assistant practice is directed by a supervising physician, and a physician assistant acts as an agent for that physician, the orders given and tasks performed by a physician assistant shall be considered the same as if they had been given and performed by the supervising physician. Unless otherwise specified in these regulations or in the delegation or protocols, these orders may be initiated without the prior patient specific order of the supervising physician. In any setting, including for example, any licensed health facility, out-patient settings, patients' residences, residential facilities, and hospices, as applicable, a physician assistant may, pursuant to a delegation and protocols where present:

(a) Take a patient history; perform a physical examination and make an assessment and diagnosis therefrom; initiate, review and revise treatment and therapy plans including plans for those services described in Section 1399.541(b) through Section 1399.541(i) inclusive; and record and present pertinent data in a manner meaningful to the physician.

(b) Order or transmit an order for x-ray, other studies, therapeutic diets, physical therapy, occupational therapy, respiratory therapy, and nursing services.

(c) Order, transmit an order for, perform, or assist in the performance of laboratory procedures, screening procedures and therapeutic procedures.

(d) Recognize and evaluate situations which call for immediate attention of a physician and institute, when necessary, treatment procedures essential for the life of the patient.

(e) Instruct and counsel patients regarding matters pertaining to their physical and mental health. Counseling may include topics such as medications, diets, social habits, family planning, normal growth and development, aging, and understanding of and long-term management of their diseases.

(f) Initiate arrangements for admissions, complete forms and charts pertinent to the patient's medical record, and provide services to patients requiring continuing care, including patients at home.

(g) Initiate and facilitate the referral of patients to the appropriate health facilities, agencies, and resources of the community.

(h) Administer medication to a patient, or transmit orally, or in writing on a patient's record, a prescription from his or her supervising physician to a person who may lawfully furnish such medication or medical device. The supervising physician's prescription, transmitted by the physician assistant, for any patient cared for by the physician assistant, shall be based either on a patient-specific order by the supervising physician or on written protocol which specifies all criteria for the use of a specific drug or device and any contraindications for the selection. A physician assistant shall not provide a drug or transmit a prescription for a drug other than that drug specified in the protocol, without a patient-specific order from a supervising physician. At the direction and under the supervision of a physician supervisor, a physician assistant may hand to a patient of the supervising physician a properly labeled prescription drug prepackaged by a physician, a manufacturer, as defined in the Pharmacy Law, or a pharmacist. In any case, the medical record of any patient cared for by the physician assistant for whom the physician's prescription has been transmitted or carried out shall be reviewed and countersigned and dated by a supervising physician within seven (7) days. A physician assistant may not administer, provide or transmit a prescription for controlled substances in Schedules II through V inclusive without patient-specific authority by a supervising physician.

(i) (1) Perform surgical procedures without the personal presence of the supervising physician which are customarily performed under local anesthesia. Prior to delegating any such surgical procedures, the supervising physician shall review documentation which indicates that the physician assistant is trained to perform the surgical procedures. All other surgical procedures requiring other forms of anesthesia may be performed by a physician assistant only in the personal presence of an approved supervising physician.

(2) A physician assistant may also act as first or second assistant in surgery under the supervision of an approved supervising physician.

CALIFORNIA CODE REGS. SEC. 1399.541

COLORADO

All licensees designated or referred to in subsection (3) of this section, who are licensed to practice a limited field of the healing arts, shall confine themselves strictly to the field for which they are licensed and to the scope of their respective licenses, and shall not use any title, word, or abbreviation mentioned in paragraph (d) of subsection (1) of this section, except to the extent and under the conditions expressly permitted by the law under which they are licensed.

(5) (a) A person licensed under the laws of this state to practice medicine may delegate to a physician assistant licensed by the board the authority to perform acts that constitute the practice of medicine to the extent and in the manner authorized by rules and regulations promulgated by the board, including the authority to prescribe medication, including controlled substances, and dispense only such drugs as designated by the board. Such acts shall be consistent with sound medical practice. Each prescription issued by a physician assistant licensed by the board shall have imprinted thereon the name of his or

her supervising physician. Nothing in this subsection (5) shall limit the ability of otherwise licensed health personnel to perform delegated acts. The dispensing of prescription medication by a physician assistant shall be subject to the provisions of section 12-22-121 (6).

(b) (I) If the authority to perform an act is delegated pursuant to paragraph (a) of this subsection (5), the act shall not be performed except under the personal and responsible direction and supervision of a person licensed under the laws of this state to practice medicine, and said person shall not be responsible for the direction and supervision of more than two physician assistants at any one time without specific approval of the board. The board may define appropriate direction and supervision pursuant to rules and regulations.

(II) For purposes of this subsection (5), "personal and responsible direction and supervision" means that the direction and supervision of a physician assistant must be personally rendered by a licensed physician practicing in the state of Colorado and not through intermediaries. The extent of direction and supervision shall be determined by rules and regulations promulgated by the board and as otherwise provided in this paragraph (b); except that, when a physician assistant is performing a delegated medical function in an acute care hospital, the board shall allow supervision and direction to be performed without the physical presence of the physician during the time the delegated medical functions are being implemented if:

(A) Such medical functions are performed where the supervising physician regularly practices or in a designated health manpower shortage area;

(B) The licensed supervising physician reviews the quality of medical services rendered by the physician assistant every two working days by reviewing the medical records to assure compliance with the physicians' directions; and

(C) The performance of the delegated medical function otherwise complies with the board's regulations and any restrictions and protocols of the licensed supervising physician and hospital.

(III) If the state board of medical examiners has a reasonable belief that additional supervision or direction may be necessary it may issue a cease and desist order to the supervising physician or physician assistant to require that a function be delegated only on a case-by-case basis, or to require that the supervising physician be present on the premises in specific types of cases that arise in an acute care hospital setting. Such a cease and desist order shall become effective upon delivery to the supervising physician or physician assistant to whom it is issued. Any supervising physician or physician assistant who receives such an order may request a hearing on the merits of the order, which request shall be promptly granted. Any restriction or requirement imposed by such an order shall not be deemed a disciplinary action, restriction, or other limitation on the physician's license or the physician assistant's licensure.

COLORADO REV. STAT. ANN. SEC. 12-36-106 (4)

CONNECTICUT

A physician assistant who has complied with the provisions of sections 20-12b and 20-12c may perform medical functions delegated by a supervising physician when: (1) The supervising physician is satisfied as to the ability and competency of the physician assistant; (2) such delegation is consistent with the health and welfare of the patient and in keeping with sound medical practice; and (3) when such functions are performed under the oversight, control and direction of the supervising physician. The functions that may be performed under such delegation are those that are within the scope of the supervising physician's license, within the scope of such physician's competence as evidenced by such physician's postgraduate education, training and experience and within the normal scope of such physician's actual practice.

Delegated functions shall be implemented in accordance with written protocols established by the supervising physician. All orders written by physician assistants shall be followed by the signature of the physician assistant and the printed name of the supervising physician. A physician assistant may, as delegated by the supervising physician within the scope of such physician's license,
(A) prescribe and administer drugs, including controlled substances in schedule IV or V in all settings,
(B) renew prescriptions for controlled substances in schedule II or III in outpatient settings, and
(C) prescribe and administer controlled substances in schedule II or III to an inpatient in a short-term hospital, chronic disease hospital, emergency room satellite of a general hospital, or after an admis-

sion evaluation by a physician, in a chronic and convalescent nursing home, as defined in the regulations of Connecticut state agencies and licensed pursuant to subsection (a) of section 19a-491, provided in all cases where the physician assistant prescribes a controlled substance in schedule II or III, the physician under whose supervision the physician assistant is prescribing shall cosign the order not later than twenty-four hours thereafter. The physician assistant may, as delegated by the supervising physician within the scope of such physician's license, dispense drugs, in the form of professional samples as defined in section 20-14c or when dispensing in an outpatient clinic as defined in the regulations of Connecticut state agencies and licensed pursuant to subsection (a) of section 19a-491 that operates on a not-for-profit basis, or when dispensing in a clinic operated by a state agency or municipality. Nothing in this subsection shall be construed to allow the physician assistant to dispense any drug the physician assistant is not authorized under this subsection to prescribe.

(b) All prescription forms used by physician assistants shall contain the printed name, license number, address and telephone number of the physician under whose supervision the physician assistant is prescribing, in addition to the signature, name, address and license number of the physician assistant.

(c) No physician assistant may:
(1) Engage in the independent practice of medicine;
(2) claim to be or allow being represented as a physician licensed pursuant to this chapter;
(3) use the title of doctor; or
(4) associate by name or allow association by name with any term that would suggest qualification to engage in the independent practice of medicine. The physician assistant shall be clearly identified by appropriate identification as a physician assistant to ensure that the physician assistant is not mistaken for a physician licensed pursuant to this chapter.

(d) A physician assistant licensed under this chapter may make the actual determination and pronouncement of death of a patient, provided:
(1) The death is an anticipated death;
(2) the physician assistant attests to such pronouncement on the certificate of death; and
(3) a physician licensed by the state of Connecticut certifies the death and signs the certificate of death within twenty-four hours of the pronouncement by the physician assistant.

CONNECTICUT GEN. STATUTE SEC. 20-12D

DELAWARE

The phrase "delegated medical acts" means the performance of health care activities and duties by a physician's assistant under the delegation and control of a supervising physician.

(b) The Board in conjunction with the Physician's Assistant Regulatory Council shall:

  (1) Adopt regulations regarding activities which may be undertaken by physician's assistants and shall license all certified physician's assistants with the Board.

  (2) Define the scope of practice of physician's assistants including:

    a. Issuance of license to physician's assistant to allow:

      1. Performance of delegated medical acts within the education and experience of the physician's assistant; and

      2. Performance of services customary to the practice of the supervising physician(s);

    b. Delegated medical services provided by a physician's assistant to include but not limited to:

      1. Performance of complete histories and physical examinations;

      2. Recording of patient progress notes in an outpatient setting;

      3. Relaying, transcribing, or executing specific diagnostic or therapeutic orders so long as all such notes, orders and other writings shall be reviewed and countersigned by the supervising physician within 24 hours, barring extraordinary events or circumstances;

      4. Delegated acts of diagnosis and prescription of therapeutic drugs and treatments within the scope of physician's assistant practice defined within the Rules and Regulations promulgated by the Physician's Assistant Regulatory Council and approved by the Board of Medical Practice;

      5. Prescriptive authority for therapeutic drugs and treatments within the scope of physician's assistant practice defined within Rules and Regulations promulgated by the Physician's Assistant Regulatory Council and approved by the Board of Medical Practice. The physician assistant's prescriptive authority and authority to make independent medical diagnoses and treatment decisions shall be subject to biennial renewal upon application to the Physician's Assistant Regulatory Council;

   c. Nothing in this chapter may be construed to authorize a physician assistant to practice independent of a supervising physician;

   d. Except as otherwise provided in this chapter or in a medical emergency, a physicianassistant may not perform any medical act which has not been delegated by a supervising physician.

TIT. 24 DELAWARE CODE SEC. 1770A-3

DISTRICT OF COLUMBIA

A physician assistant may, in accordance with this chapter and the act, perform health care tasks that are consistent with sound medical practice, taking into account the following:

(a) The physician assistant's education, skill, training, and experience;
(b) The patient's health and safety;
(c) The degree of supervision by the supervising physician;
(d) The qualifications of the supervising physician; and
(e) The nature of the supervising physician's practice.

A physician assistant in collaboration with a licensed physician shall perform health care tasks only if the following requirements are met:

(a) The health care tasks are authorized by a standard or advanced job description registered by the Board; or
(b) The health care tasks are undertaken in immediate collaboration as defined in § 101(2)(c) of the Act, D.C. Official Code § 3-1201.01(2)(C) (1985) with a supervising physician.

A standard job description registered by the Board authorizes a physician assistant to perform those health care tasks listed in the job description at a supervising physician's primary location and may include the following:

(a) Screening patients to determine the need for medical attention;
(b) Taking a patient history;
(c) Performing a physical examination;
(d) Recording patient data in patient medical records;
(e) Performing the following diagnostic, therapeutic, and clinical procedures:
   (1) Cultures;
   (2) Venipuncture;
   (3) Intradermal tests;
   (4) Electrocardiograms;
   (5) Pulmonary function tests, excluding endoscopic procedures;
   (6) Arterial blood gases;

(7) Tonemetry screening;

(8) Audiometry screening;

(9) Visual screening;

(10) Catheterization of the bladder;

(11) Nasogastric intubation and gastric lavage;

(12) Administration of injections, medications, immunizations, and intravenous fluids;

(13) Strapping, splinting, and casting of sprains and non-displaced fractures;

(14) Removal of casts;

(15) Care of superficial wounds, burns, and skin infections, including suturing;

(16) Application of dressings and bandages;

(17) Cardiopulmonary resuscitation;

(18) Removal of impacted cerumen;

(19) Initiating treatment procedures essential for the life of the patient in emergency circumstances;

(20) Prescribing and dispensing drugs as specified in § 4912; and

(f) Assisting in patient care and management, as follows:

(1) Arranging admissions to a hospital or health care facility under specific orders from a supervising physician;

(2) Providing counseling and instruction regarding common patient problems such as nutrition, family planning, exercise, and human development;

(3) Attending rounds consistent with the policies of a hospital or health care facility;

(4) Referring patients to community resources and health care services; and

(5) Assisting in office management by keeping records, ordering supplies and drugs, and maintaining equipment.

A physician assistant shall obtain authorization in an advanced job description registered by the Board to perform health care tasks that:

(a) Are undertaken in a location which is geographically separate from the supervising physician's primary location for seeing patients; or

(b) Are not expressly enumerated in § 4911.3.

4911.5 A physician assistant may perform health care tasks that are authorized by a standard job description before the Board registers the standard job description for a period of sixty (60) days from the date of application if the following occurs:

(a) An application to register the standard job description is pending before the Board;

  (b) The physician assistant is licensed in good standing in the District of Columbia with no pending disciplinary charges and no pending criminal charges in any jurisdiction relating to the physician's assistant's fitness to practice;

  (c) The supervising and back-up supervising physicians are licensed in good standing in the District of Columbia with no pending disciplinary charges and no pending criminal charges in any jurisdiction relating to their fitness to practice medicine;

  (d) The health care tasks are performed at the supervising physician's primary location for seeing patients; and

  (e) The health care tasks are performed in accordance with the limitations of this chapter and the act.

A physician assistant whose application for registration of a standard job description is pending before the Board shall not administer, dispense, or prescribe prescription drugs unless these tasks are undertaken in immediate collaboration with a supervising physician.

A physician assistant performing health care tasks shall cease to perform health care tasks immediately upon notification from the Board that the Board has decided not to register the standard job description.

A physician assistant shall wear an identification badge with lettering clearly visible to a patient bearing the name of the physician assistant and the title "Physician Assistant." In addition, a physician assistant shall, upon introduction to a patient and prior to rendering services, explain that the physician assistant is not a physician and that the supervising physician is ultimately responsible for the patient's care.

A physician assistant may give medical orders to health professionals and personnel consistent with the following:

  (a) The scope of the physician assistant's registered job description; and

  (b) The policies of a hospital or health care facility where the orders are to be executed.

A physician assistant shall not perform health care tasks if a supervising physician is not available to provide supervision in accordance with the general provisions of this chapter and the specific provisions of a registered job description unless the supervising physician has designated a back-up physician to provide substitute supervision pursuant to § 4914.6.

TIT. 17 DISTRICT OF COLUMBIA MUN. REG. SEC. 4911

FLORIDA

A supervisory physician may delegate to a licensed physician assistant, pursuant to a written protocol, the authority to act according to s. 154.04(1)(c). Such delegated authority is limited to the supervising physician's practice in connection with a county health department as defined and established pursuant to chapter 154. The boards shall adopt rules governing the supervision of physician assistants by physicians in county health departments.

FLORIDA STATE CH. 458.347(1)(D)

GEORGIA

On receipt of notice of the board's approval, a physician's assistant, under the direction of the applying physician, may perform the tasks described in the job description, provided that nothing in this Code section shall make unlawful the performance of a medical task by the physician's assistant, whether or not such task is specified in the general job description, when it is performed under the direct supervision and in the presence of the physician utilizing him.

GEORGIA CODE ANN. SEC. 43-34-105

HAWAII

A physician assistant shall be considered the agent of the physician assistant's supervising physician in the performance of all practice-related activities as established in writing by the employer.
(b) Medical services rendered by the physician assistants may include, but are not limited to:
   (1) Obtaining patient histories and performing physical examinations;
   (2) Ordering, interpreting, or performing diagnostic and therapeutic procedures;
   (3) Formulating a diagnosis;
   (4) Developing and implementing a treatment plan;
   (5) Monitoring the effectiveness of therapeutic interventions;
   (6) Assisting at surgery;
   (7) Offering counseling and education to meet patient needs; and
   (8) Making appropriate referrals.
(c) Physician assistants may not advertise in any manner without the name or names of the supervising physician or physicians, as the case may be, or in any manner which implies that the physician assistant is an independent practitioner.

HAWAII ADMIN. R. SEC. 16-85-49.1

IDAHO

Delegation Of Services (DOS) Agreement. A written document mutually agreed upon and signed and dated by the physician assistant and supervising physician that defines the working relationship and delegation of duties between the supervising physician and the physician assistant as specified by Board rule. The Board of Medicine may review the written delegation of services agreement, job descriptions, policy statements, or other documents that define the responsibilities of the physician assistant in the practice setting, and may require such changes as needed to achieve compliance with these rules, and to safeguard the public.

IDAHO ADMIN. CODE SEC. 22.01.01.06

Scope of Practice

Physical Examination. A physician assistant may evaluate the physical and psychosocial health status through a comprehensive health history and physical examination. This may include the performance of pelvic examinations and pap smears; and:

Screening And Evaluating. Initiate appropriate laboratory or diagnostic studies, or both, to screen or evaluate the patient health status and interpret reported information in accordance with knowledge of the laboratory or diagnostic studies, provided such laboratory or diagnostic studies are related to and consistent with the physician assistant's scope of practice.

Minor Illness. Diagnose and manage minor illnesses or conditions.

Manage Care. Manage the health care of the stable chronically ill patient in accordance with the medical regimen initiated by the supervising physician.

Emergency Situations. Institute appropriate care which might be required to stabilize a patient's condition in an emergency or potentially life threatening situation until physician consultation can be obtained.

Surgery. The acts of surgery which may be performed by a physician assistant are minor office surgical procedures such as punch biopsy, sebaceous cyst and ingrown toenail removal, cryotherapy for wart removal; assist in surgery with retraction, surgical wound exposure, and skin closure with direct personal supervision of the supervising physician; use non-ablative lasers under supervision; and the repair of lacerations, not involving nerve, tendon, or major vessel.

Casting. Manage the routine care of non-displaced fractures and sprains.

Hospital Discharge Summary. May complete hospital discharge summaries and the discharge summary shall be co-signed by the supervising physician.

IDAHO ADMIN. CODE SEC. 22.01.01.028

ILLINOIS

a) A physician assistant may provide medical/surgical services delegated to him/her by the supervising physician(s) when such services are within his/her skills and within the current scope of practice of the supervising physician/alternate supervising physician and are provided under the supervision and direction of the supervising physician/alternate supervising physician.

b) The physician/physician assistant team shall establish written guidelines that are individual to the physician assistant in the practice setting and keep those guidelines current and available in the supervising physician's office or location where the physician assistant is practicing.

ILLINOIS ADMIN. CODE TIT. 68 SEC. 1350.90

INDIANA

(a) When engaged in the physician assistant's professional activities, a physician assistant shall wear a name tag identifying the individual as a physician assistant and shall inform patients that he or she is a physician assistant. A physician assistant shall not portray himself or herself as a licensed physician.

(b) A physician assistant shall make available for inspection at his or her primary place of business:
  (1) the physician assistant's certificate issued by the committee;
  (2) a statement from the supervising physician that the physician assistant is, or will be, supervised by that physician;
  (3) a description of the setting in which the physician assistant shall be working under the physician supervision;
  (4) a job description with duties to be performed by the physician assistant and to be signed by both the physician and physician assistant; and
  (5) the name, business address, and telephone number of the physician under whose supervision the physician assistant will be supervised.

(c) The physician assistant may perform, under the supervision of the supervising physician, such duties and responsibilities within the scope of the supervising physician's practice.

INDIANA ADMIN. CODE TIT. 844 R. 2.2-2-5

IOWA

The medical services to be provided by the physician assistant are those delegated by a supervising physician. The ultimate role of the physician assistant cannot be rigidly defined because of the variations in practice requirements due to geographic, economic, and sociologic factors. The high degree of responsibility a physician assistant may assume requires that, at the conclusion of the formal education, the physician assistant possess the knowledge, skills and abilities necessary to provide those services appropriate to the practice setting. The physician assistant's services may be utilized in any clinical settings including, but not limited to, the office, the ambulatory clinic, the hospital, the patient's home, extended care facilities and nursing homes. Diagnostic and therapeutic medical tasks common to the physician's practice may be assigned to the physician assistant by a supervising physician after demonstration of proficiency and competence. The medical services to be provided by the physician assistant include, but are not limited to, the following:

a. The initial approach to a patient of any age group in any setting to elicit a medical history and perform a physical examination.

b. Assessment, diagnosis and treatment of medical or surgical problems and recording the findings.

c. Order, interpret, or perform laboratory tests, X-rays or other medical procedures or studies.

d. Performance of therapeutic procedures such as injections, immunizations, suturing and care of wounds, removal of foreign bodies, ear and eye irrigation and other clinical procedures.

e. Performance of office surgical procedures including, but not limited to, skin biopsy, mole or wart removal, toenail removal, removal of a foreign body, arthrocentesis, incision and drainage of abscesses.

f. Assisting in surgery.

g. Prenatal and postnatal care and assisting a physician in obstetrical care.

h. Care of orthopedic problems.

i. Performing and screening the results of special medical examinations including, but not limited to, electrocardiogram or Holter monitoring, radiography, audiometric and vision screening, tonometry, and pulmonary function screening tests.

j. Instruction and counseling of patients regarding physical and mental health on matters such as diets, disease, therapy, and normal growth and development.

k. Assisting a physician in the hospital setting by performing medical histories and physical examinations, making patient rounds, recording patient progress notes and other appropriate medical records, assisting in surgery, performing or assisting with medical procedures, providing emergency medical services and issuing, transmitting and executing patient care orders of the supervising physician.

l. Providing services to patients requiring continuing care (i.e., home, nursing home, extended care facilities).

m. Referring patients to specialty or subspecialty physicians, medical facilities or social agencies as indicated by the patients' problems.

n. Immediate evaluation, treatment and institution of procedures essential to providing an appropriate response to emergency medical problems.

o. Order drugs and supplies in the office, and assist in keeping records and in the upkeep of equipment.

p. Admit patients to a hospital or health care facility.

q. Order diets, physical therapy, inhalation therapy, or other rehabilitative services as indicated by the patient's problems.

r. Administer any drug (a single dose).

s. Prescribe drugs and medical devices under the following conditions:

(1) The physician assistant shall have passed the national certifying examination conducted by the National Commission on the Certification of Physician Assistants or its successor examination approved by the board. Physician assistants with a temporary license may order drugs and medical devices only with the prior approval and direction of a supervising physician. Prior approval may include discussion of the specific medical problems with a supervising physician prior to the patient's being seen by the physician assistant.

(2) The physician assistant may not prescribe Schedule II controlled substances which are listed as stimulants or depressants in Iowa Code chapter 124. The physician assistant may order Schedule II controlled substances which are listed as stimulants or depressants in Iowa Code chapter 124 only with the prior approval and direction of a physician. Prior approval may include discussion of the specific medical problems with a supervising physician prior to the patient's being seen by the physician assistant.

(3) The physician assistant shall inform the board of any limitation on the prescriptive authority of the physician assistant in addition to the limitations set out in 327.1(1)"s"(2).

(4) A physician assistant shall not prescribe substances that the supervising physician does not have the authority to prescribe except as allowed in 327.1(1)"n."

(5) The physician assistant may prescribe, supply and administer drugs and medical devices in all settings including, but not limited to, hospitals, health care facilities, health care institutions, clinics, offices, health maintenance organizations, and outpatient and emergency care settings except as limited by 327.1(1)"s"(2).

(6) A physician assistant who is an authorized prescriber may request, receive, and supply sample drugs and medical devices except as limited by 327.1(1)"s"(2).

(7) The board of physician assistant examiners shall be the only board to regulate the practice of physician assistants relating to prescribing and supplying prescription drugs, controlled substances and medical devices.

t. Supply properly packaged and labeled prescription drugs, controlled substances or medical devices when pharmacist services are not reasonably available or when it is in the best interests of the patient as delegated by a supervising physician.

(1) When the physician assistant is the prescriber of the medications under 327.1(1)"s," these medications shall be supplied for the purpose of accommodating the patient and shall not be sold for more than the cost of the drug and reasonable overhead costs as they relate to supplying prescription drugs to the patient and not at a profit to the physician or physician assistant.

(2) When a physician assistant supplies medication on the direct order of a physician, subparagraph (1) does not apply.

(3) A nurse or staff assistant may assist the physician assistant in supplying medications when prescriptive drug supplying authority is delegated by a supervising physician to the physician assistant under 327.1(1)"s."

u. When a physician assistant supplies medications as delegated by a supervising physician in a remote site, the physician assistant shall secure the regular advice and consultation of a pharmacist regarding the distribution, storage and appropriate use of prescription drugs, controlled substances, and medical devices.

v. May, at the request of the peace officer, withdraw a specimen of blood from a patient for the purpose of determining the alcohol concentration or the presence of drugs.

w. Direct medical personnel, health professionals and others involved in caring for patients in the execution of patient care.

x. May authenticate medical forms by signing the form and including a supervising physician's name.

y. Perform other duties appropriate to a physician's practice.

z. Health care providers shall consider the instructions of the physician assistant to be instructions of a supervising physician if the instructions concern duties delegated to the physician assistant by the supervising physician.

IOWA ADMIN. CODE R. 645-327.1

KANSAS

(a) The practice of a physician assistant shall include medical services within the education, training and experience of the physician assistant that are delegated by the responsible physician. Physician assistants practice in a dependent role with a responsible physician, and may perform those duties and responsibilities through delegated authority or written protocol. Medical services rendered by physician assistants may be performed in any setting authorized by the responsible physician, including but not limited to, clinics, hospitals, ambulatory surgical centers, patient homes, nursing homes and other medical institutions.

(b) A person licensed as a physician assistant may perform, only under the direction and supervision of a physician, acts which constitute the practice of medicine and surgery to the extent and in the manner authorized by the physician responsible for the physician assistant and only to the extent such acts are consistent with rules and regulations adopted by the board which relate to acts performed by a physician assistant under the responsible physician's direction and supervision. A physician assistant may prescribe drugs pursuant to a written protocol as authorized by the responsible physician.

(c) Before a physician assistant shall perform under the direction and supervision of a physician, such physician assistant shall be identified to the patient and others involved in providing the patient services as a physician assistant to the responsible physician. Physician assistants licensed under the provisions of this act shall keep their license available for inspection at their primary place of business. A physician assistant may not perform any act or procedure performed in the practice of optometry except as provided in K.S.A. 65-1508 and 65-2887 and amendments thereto.

(d) The board shall adopt rules and regulations governing the prescribing of drugs by physician assistants and the responsibilities of the responsible physician with respect thereto. Such rules and regulations shall establish such conditions and limitations as the board determines to be necessary to protect the public health and safety. In developing rules and regulations relating to the prescribing of drugs by physician assistants, the board shall take into consideration the amount of training and capabilities of physician assistants, the different practice settings in which physician assistants and responsible physicians practice, the degree of direction and supervision to be provided by a responsible physician and the needs of the geographic area of the state in which the physician's physician assistant and the responsible physician practice. In all cases in which a physician assistant is authorized to prescribe drugs by a responsible physician, a written protocol between the responsible physician and the physician assistant containing the essential terms of such authorization shall be in effect. Any written prescription order shall include the name, address and telephone number of the responsible physician. In no case shall the scope of the authority of the physician assistant to prescribe drugs exceed the normal and customary practice of the responsible physician in the prescribing of drugs.

(e) The physician assistant may not dispense drugs, but may request, receive and sign for professional samples and may distribute professional samples to patients pursuant to a written protocol as authorized by the responsible physician. In order to prescribe controlled substances, the physician assistant shall register with the federal drug enforcement administration.

(f) As used in this section, "drug" means those articles and substances defined as drugs in K.S.A. 65-1626 and 65-4101 and amendments thereto.

Kansas Stat. Ann. sec. 65-28a08

Scope of practice. A physician assistant may perform acts that constitute the practice of medicine and surgery in the following instances:

(a) If directly ordered, authorized, and coordinated by the responsible or designated physician through the physician's immediate or physical presence;

(b) if directly ordered, authorized, and coordinated by the responsible or designated physician through radio, telephone, or other form of telecommunication;

(c) if authorized on the form provided by, and presented to, the board by the responsible physician pursuant to K.S.A. 2000 Supp. 65-28a03 and amendments thereto; or

(d) if an emergency exists. (Authorized by K.S.A. 2000 Supp. 65-28a03; implementing K.S.A. 2000 Supp. 65-28a08; effective, T-100-2-13.)

KANSAS ADMIN. REGS. 100-28A-6

KENTUCKY

Services and procedures that may be performed by physician assistant—Restrictions.

(1) A physician assistant may perform medical services and procedures within the scope of medical services and procedures described in the initial or any supplemental application received by the board under KRS 311.854.

(2) A physician assistant shall be considered an agent of the supervising physician in performing medical services and procedures described in the initial application or any supplemental application received by the board under KRS 311.854.

(3) A physician assistant may initiate evaluation and treatment in emergency situations without specific approval.

(4) A physician assistant may prescribe and administer all nonscheduled legend drugs and medical devices as delegated by the supervising physician. A physician assistant who is delegated prescribing authority may request, receive, and distribute professional sample drugs to patients.

(5) A physician assistant shall not submit direct billing for medical services and procedures performed by the physician assistant.

(6) A physician assistant may perform local infiltrative anesthesia under the provisions of subsection (1) of this section, but a physician assistant shall not administer or monitor general or regional anesthesia unless the requirements of KRS 311.862 are met.

(7) A physician assistant may perform services in the offices or clinics of the supervising physician. A physician assistant may also render services in hospitals or other licensed health care facilities only with written permission of the facility's governing body, and the facility may restrict the physician assistant's scope of practice within the facility as deemed appropriate by the facility.

(8) A physician assistant shall not practice medicine or osteopathy independently. Each physician assistant shall practice under supervision as defined in KRS 311.840.

KENTUCKY REV. STAT. SEC. 311.858

Practice as anesthesiology assistant.

(1) A physician assistant who was practicing as an anesthesiology assistant in Kentucky prior to July 15, 2002, may continue to practice if the physician assistant:

    (a) Met the practice, education, training, and certification requirements specified in KRS 311.844 and 311.846;

    (b) Is a graduate of an approved program accredited by the Committee on Allied Health Education and Accreditation or the Commission on Accreditation of Allied Health Education Programs that is specifically designed to train an individual to administer general or regional anesthesia; and

    (c) Is employed by a supervising physician in anesthesia.

(2) A physician assistant who has not practiced as an anesthesiology assistant in Kentucky prior to the July 15, 2002, shall meet the following requirements prior to practicing as an anesthesiology assistant:

    (a) Graduation from an approved four (4) year physician assistant program as specified in subsection (1)(b) of this section and graduation from another two (2) year approved and accredited program that consists of academic and clinical training in anesthesiology;

    (b) Compliance with the practice, education, training, and certification requirements specified in KRS 311.844 and 311.846; and

    (c) Employment with a supervising physician in anesthesia.

(3) A physician assistant practicing as an anesthesiology assistant shall not administer or monitor general or regional anesthesia unless the supervising physician in anesthesia:

    (a) Is physically present in the room during induction and emergence;

    (b) Is not concurrently performing any other anesthesiology procedure; and

    (c) Is available to provide immediate physical presence in the room.

Kentucky Rev. Stat. sec. 311.862

Services performed in location separate from supervising physician.

(1) A supervising physician who uses the services of a physician assistant in an office or clinic separate from the physician's primary office shall submit for board approval a specific written

request that describes the services to be provided by the physician assistant in the separate office or clinic, the distance between the primary office and the separate location, and the means and availability of direct communication at all times with the supervising physician.

(2) A physician assistant shall not practice medicine or osteopathy in an office, clinic, or separate location from the supervising physician unless the physician assistant has two (2) continuous years of experience in a non-separate location. The board in its discretion may modify or waive the requirements of this subsection.

(3) Except as provided by KRS 311.862, a physician assistant may perform services when the supervising physician is not physically present in the supervising physician's office or clinic when a reliable means of direct communication with the supervising physician is available at all times.

(4) Except as provided by KRS 311.862, a physician assistant may perform services when the supervising physician is not physically present in a hospital or other licensed health care facility when a reliable means of direct communication with the supervising physician is available at all times and the hospital or facility has given specific approval for the provision of physician assistant services without the physical presence of the supervising physician.

KENTUCKY REV. STAT. SEC. 311.860

LOUISIANA

A physician assistant performs medical services when such services are rendered under the supervision of a supervising physician. A physician assistant may have multiple supervising physicians in no more than five medical specialties or subspecialties, provided all of the physician assistant's supervising physicians are properly registered with the board in accordance with the provisions of this Part. A physician assistant may perform those duties and responsibilities that are delegated to him by his supervising physician. A physician assistant is considered to be and is deemed the agent of his supervising physician in the performance of all practice-related activities, including but not limited to assisting in surgery and the ordering of diagnostic and other medical services. A physician assistant shall not practice without supervision except in life-threatening emergencies and in emergency situations such as man-made and natural disaster relief efforts.

(2) A physician assistant may inject local anesthetic agents subcutaneously, including digital blocks or apply topical anesthetic agents when delegated to do so by a supervising physician. However,

nothing in this Part shall otherwise permit a physician assistant to administer local anesthetics perineurally, peridurally, epidurally, intrathecally, or intravenously unless such physician assistant is a certified registered nurse anesthetist and meets the requirements in R.S. 37:930.

(B) The practice of a physician assistant shall include the performance of medical services within the scope of his education, training, and experience, which are delegated by the supervising physician. Medical services rendered by a physician assistant may include but are not limited to:

    (1) Obtaining patient histories and performing physical examinations.

    (2) Ordering or performing diagnostic procedures as delegated by the supervising physician.

    (3) Developing and implementing a treatment plan in accordance with written clinical practice guidelines and protocols set forth by the supervising physician.

    (4) Monitoring the effectiveness of therapeutic intervention.

    (5) Suturing wounds as delegated by the supervising physician.

    (6) Offering counseling and education to meet patient needs.

    (7) Making appropriate referrals.

(C) The activities listed above may be performed in any setting authorized by the supervising physician including: clinics, hospitals, ambulatory surgical centers, patient homes, nursing homes, other institutional settings, and health manpower shortage areas.

LOUISIANA REV. STAT. SEC. 1360.31

MAINE

Physician assistants practice medicine with physician supervision.

(A) DELEGATED AUTHORITY

Physician assistants may perform only those medical activities that have been delegated to the physician assistant by a supervising physician. Medical activities that may be delegated include the following:

    1. the ordering of diagnostic, therapeutic and other medical services;

    2. the prescribing and dispensing of drugs and medical devices to the extent permitted by state and federal law. Prescribing and dispensing drugs may include Schedule III through V

substances and all legend drugs. A Physician Assistant and primary supervising physician may together request individual consideration for authorization to prescribe schedule II drugs under specific individual guidelines detailed by the Board. Physician assistants may request, receive, and sign for professional samples and may distribute professional samples to patients; and

3. the performance of tasks that are not routinely within the practice or regularly performed by the primary supervising physician so long as adequate oversight, secondary supervisory, and referral arrangements are in place to ensure competent provision of services by the physician assistant.

B. PRACTICE SETTING
A physician assistant may perform medical activities only in a practice setting in which the supervising physician agrees to provide supervision.

CODE MAINE R. SEC. 02 373 6

MASSACHUSETTS

(1) A physician assistant may, under the supervision of a licensed physician, perform any and all services which are:
   (a) Within the competence of the physician assistant in question, as determined by the supervising physician's assessment of his or her training and experience; and
   (b) Within the scope of services for which the supervising physician can provide adequate supervision to ensure that accepted standards of medical practice are followed.

(2) A physician assistant may approach patients of all ages and with all types of conditions; elicit histories; perform examinations; order, perform and interpret diagnostic studies; order and perform therapeutic procedures; instruct and counsel patients regarding physical and mental health issues; respond to life-threatening situations; and facilitate the appropriate referral of patients; consistent with his or her supervising physician's scope of expertise and responsibility and the level of authority and responsibility delegated to him or her by the supervising physician.

(3) Nothing contained herein shall be construed to allow a physician assistant to:
   (a) Give general anesthesia;
   (b) Perform any procedure involving ionizing radiation, except in an emergency situation where the procedure is performed

under the direction and control of a licensed physician; or
(c) Render a formal medical opinion on procedures involving ion-izing radiation.

Where a physician assistant is involved in the performance of major invasive procedures, such procedures shall be undertaken under specific written protocols, available to the Board upon request, which have been developed between the supervising physician and the physician assistant and which specify, inter alia, the level of supervision the service requires, e.g., direct (physician in room), personal (physician in building), or general (physician available by telephone).

CODE MASSACHUSETTS REGS. TIT. 263 SEC. 5.04

MICHIGAN

(1) Except in an emergency situation, a physician's assistant shall provide medical care services only under the supervision of a physician or properly designated alternative physician, and only if those medical care services are within the scope of practice of the supervising physician and are delegated by the supervising physician.

(2) A physician's assistant shall provide medical care services only in a medical care setting where the supervising physician regularly sees patients. However, a physician's assistant may make calls or go on rounds under the supervision of a physician in private homes, public institutions, emergency vehicles, ambulatory care clinics, hospitals, intermediate or extended care facilities, health maintenance organizations, nursing homes, or other health care facilities to the extent permitted by the bylaws, rules, or regulations of the governing facility or organization, if any.

(3) A physician's assistant may prescribe drugs as a delegated act of a supervising physician, but shall do so only in accordance with procedures and protocol for the prescription established by rule of the appropriate board. Until the rules are promulgated, a physician's assistant may prescribe a drug other than a controlled substance as defined by article 7 or federal law, as a delegated act of the supervising physician. When delegated prescription occurs, the supervising physician's name shall be used, recorded, or otherwise indicated in connection with each individual prescription so that the individual who dispenses or administers the prescription knows under whose delegated authority the physician's assistant is prescribing.

(4) A physician's assistant may order, receive, and dispense complimentary starter dose drugs other than controlled substances as defined by article 7 or federal law as a delegated act of a supervis-

ing physician. When the delegated ordering, receipt, or dispensing of complimentary starter dose drugs occurs, the supervising physician's name shall be used, recorded, or otherwise indicated in connection with each order, receipt, or dispensing so that the individual who processes the order or delivers the complimentary starter dose drugs or to whom the complimentary starter dose drugs are dispensed knows under whose delegated authority the physician's assistant is ordering, receiving, or dispensing. As used in this subsection, "complimentary starter dose" means that term as defined in section 17745. It is the intent of the legislature in enacting this subsection to allow a pharmaceutical manufacturer or wholesale distributor, as those terms are defined in part 177, to distribute complimentary starter dose drugs to a physician's assistant, as described in this subsection, in compliance with section 503(d) of the federal food, drug, and cosmetic act, chapter 675, 52 Stat. 1051, 21 U.S.C. 353.

MICHIGAN COMPLIED LAWS SEC. 333.17076

MINNESOTA

Physician assistants shall practice medicine only with physician supervision. Physician assistants may perform those duties and responsibilities as delegated in the physician-physician assistant agreement and delegation forms maintained at the address of record by the supervising physician and physician assistant, including the prescribing, administering, and dispensing of medical devices and drugs, excluding anesthetics, other than local anesthetics, injected in connection with an operating room procedure, inhaled anesthesia and spinal anesthesia.

Patient service must be limited to:

(1) services within the training and experience of the physician assistant;

(2) services customary to the practice of the supervising physician;

(3) services delegated by the supervising physician; and

(4) services within the parameters of the laws, rules, and standards of the facilities in which the physician assistant practices.

Nothing in this chapter authorizes physician assistants to perform duties regulated by the boards listed in section 214.01, subdivision 2, other than the Board of Medical Practice, and except as provided in this section.

Delegation. Patient services may include, but are not limited to, the following, as delegated by the supervising physician and authorized in the agreement:

(1) taking patient histories and developing medical status reports;

(2) performing physical examinations;

(3) interpreting and evaluating patient data;

(4) ordering or performing diagnostic procedures;

(5) ordering or performing therapeutic procedures;

(6) providing instructions regarding patient care, disease prevention, and health promotion;

(7) assisting the supervising physician in patient care in the home and in health care facilities;

(8) creating and maintaining appropriate patient records;

(9) transmitting or executing specific orders at the direction of the supervising physician;

(10) prescribing, administering, and dispensing legend drugs and medical devices if this function has been delegated by the supervising physician pursuant to and subject to the limitations of section 147.34 and chapter 151. Physician assistants who have been delegated the authority to prescribe controlled substances shall maintain a separate addendum to the delegation form which lists all schedules and categories of controlled substances which the physician assistant has the authority to prescribe. This addendum shall be maintained with the physician-physician assistant agreement, and the delegation form at the address of record;

(11) for physician assistants not delegated prescribing authority, administering legend drugs and medical devices following prospective review for each patient by and upon direction of the supervising physician;

(12) functioning as an emergency medical technician with permission of the ambulance service and in compliance with section 144E.127, and ambulance service rules adopted by the commissioner of health;

(13) initiating evaluation and treatment procedures essential to providing an appropriate response to emergency situations; and

(14) certifying a physical disability under section 169.345, subdivision 2a.

Orders of physician assistants shall be considered the orders of their supervising physicians in all practice-related activities, including, but not limited to, the ordering of diagnostic, therapeutic, and other medical services.

MINNESOTA STAT. ANN. SEC. 147A.09

MISSISSIPPI

1. Physician Assistants shall practice according to a Board-approved protocol which has been mutually agreed upon by the Physician

Assistant and the supervising physician. Each protocol shall be prepared taking into consideration the specialty of the supervising physician, and must outline diagnostic and therapeutic procedures and categories of pharmacologic agents which may be ordered, administered, dispensed and/or prescribed for patients with diagnoses identified by the Physician Assistant. Each protocol shall contain a detailed description of back-up coverage if the supervising physician is away from the primary office. Although licensed by the Mississippi State Board of Medical Licensure, no Physician Assistant shall practice until a duly executed protocol has been approved by the Board.

2. Physician Assistants may not write prescriptions for or dispense controlled substances or any other drug having addiction-forming or addiction-sustaining liability. A Physician Assistant may, however, administer such medications pursuant to an order by the supervising physician according to the protocol worked out with the physician.

MISSISSIPPI RULES CH. XXII SEC. 4(D)

MISSISSIPPI

The scope of practice of a physician assistant shall consist only of the following services and procedures:

(1) Taking patient histories;

(2) Performing physical examinations of a patient;

(3) Performing or assisting in the performance of routine office laboratory and patient screening procedures;

(4) Performing routine therapeutic procedures;

(5) Recording diagnostic impressions and evaluating situations calling for attention of a physician to institute treatment procedures;

(6) Instructing and counseling patients regarding mental and physical health using procedures reviewed and approved by a licensed physician;

(7) Assisting the supervising physician in institutional settings, including reviewing of treatment plans, ordering of tests and diagnostic laboratory and radiological services, and ordering of therapies, using procedures reviewed and approved by a licensed physician;

(8) Assisting in surgery;

(9) Performing such other tasks not prohibited by law under the supervision of a licensed physician as the physician's assistant has been trained and is proficient to perform;

(10) Physician assistants shall not perform abortions.

MISSOURI REV. STAT. SEC. 334.75.2

MONTANA

(1) A physician, office, firm, state institution, or professional service corporation may not employ or make use of the services of a physician assistant-certified in the practice of medicine, as defined in 37-3-102, and a physician assistant-certified may not be employed or practice as a physician assistant-certified unless the physician assistant-certified:

 (a) is supervised by a licensed physician;

 (b) is licensed by the Montana state board of medical examiners; and

 (c) has received board approval of a physician assistant-certified utilization plan.

(2) A physician assistant-certified utilization plan must set forth in detail the following information:

 (a) the name and qualifications of the supervising physician, as provided in 37-20-101, and the name and license number of the physician assistant-certified;

 (b) the nature and location of the physician's medical practice;

 (c) the scope of practice of the physician assistant-certified and the locations where the physician assistant-certified will practice;

 (d) the name and qualifications of a second physician meeting the requirements of 37-20-101 to act as an alternate supervising physician in the absence of the primary supervising physician;

 (e) necessary guidelines describing the intended availability of the supervising or alternate physician for consultation by the physician assistant-certified; and

 (f) other information the board may consider necessary.

(3) The board shall approve the utilization plan if it finds that the practice of the physician assistant-certified is:

 (a) assigned by the supervising physician;

 (b) within the scope of the training, knowledge, experience, and practice of the supervisory physician; and

 (c) within the scope of the training, knowledge, education, and experience of the physician assistant-certified.

(4) A supervising physician and a physician assistant-certified may submit a new or additional utilization plan to the board for approval without reestablishing the criteria set out in 37-20-402, so long as the information requirements of subsection (2) have been met and the appropriate fee provided for in 37-20-302(1) has been paid.

(5) A utilization plan may provide that a physician assistant-certified be allowed to furnish services on a locum tenens basis at a location other than the physician assistant-certified's primary place of practice. A locum tenens utilization plan may be approved by a single board member.

MONTANA CODE ANN. SEC. 37-20-301

NEBRASKA

The supervising physician and the physician assistant must have a written scope of practice agreement which is kept on file at the primary practice site and available for review by the Department upon request.
1. The scope of practice agreement must delineate:
   (a) The activities of the physician assistant; and
   (b) The limits of the physician assistant.

172 NEBRASKA CODE ANN. SEC. 90-006

Physician assistants; services performed; supervision requirements. (1) Notwithstanding any other provision of law, a physician assistant may perform medical services when he or she renders such services under the supervision of a licensed physician or group of physicians approved by the board, in the specialty area or areas for which the physician assistant shall be trained or experienced. Any physician assistant licensed under sections 71-1,107.15 to 71-1,107.30 to perform services may perform those services only:
(a) In the office of the supervising physician where such physician maintains his or her primary practice;
(b) In any other office which is operated by the supervising physician with the personal presence of the supervising physician. The physician assistant may function without the personal presence of the supervising physician in an office other than where such physician maintains his or her primary practice as provided in subsection (2) of this section and when approved on an individual basis by the board. Any such approval shall require site visits by the supervising physician, regular reporting to the supervising physician by the physician assistant, and arrangements for supervision at all times by the supervising physician which are sufficient to provide quality medical care;
(c) In a hospital, with the approval of the governing board of such hospital, where the supervising physician is a member of the staff and the physician assistant is subject to the rules and regulations of the hospital. Such rules and regulations may include, but need

not be limited to, reasonable requirements that physician assistants and the supervising physician maintain professional liability insurance with such coverage and limits as may be established by the hospital governing board, upon the recommendation of the medical staff; or

(d) On calls outside such offices, when authorized by the supervising physician and with the approval of the governing board of any affected hospital.

(2) The board shall adopt and promulgate rules and regulations establishing minimum requirements for the personal presence of the supervising physician, stated in hours or percentage of practice time. The board may provide different minimum requirements for the personal presence of the supervising physician based on the geographic location of the supervising physician's primary and other practice sites and other factors the board deems relevant.

NEBRASKA REV. STAT. SEC. 71-1.107.17

NEVADA

1. The medical services which a physician assistant is authorized to perform must be:
    (a) Commensurate with his education, training, experience and level of competence; and
    (b) Within the scope of the practice of his supervising physician.
2. The physician assistant shall wear at all times while on duty a placard, plate or insignia which identifies him as a physician assistant.
3. No physician assistant may represent himself in any manner which would tend to mislead the general public or the patients of the supervising physician.
4. A physician assistant shall notify the board in writing within 72 hours after any change relating to his supervising physician.

NEVADA ADMIN. CODE SEC. 630.360

NEW HAMPSHIRE

(a) Medical services delegated by a supervising physician may be performed by the physician assistant in any setting authorized by the supervising physician, including but not limited to:
    (1) Clinics;
    (2) Hospitals, including emergency departments;
    (3) Ambulatory surgical centers;
    (4) Patient homes;

(5) Nursing homes, or other extended care facilities; and

(6) Other institutional settings.

    (b) A physician assistant may write orders for patients in the in-patient setting as delegated by the supervising physician or alternate. Such orders shall be countersigned by the RSP or ARSP as required by institutional policy, however, such countersignature shall not be required prior to the order being executed.

    (c) Physician assistants shall perform all practice-related activities, including but not limited to, the ordering of diagnostic or therapeutic services to be implemented by other health professionals, as the agent of the RSP or ARSP.

NEW HAMPSHIRE CODE ADMIN. R. ANN. (MED) SEC. 603.01

NEW JERSEY

a. A physician assistant may practice in all medical care settings, including, but not limited to, a physician's office, a health care facility, an institution, a veterans home or a private home, provided that:

(1) the physician assistant is under the direct supervision of a physician pursuant to section 9 of this act;

(2) the practice of the physician assistant is limited to those procedures authorized under section 7 of this act;

(3) an appropriate notice of employment has been filed with the board pursuant to subsection b. of section 5 of this act;

(4) the supervising physician or physician assistant advises the patient at the time that services are rendered that they are to be performed by the physician assistant;

(5) the physician assistant conspicuously wears an identification tag using the term "physician assistant" whenever acting in that capacity; and

(6) any entry by a physician assistant in a clinical record is appropriately signed and followed by the designation, "PAC."

b. Any physician assistant who practices in violation of any of the conditions specified in subsection a. of this section shall be deemed to have engaged in professional misconduct

NEW JERSEY STAT. ANN. SEC. 45: 9-27.15

A physician assistant may perform the following procedures:

(1) Approaching a patient to elicit a detailed and accurate history, perform an appropriate physical examination, identify problems,

record information and interpret and present information to the supervising physician;

(2) Suturing and caring for wounds including removing sutures and clips and changing dressings, except for facial wounds, traumatic wounds requiring suturing in layers and infected wounds;

(3) Providing patient counseling services and patient education consistent with directions of the supervising physician;

(4) Assisting a physician in an inpatient setting by conducting patient rounds, recording patient progress notes, determining and implementing therapeutic plans jointly with the supervising physician and compiling and recording pertinent narrative case summaries;

(5) Assisting a physician in the delivery of services to patients requiring continuing care in a private home, nursing home, extended care facility or other setting, including the review and monitoring of treatment and therapy plans;

(6) Facilitating the referral of patients to, and promoting their awareness of, health care facilities and other appropriate agencies and resources in the community; and

(7) Such other procedures suitable for discretionary and routine performance by physician assistants as designated by the board pursuant to subsection a. of section 15 of this act.1 or

(8) A physician assistant may perform the following procedures only when directed, ordered or prescribed by the supervising physician or specified in accordance with protocols promulgated pursuant to subsection c. of section 15 of this act:

    (a) Performing non-invasive laboratory procedures and related studies or assisting duly licensed personnel in the performance of invasive laboratory procedures and related studies;

    (b) Giving injections, administering medications and requesting diagnostic studies;

    (c) Suturing and caring for facial wounds, traumatic wounds requiring suturing in layers and infected wounds;

    (d) Writing prescriptions or ordering medications in an inpatient or outpatient setting in accordance with section 10 of this act; or and

    (e) Such other procedures as may be specified in accordance with protocols promulgated in accordance with subsection b. of section 15 of this act.

(9) A physician assistant may assist a supervising surgeon in the operating room when a qualified assistant physician is not required by the board and a second assistant is deemed necessary by the supervising surgeon.

NEW JERSEY STAT. ANN. SEC. 45: 9-27.16

NEW MEXICO

A physician assistant shall perform only the acts and duties assigned to the physician assistant by a supervising licensed physician that are within the scope of practice of the supervising licensed physician.

NEW MEXICO STAT. ANN. SEC. 61-6-7

NEW YORK

1. Notwithstanding any other provision of law, a physician assistant may perform medical services, but only when under the supervision of a physician and only when such acts and duties as are assigned to him are within the scope of practice of such supervising physician.

2. Notwithstanding any other provision of law, a specialist assistant may perform medical services, but only when under the supervision of a physician and only when such acts and duties as are assigned to him are related to the designated medical specialty for which he is registered and are within the scope of practice of his supervising physician.

3. Supervision shall be continuous but shall not be construed as necessarily requiring the physical presence of the supervising physician at the time and place where such services are performed.

4. No physician shall employ or supervise more than two physician assistants and two specialist assistants in his private practice.

5. Nothing in this article shall prohibit a hospital from employing physician assistants or specialist assistants provided they work under the supervision of a physician designated by the hospital and not beyond the scope of practice of such physician. The numerical limitation of subdivision 4 of this section shall not apply to services performed in a hospital.

6. Notwithstanding any other provision of this article, nothing shall prohibit a physician employed by or rendering services to the department of correctional services under contract from supervising no more than four physician assistants or specialist assistants in his practice for the department of correctional services.

7. Notwithstanding any other provision of law, a trainee in an approved program may perform medical services when such services are performed within the scope of such program.

8. Nothing in this article, or in article 37 of the public health law, shall be construed to authorize physician assistants or specialist assistants to perform those specific functions and duties specifi-

cally delegated by law to those persons licensed as allied health professionals under the public health law or the education law.

NEW YORK STAT. C. L. SEC. 6542

NORTH CAROLINA

(a) Physician assistants perform medical acts, tasks or functions with physician supervision. Physician assistants perform those duties and responsibilities, including the prescribing and dispensing of drugs and medical devices, that are delegated by their supervising physician(s).

(b) Physician assistants shall be considered the agents of their supervising physicians in the performance of all medical practice-related activities, including but not limited to, the ordering of diagnostic, therapeutic and other medical services.

21 NORTH CAROLINA ANN. CODE 32 SEC. .0108

NORTH DAKOTA

Physician assistants may perform only those duties and responsibilities that are delegated by their supervising physicians. No supervising physician may delegate to a physician assistant any duty or responsibility for which the physician assistant has not been adequately trained. Physician assistants are the agents of their supervising physicians in the performance of all practice-related activities. A physician assistant may provide patient care only in those areas of medical practice where the supervising physician provides patient care.

NORTH DAKOTA ADMIN. CODE SEC. 50-03-01-06

OHIO

(A) The physician assistant shall perform only in the manner and to the extent set forth in the standard utilization plan and any supplemental plans of the supervising physician as approved by the state medical board. Further, the physician assistant shall perform only within the degree of supervision specified in the standard utilization plan and any supplemental plans of the supervising physician as approved by the state medical board.

(B) Pursuant to a standard utilization plan as approved by the board, a supervising physician may authorize a physician assistant to perform the following functions:

    (1) Under "off-site supervision, on-site supervision, or direct supervision" as defined by rule 4731-4-03 of the Administrative Code:

(a) Obtaining comprehensive patient histories;

(b) Performing physical examinations, including audiometry screening, routine visual screening, and pelvic, rectal, and genital-urinary examinations when indicated;

(c) Initiating, requesting and/or performing routine laboratory, radiologic and diagnostic studies as indicated;

(d) Identifying normal and abnormal findings on histories, physical examinations, and commonly performed initial laboratory studies;

(e) Assessing patients;

(f) Developing treatment plans for patients;

(g) Implementing treatment plans that have been reviewed and approved by the supervising physician, subject to the supervision requirements of rule 4731-4-03(D) of the Administrative Code;

(h) Monitoring the effectiveness of therapeutic interventions;

(i) Providing patient education;

(j) Instituting and changing orders on patient charts as directed by the supervising physician, with any such orders written by the physician assistant to be reviewed by a supervising physician within twenty-four (24) hours after the order is written and countersigned if the order is appropriate;

(k) Screening patients to aid the supervising physician in determining need for further medical attention;

(l) Performing developmental screening examinations on children as relating to neurological, motor and mental functions;

(m) Performing care and suturing and removal of sutures of minor lacerations;

(n) Applying cast or splint and removing such cast or splint under direction of the supervising physician. Such application shall be made only after examination by the supervising physician;

(o) Administering medication and intravenous fluids upon order of the supervising physician;

(p) Removing superficial foreign bodies after consultation with the supervising physician and under his direction;

(q) Inserting a Foley or Cudae catheter into the urinary bladder or removing the catheter;

(r) Performing cardio-pulmonary resuscitation;

(s) Carrying out or relaying the supervising physician's orders for medication, to the extent permitted under laws pertaining to drugs;

    (t) Noninvasive application of skeletal traction under physician order;

    (u) Removing intrauterine devices;

    (v) Performing punch biopsies of superficial lesions;

   (w) Removing arterial lines;

    (x) Removing central venous catheter;

    (y) Inserting and removing nasogastric tube; and

    (z) Adjusting skeletal traction, excluding cervical traction, as ordered by the supervising physician.

(2) Under "on-site or direct supervision" as defined by rule 4731-4-03 of the Administrative Code:

    (a) Injection of contrast for IVP under direct supervision.

(3) Assisting in surgery in a hospital, as defined in section 3727.01 of the Revised Code, or an outpatient surgical care center affiliated with the hospital if the center meets the same credential, quality assurance and plan review standards as the hospital, provided that these physician-supervised procedures have been delineated within the scope of practice of a physician assistant and approved by the appropriate committee of the hospital or outpatient surgical care center where such services are to be rendered.

    (a) A physician assistant shall function as a physician assistant assisting in surgery only when under the direct supervision of the surgeon who is present during the surgery and only when the participation of a physician assistant assisting in surgery is indicated on the informed consent form. The performance of the following listed tasks is solely for the purpose of assisting the surgeon in performing a safe operation and shall not be construed to allow the physician assistant to perform surgery. The tasks a physician assistant assisting in surgery may perform include, but are not limited to, the following:

       (i)   handling of tissue;

      (ii) using instruments (e.g., retractors);

     (iii) providing hemostasis; and

     (iv) placing sutures as part of the surgical procedure;

    (b) A physician assistant functioning as a physician assistant assisting in surgery may close subcutaneous tissue and skin when the surgeon who performed the surgery provides supervision in close proximity within the surgical suite.

    (c) No physician assistant shall otherwise perform surgery, act as a surgeon, hold himself or herself out as a surgeon, practice medicine independently, or hold himself or herself out as a physician as defined in Chapter 4731. of the Revised Code.

(d) No person registered as a physician assistant under Chapter 4730. of the Revised Code shall engage in the practice of assisting in surgery unless the physician assistant meets the requirements of Chapter 4730. of the Revised Code and this Chapter of the Administrative Code.

(e) No physician assistant shall perform a surgical task or procedure which is the primary purpose of the surgery.

OHIO ADMIN. RULES SEC. 4731-4.01

A physician assistant shall not perform services or acts including, but not limited to, the following:

(A) Make a diagnosis of a disease or ailment or the absence thereof independent of the supervising physician;

(B) Prescribe any treatment or regimen not previously set forth by the supervising physician;

(C) Prescribe medication; sign or stamp prescriptions on behalf of the supervising physician; have prescription blanks available that have been presigned or stamped by the physician; or dispense or order medication, although the supervising physician's order for medication may be carried out or relayed by the physician assistant in accordance with existing drug laws;

(D) Sign a physician's name for the purpose of authenticating any prescriptions, orders, or recordings; or sign the physician's name in any situation where the physician's signature gives the appearance of the physician's approval;

(E) Maintain an office independent from the offices of the supervising physician;

(F) Admit patients to or release patients from a hospital independent of the supervising physician;

(G) Represent himself or herself in any way as being able to perform beyond the specific functions set forth in the supervising physician's board approved standard or supplemental physician assistant utilization plan;

(H) Hold himself or herself out as being able to function as a physician assistant, or use any words or letters indicating or implying that the person is a physician assistant, without a current, valid certificate of registration or temporary certificate of registration as a physician assistant issued pursuant to Chapter 4730. of the Revised Code;

(I) Practice as a physician assistant without the supervision and direction of a physician;

(J) Practice as a physician assistant without having entered into a supervision agreement that has been approved by the board;

(K) Practice as a physician assistant in a manner that is inconsistent with the standard or supplemental physician assistant utilization plan approved for the physician who is responsible for supervising the physician assistant;

(L) Independently advertise, except for the purpose of seeking employment;

(M) Practice as a physician assistant while failing to wear at all times when on duty a placard, plate, or other device identifying himself or herself as a "physician assistant."

(N) Represent himself or herself in any way as being able to function as a physician.

OHIO ADMIN. RULES SEC. 4731-4.04

OKLAHOMA

A physician assistant may perform the following health care services under the supervision and at the direction of the supervising physician. Such services include, but are not limited to:

(1) Initially approach a patient of any age group in a patient care setting to elicit a detailed history, perform a physical examination, delineate problems, and record the data.

(2) Assist the physician in conducting rounds in acute and long-term inpatient care settings, develop and implement patient management plans, record progress notes, and assist in the provision of continuity of care in other patient care settings.

(3) Order, perform, and/or interpret, at least to the point of recognizing deviations from the norm, common laboratory, radiological, cardiographic, and other routine diagnostic procedures used to identify pathophysiologic processes.

(4) Order or perform routine procedures such as injections, immunizations, suturing and wound care, and manage simple conditions produced by infection or trauma.

(5) Issue written and oral prescriptions and orders for medical supplies, services and drugs, including controlled medications in Schedules III, IV, and V under 63 O.S. ss 2-312 as approved in the Physician Drug Formulary and Board rules.

(6) A physician assistant may write an order for a Schedule II drug for immediate or ongoing administration on site under 63 O.S. ss 2-312 as approved in the Physician Assistant Drug Formulary and Board rules.

(7) Assist in the management of more complex illness and injuries, which may include assisting surgeons in the conduct of operations and taking initiative in performing evaluation and therapeutic procedures in response to life-threatening situations. In patients with newly diagnosed chronic or complex illness, the physician assistant shall contact the supervising physician within forty-eight (48) hours of the physician assistant's initial examination or treatment, and schedule the patient for appropriate evaluation by the supervising physician as directed by the physician.

(8) Instruct and counsel patients regarding compliance with prescribed therapeutic regimens, normal growth and development, family planning, emotional problems of daily living and health maintenance.

(9) Facilitate the referral of patients to the community's health and social service agencies when appropriate.

(10) Provide health care services which are delegated by the supervising physician when the service:

    (A) is within the physician assistant's skill,

    (B) forms a component of the physician's scope of practice, and

    (C) is provided with supervision, including authenticating with the signature any form that may be authenticated by the supervising physician's signature with prior delegation by the physician.

(b) Heath care services prohibited.

(1) No health care services may be performed in any of the following areas:

    (A) The measurement of the powers of human vision, or the determination of the accommodation and refractive states of the human eye or the scope of its functions in general, or the fitting or adaptation of lenses or frames for the aid thereof.

    (B) The prescribing or directing the use of, or using, any optical device in connection with ocular exercises, visual training, vision training or orthoptics.

    (C) The prescribing of contact lenses for, or the fitting or adaptation of contact lenses to, the human eye.

(2) Nothing in this section shall preclude the performance of routine visual screening.

OKLAHOMA ADMIN. CODE SEC. 435:15-5-1.1

OREGON

(1) The physician assistant may perform at the direction of the supervising physician and/or agent only those medical services as included in the Board-approved practice description.

(2) The physician assistant must clearly identify himself/herself as such when performing duties. The physician assistant shall at all times when on duty wear a name tag with the designation of "physician assistant" thereon.

(3) The supervising physician shall furnish reports, as required by the Board, on the performance of the physician assistant or trainee.

(4) All additions must be pre-approved. Requests for any change in the practice description of a physician assistant licensed in Oregon shall be submitted to the Board by the supervising physician in writing. The Board may require an examination prior to the approval of any such changes.

OREGON ADMIN. RULES SEC. 847-050-0040

PENNSYLVANIA

The physician assistant shall, under appropriate direction and supervision by a physician assistant supervisor, augment the physician's data gathering abilities in order to assist the physician in reaching decisions and instituting care plans for the physician's patients. Physician assistants may be permitted to perform the following functions. This list is not intended to be all-inclusive.

(1) Screen patients to determine need for medical attention.

(2) Review patient records to determine health status.

(3) Take a patient history.

(4) Perform a physical examination.

(5) Perform developmental screening examination on children.

(6) Record pertinent patient data.

(7) Make decisions regarding data gathering and appropriate management and treatment of patients being seen for the initial evaluation of a problem of the follow-up evaluation of a previously diagnosed and stabilized condition.

(8) Prepare patient summaries.

(9) Initiate requests for commonly performed initial laboratory studies.

(10) Collect specimens for and carry out commonly performed blood, urine and stool analyses and cultures.

(11) Identify normal and abnormal findings on history, physical examination and commonly performed laboratory studies.

(12) Initiate appropriate evaluation and emergency management for emergency situations, for example, cardiac arrest, respiratory distress, injuries, burns and hemorrhage.

(13) Perform clinical procedures such as:

    (i) Venipuncture.

    (ii) Intradermal tests.

      (iii) Electrocardiogram.

      (iv) Care and suturing of minor lacerations.

      (v) Casting and splinting.

      (vi) Control of external hemorrhage.

      (vii) Application of dressings and bandages.

      (viii) Administration of medications, except as specified in § 18.158 (relating to prescribing and dispensing drugs), intravenous fluids, whole blood and blood components except as specified in § 18.157 (relating to administration of controlled substances and whole blood and blood components).

      (ix) Removal of superficial foreign bodies.

      (x) Cardio-pulmonary resuscitation.

      (xi) Audiometry screening.

      (xii) Visual screening.

      (xiii) Carrying out aseptic and isolation techniques.

(14) Provide counseling and instruction regarding common patient problems.

PENNSYLVANIA ADMIN. CODE SEC. 18.151

Prohibitions.

(a) A physician assistant may not:

    (1) Provide medical services except as described in the written agreement.

    (2) Prescribe or dispense drugs except as described in the written agreement.

    (3) Maintain or manage a satellite location under § 18.155 (relating to satellite locations) unless approved by the Board.

    (4) Independently bill patients for services provided.

    (5) Independently delegate a task specifically assigned to him by the supervising physician to another health care provider.

    (6) List his name independently in a telephone directory or other directory for public use in a manner which indicates that he functions as an independent practitioner.

    (7) Perform acupuncture except as permitted by section 13(k) of the act (63 P. S. § 422.13(k)).

    (8) Pronounce a patient dead.

    (9) Perform a medical service without the supervision of a physician assistant supervisor.

(b) A physician assistant supervisor may not:

    (1) Permit a physician assistant to engage in conduct proscribed in subsection (a).

    (2) Have primary responsibility for more than two physician assistants.

PENNSYLVANIA ADMIN. CODE SEC. 18.152

Executing and relaying medical regimens.

(a) A physician assistant may execute a medical regimen or may relay a medical regimen to be executed by a health care practitioner subject to the requirements of this section.

(b) The physician assistant shall report orally or in writing, to a physician assistant supervisor, within 12 hours, medical regimens executed or relayed by him while the physician assistant supervisor was not physically present, and the basis for each decision to execute or relay a medical regimen.

(c) The physician assistant shall record, date and authenticate the medical regimen on the patient's chart at the time it is executed or relayed. The physician assistant supervisor shall countersign the patient's record within a reasonable time, not to exceed 3 days, unless countersignature is required sooner by regulation, policy within the medical care facility or the requirements of a third-party payor.

(d) A physician assistant or physician assistant supervisor shall provide immediate access to the written agreement to anyone seeking to confirm the physician assistant's authority to relay a medical regimen or administer a therapeutic or diagnostic measure.

PENNSYLVANIA ADMIN. CODE SEC. 18.153

Osteopathic.

(a) The physician assistant shall, under appropriate direction and supervision by a physician, augment the physician's data gathering abilities to assist the supervising physician in reaching decisions and instituting care plans for the physician's patients. The physician assistant shall have as a minimum, the knowledge and competency to perform the following functions and should under appropriate supervision be permitted by the Board to perform them. This list is not intended to be specific or all-inclusive:

(1) Screen patients to determine need for medical attention.

(2) Review patient records to determine health status.

(3) Take patient history.

(4) Perform a physical examination.

(5) Perform a development screening examination on children.

(6) Record pertinent information data.

(7) Make decisions regarding data gathering and appropriate management and treatment of patients being seen for the initial evaluation of a problem or the follow-up evaluation of a previously diagnosed and stabilized condition.

(8) Prepare patient summaries.

(9) Initiate request for commonly performed initial laboratory studies.

(10) Collect specimens for and carry out commonly performed blood, urine and stool analyses and cultures.

(11) Identify normal and abnormal findings on history, physical examination and commonly performed laboratory studies.

(12) Initiate appropriate evaluation and emergency management for emergency situations, for example, cardiac arrest, respiratory distress, injuries, burns, hemorrhage.

(13) Perform clinical procedures such as:

    (i) Venipuncture.

    (ii) Intradermal tests.

    (iii) Electrocardiogram.

    (iv) Care and suturing of minor lacerations.

    (v) Casting and splinting.

    (vi) Control of external hemorrhage.

    (vii) Application of dressings and bandages.

    (viii) Administration of medications with the exception of controlled substances, whole blood and blood components.

    (ix) Removal of superficial foreign bodies.

    (x) Cardio-pulmonary resuscitation.

    (xi) Audiometry screening.

    (xii) Visual screening.

    (xiii) Carrying out aseptic and isolation techniques.

(14) Provide counseling and instruction regarding common patient problems.

(b) The tasks physician assistants may perform are those which require technical skills, execution of standing orders, routine patient care tasks and such diagnostic and therapeutic procedures as the supervising physician may wish to delegate to the physician assistant after the supervising physician has satisfied himself as to the ability and competence of the physician assistant. The supervising physician may, with due regard to the safety of the patient and in keeping with sound medical practice, delegate to the physician assistant, subject to prior approval by the Board, such medical procedures and other tasks as are usually performed within the normal scope of the supervising physician's practice and subject to the limitations set forth in this subchapter, the act and the training and expertise of the physician assistant.

PENNSYLVANIA OSTEO. ADMIN. CODE SEC. 25.171

Prohibitions.

(a) A supervising physician may not permit a physician assistant to independently practice medicine. Supervision shall be maintained at all times.

(b) A physician assistant may not:

    (1) Maintain or manage an office separate and apart from the supervising physician's primary office for treating patients unless the Board has granted the supervising physician specific permission to establish a satellite operation under § 25.175 (relating to physician assistants and satellite operations).

    (2) Independently bill patients for services provided.

    (3) Independently delegate a task assigned to him by his supervising physician to another individual; list his name independently in a telephone directory or otherwise advertise, using the title "Physician Assistant" or "P.A." or another term in a manner which would indicate that he functions as an independent health care provider.

    (4) Perform acupuncture.

    (5) Pronounce a patient dead.

PENNSYLVANIA OSTEO. ADMIN. CODE SEC. 25.172

Physician assistants and satellite operations.

(a) No physician assistant may be permitted to be utilized in an office or clinic separate and apart from the supervising physician's primary place for meeting patients unless the supervising physician has obtained specific approval from the Board. A supervising physician may supervise only one satellite operation. The criteria for granting approval is that the supervising physician demonstrate the following to the satisfaction of the Board:

    (1) That the physician assistant will be utilized in an area of medical need recognized by the Board.

    (2) That there is adequate provision for direct communication between the physician assistant and the supervising physician and that the distance between the main office and the satellite operation is not so great as to prohibit or impede appropriate support services.

    (3) That provision is made for the supervising physician to see each regular patient every fifth visit, except for those patients referred to in paragraph (5).

    (4) That the supervising physician will visit the remote office at least weekly and spend enough time on-site to provide super-

vision and personally review the records of each patient seen by the physician assistant in this setting.

(5) That the supervising physician will see every child patient from infancy to 2 years of age at least every third visit, and from 2 years of age to 18 years of age, at least every other visit.

(6) That the physician assistant to be utilized in the satellite office has been employed by a Pennsylvania Board approved supervising physician in his primary office for at least 1 year.

(b) Appropriate records of patient and supervisory contact shall be maintained and available for Board review. Failure to maintain the standards required for such an operation under the criteria listed in subsection (a) may result not only in the loss of the privilege to maintain a satellite operation but may result in the revocation of the supervising physician's registration and license.

PENNSYLVANIA OSTEO. ADMIN. CODE SEC. 25.175

Physician assistants in medical care facilities.

(a) This chapter may not be construed to require medical care facilities to accept physician assistants or to use them within their premises. It is appropriate for the physician assistant to provide services to the hospitalized patients of the supervising physician under the supervision of that physician, if the medical care facility permits it.

(b) The medical staff of the facility should recommend to the facility's governing authority the establishment of a standing committee to develop standards and procedures for physician assistants provided they are consistent with this chapter governing physician assistant utilization and prohibition.

(c) Physician assistants employed directly by medical care facilities shall perform services only under the supervision of a clearly identified and registered supervising physician and physician shall supervise no more than two physician assistants.

PENNSYLVANIA OSTEO. ADMIN. CODE SEC. 25.181

Physician assistants and emergency departments.

A physician assistant may provide medical care or services in an emergency department so long as he has training in emergency medicine, functions under specific protocols which govern his performance, and is under the direct supervision of a physician with whom he has ready contact and who is willing to assume full responsibility for the physician assistant's performance. A physician assistant may not substitute for a physician who is "on call" in the emergency department.

PENNSYLVANIA OSTEO. ADMIN. CODE SEC. 25.182

RHODE ISLAND

Physician assistants, depending upon their level of professional training and experience, as determined by a supervising physician, may perform health care services consistent with their expertise and that of the supervising physician who is a licensed physician in solo practice, in group practice, or in health care facilities.

RHODE ISLAND R5-54-PA-6.2

SOUTH CAROLINA

Physician assistants may perform:
(1) medical acts, tasks, or functions with written scope of practice guidelines under physician supervision;
(2) those duties and responsibilities, including the prescribing and dispensing of drugs and medical devices, that are lawfully delegated by their supervising physicians.

A physician assistant is an agent of his or her supervising physician in the performance of all practice related activities including, but not limited to, the ordering of diagnostic, therapeutic, and other medical services.

SOUTH CAROLINA PA PRAC. ACT SEC. 40-47-935

Scope of practice guidelines; signature and filing requirements; contents.

A physician assistant practicing at all sites shall practice pursuant to written scope of practice guidelines signed by all supervisory physicians and the physician assistant. Copies of the guidelines must be on file at all practice sites. The guidelines shall include at a minimum the:
(1) name, license number, and practice addresses of all supervising physicians;
(2) name and practice address of the physician assistant;
(3) date the guidelines were developed and dates they were reviewed and amended;
(4) medical conditions for which therapies may be initiated, continued, or modified;
(5) treatments that may be initiated, continued, or modified;
(6) drug therapy, if any, that may be prescribed with drug-specific classifications; and

(7) situations that require direct evaluation by or immediate referral to the physician.

SOUTH CAROLINA PA PRAC. ACT SEC. 40-47-960

Limitations on permissible tasks for physician assistants.

A physician assistant may not:
(1) perform a task which has not been listed and approved on the scope of practice guidelines currently on file with the board;
(2) prescribe drugs, medications, or devices not specifically authorized by the supervising physician and documented in the written scope of practice guidelines;
(3) prescribe, under any circumstances, controlled substances in Schedules II through IV.

SOUTH CAROLINA PA PRAC. ACT SEC. 40-47-97

SOUTH DAKOTA

Tasks allowed to primary care physician assistant. An assistant to the primary care physician may perform, under the responsibility and supervision of the primary care physician, selected diagnostic and therapeutic tasks in each of five major clinical disciplines (medicine, surgery, pediatrics, psychiatry, and obstetrics).

SOUTH DAKOTA CODIFIED LAWS 36-4A-21

Practice agreement not to include abortion. The board may not approve any practice agreement that includes abortion as a permitted procedure.

SOUTH DAKOTA CODIFIED LAWS 36-4A-21.1

Specific tasks allowed to assistant to primary care physician. Specifically, and by way of limitations, an assistant to the primary care physician may:
(1) Take a complete, detailed, and accurate history; do a complete physical examination, when appropriate, to include pelvic and breast examinations specifically excluding endoscopic examinations; record pertinent data in acceptable medical form; and, if the physical examination is for participation in athletics, certify that the patient is healthy and able to participate;
(2) Perform or assist in the performance of the following routine laboratory and governing techniques:
    (a) The drawing of venous or peripheral blood and the routine examination of the blood;

    (b) Urinary bladder catheterization and routine urinalysis;

    (c) Nasogastric intubation and gastric lavage;

    (d) The collection of and the examination of the stool;

    (e) The taking of cultures;

    (f) The performance and reading of skin tests;

    (g) The performance of pulmonary function tests excluding endoscopic procedures;

    (h) The performance of tonometry;

    (i) The performance of hearing screenings;

    (j) The taking of EKG tracings;

(3) Make a tentative medical diagnosis and institute therapy or referral; prescribe medications and provide drug samples or a limited supply of labeled medications, including controlled drugs or substances listed on Schedule II in chapter 34-20B for one period of not more than forty-eight hours, for symptoms and temporary pain relief; treat common childhood diseases; to assist in the follow-up treatment of geriatric and psychiatric disorders referred by the physicians. Medications or sample drugs provided to patients shall be accompanied with written administration instructions and appropriate documentation shall be entered in the patient's medical record;

(4) Perform the following routine therapeutic procedures:

    (a) Injections;

    (b) Immunizations;

    (c) Debridement, suture, and care of superficial wounds;

    (d) Debridement of minor superficial burns;

    (e) Removal of foreign bodies from the external surface of the skin (specifically excluding foreign bodies of the cornea);

    (f) Removal of sutures;

    (g) Removal of impacted cerumen;

    (h) Subcutaneous local anesthesia, excluding any nerve blocks;

    (i) Strapping, casting, and splinting of sprains;

    (j) Anterior nasal packing for epistaxis;

    (k) Removal of cast;

    (l) Application of traction;

    (m) Application of physical therapy modalities;

    (n) Incision and drainage of superficial skin infections;

(5) Assist the primary care physician in health maintenance of patients by:

    (a) Well-baby and well-child clinics to include initial and current booster immunization for communicable disease;

    (b) Pre- and post-natal surveillance to include clinics and home visits;

(c) Family planning, counseling, and management;

(6) Institute emergency measures and emergency treatment or appropriate measures in situations such as cardiac arrest, shock, hemorrhage, convulsions, poisonings, and emergency obstetric delivery.
Emergency measures includes writing a chemical or physical
restraint order when the patient may do personal harm or harm
others;

(7) Assist the primary care physician in the management of long-term
care to include:

(a) Ordering indicated laboratory procedures;

(b) Managing a medical care regimen for acute and chronically
ill patients within established standing orders. (Prescription
of modifications needed by patients coping with illness or
maintaining health, such as in diet, exercise, relief from pain,
medication, and adaptation to handicaps or impairments);

(c) Making referrals to appropriate agencies;

(8) Assist the primary care physician in the hospital setting by arranging hospital admissions under the direction of the physician, by
accompanying the primary care physician on rounds, and recording the physician's patient progress notes; by accurately and
appropriately transcribing and executing specific orders at the
direction of the physician; by assistance at surgery; by compiling detailed narrative and case summaries; by completion of the
forms pertinent to the patient's medical record;

(9) Assist the primary care physician in the office in the ordering of
drugs and supplies, in the keeping of records, and in the upkeep
of equipment;

(10) Assist the primary care physician in providing services to patients
requiring continuing care (nursing home, extended care, and
home care) including follow-up visits after the initial treatment by
the physician;

(11) Assist the primary care physician in the completion of official
documents such as death certificates, birth certificates, and similar
documents required by law, including signing the documents;

(12) Take X-rays to be read by a physician. A physician's assistant may
not administer injections in conjunction with the taking of any
X-rays.

SOUTH DAKOTA CODIFIED LAWS 36-4A-22

Additional tasks when qualification demonstrated. In addition to the
tasks performable listed in § 36-4A-22 an assistant to the primary care
physician may be permitted to perform, under the supervision of

the primary care physician, such other tasks, except those expressly excluded herein, for which adequate training and proficiency can be demonstrated in a manner satisfactory to the board.

SOUTH DAKOTA CODIFIED LAWS 36-4A-23

Tasks allowed to assistant to specialist. An assistant to the specialist physician may perform, under the responsibility and supervision of the specialist physician, selected diagnostic and therapeutic tasks in the major clinical disciplines.

SOUTH DAKOTA CODIFIED LAWS 36-4A-24

Specific tasks allowed to assistant to specialist. Specifically, and by way of limitations, an assistant to the specialist physician may perform those tasks authorized for the assistant to the primary care physician under subdivisions 36-4A-22(1), (2), (4), and (6), provided, however, that the assistant to the specialist physician may remove superficial foreign bodies of the cornea. An assistant to the specialist physician may also assist at major surgery.

SOUTH DAKOTA CODIFIED LAWS 36-4A-25

Additional tasks allowed assistant to specialist when qualification demonstrated. In addition to the tasks performable listed in § 36-4A-25 an assistant to the specialist physician may be permitted to perform, under the supervision of the specialist physician, such other tasks, except those expressly excluded herein, for which adequate training and proficiency can be demonstrated in a manner satisfactory to the board.

SOUTH DAKOTA CODIFIED LAWS 36-4A-26

TENNESSEE

A physician assistant who holds state license in accordance with T.C.A. § 63-19-105 may provide selected medical/surgical services as outlined in a written protocol according to T.C.A. § 63-19-106, and when such services are within his skills. The services delegated to the physician assistant must form a usual component of the supervising physician's scope of practice. Services rendered by the physician assistant must be provided under the supervision, direction, and ultimate responsibility of a licensed physician accountable to the Board of Medical Examiners or the Board of Osteopathic Examination under the provision of T.C.A. § 63-19-109.

RRT SEC.0880-3-02

(1) The range of services which may be provided by a physician assistant shall be set forth in a written protocol, jointly developed and signed by the physician assistant and the supervising physician and maintained at the physician assistant's practice location.

(2) A physician assistant is authorized to perform the services outlined in his or her protocol under the supervision of a supervising physician who complies with all the requirements of 0880-2-.18.

(3) Each physician assistant shall have a designated primary supervising physician and shall notify the Committee of the name, address, and license number of his/her primary supervising physician and shall notify the Committee of any change in such primary supervising physician within fifteen (15) days of the change.

RRT SEC.0880-3-10

TEXAS

The physician assistant shall provide, within the education, training, and experience of the physician assistant, medical services that are delegated by the supervising physician. The activities listed in paragraphs (1)–(9)of this subsection may be performed in any place authorized by a supervising physician, including, but not limited to a clinic, hospital, ambulatory surgical center, patient home, nursing home, or other institutional setting. Medical services provided by a physician assistant may include, but are not limited to:

(1) obtaining patient histories and performing physical examinations;

(2) ordering and/or performing diagnostic and therapeutic procedures;

(3) formulating a working diagnosis;

(4) developing and implementing a treatment plan;

(5) monitoring the effectiveness of therapeutic interventions;

(6) assisting at surgery;

(7) offering counseling and education to meet patient needs;

(8) requesting, receiving, and signing for the receipt of pharmaceutical sample prescription medications and distributing the samples to patients in a specific practice setting where the physician assistant is authorized to prescribe pharmaceutical medications and sign prescription drug orders at a site, as provided by the Medical Practice Act, Chapter 157, and its subsequent amendments, or as otherwise authorized by this Act or board rule;

(9) the signing or completion of a prescription as provided by the Medical Practice Act, Chapter 157; and

(10) making appropriate referrals.

TEXAS CODE ANN. SEC. 185.10

Tasks not permitted to be delegated to a physician assistant.

Except at sites designated by the Medical Practice Act, Chapter 157, the supervising physician shall not allow a physician assistant to prescribe or supply medication.

TEXAS CODE ANN. SEC. 185.11

UTAH

(1) A physician assistant may provide any medical services that are not specifically prohibited under this chapter or rules adopted under this chapter, and that are:

    (a) within the physician assistant's skills and scope of competence;

    (b) within the usual scope of practice of the physician assistant's supervising physician; and

    (c) provided under the supervision of a supervising physician and in accordance with a delegation of services agreement.

(2) A physician assistant, in accordance with a delegation of services agreement, may prescribe or administer an appropriate controlled substance if:

    (a) the physician assistant holds a Utah controlled substance license and a DEA registration;

    (b) the prescription or administration of the controlled substance is within the prescriptive practice of the supervising physician and also within the delegated prescribing stated in the delegation of services agreement; and

    (c) the supervising physician cosigns any medical chart record of a prescription of a Schedule 2 or Schedule 3 controlled substance made by the physician assistant.

(3) A physician assistant shall, while practicing as a physician assistant, wear an identification badge showing his license classification as a practicing physician assistant.

(4) A physician assistant may not

    (a) independently charge or bill a patient, or others on behalf of the patient, for services rendered;

    (b) identify himself to any person in connection with activities allowed under this chapter other than as a physician assistant; or

    (c) use the title "doctor" or "physician," or by any knowing act or omission lead or permit anyone to believe he is a physician.

UTAH CODE ANN. SEC. 58-70A-501

VERMONT

The scope of practice document shall cover at least the following:

(a) Narrative: A brief description of practice setting, the types of patients and patient encounters common to this practice in a general overview of the role of the physician assistant in that practice.

(b) Supervision:

    (1) The mechanisms for on-site and offsite physician supervision and communication

    (2) How back-up and secondary supervising physicians will be utilized, and the means by which communication with them will be managed

    (3) How emergency conditions will be handled in the absence of an on-site physician including:

        (A)   plans for immediate care,

        (B)   means of accessing emergency transport;

    (4) How ongoing supervision of the PA's activities are reviewed;

    (5) Provisions for retrospective review of PA charts:

        (A)   the frequency with which these reviews will be conducted,

        (B)   methods to be used to document his/her review;

    (6) The practice referral patterns to non-supervising physicians and other health-care providers. If a referral is to be made out of the usual referral pattern of the practice describe:

        (A)   the supervising physician's role in decision,

        (B)   the method to be used to document his/her involvement

    (7) The methods for in-practice consultation for patients who are not improving in a reasonable manner or time frame, including the ways in which the PA will access the supervising physician's expertise in determining diagnostic treatment and referral plans for patients who are not progress is not satisfactorily;

(c) Sites of Practice: A description of any and all practice sites (e.g. office, clinic, hospital outpatient, hospital inpatient, industrial sites, schools). For each site a description of the PA's activities

(d) Tasks/Duties: A list of the PA's assigned duties in the supervising physician's scope of practice. The supervising physician may only delegate those tasks for which the physician assistant is qualified by education training and experience to perform. Notwithstanding the above, the physician assistant should initiate emergency care when required, while accessing a backup system. At no time should a particular task assigned to the PA fall outside the scope of practice of the supervising physician.

(e) An Authorization to Prescribe medication which shall include the following statement verbatim:

   (1) "[Insert physician assistant name] is authorized to prescribe medications in accordance with as scope of practice submitted to and approved by the Vermont Board of Medical Practice."

   (2) "[Insert physician assistant name] is authorized to prescribe controlled drugs in accordance with as scope of practice submitted to and approved by the Vermont Board of Medical Practice. [insert physician assistant name] has obtained a DEA number, which is [insert number]."

VERMONT RULES OF THE BD. OF MED. SEC. II.7.3

VIRGINIA

(A) Prior to initiation of practice, a physician assistant and his supervising physician shall submit a written protocol which spells out the roles and functions of the assistant. Any such protocol shall take into account such factors as the physician assistant's level of competence, the number of patients, the types of illness treated by the physician, the nature of the treatment, special procedures, and the nature of the physician availability in ensuring direct physician involvement at an early stage and regularly thereafter. The protocol shall also provide an evaluation process for the physician assistant's performance, including a requirement specifying the time period, proportionate to the acuity of care and practice setting, within which the supervising physician shall review the record of services rendered by the physician assistant.

B. The board may require information regarding the level of supervision; "direct," "personal" or "general," with which the supervising physician plans to supervise the physician assistant for selected tasks. The board may also require the supervising physician to document the assistant's competence in performing such tasks.

C. If the role of the assistant includes prescribing for drugs and devices, the written protocol shall include those schedules and categories of drugs and devices that are within the scope of practice and proficiency of the supervising physician.

18 VIRGINIA ADMIN. CODE SEC. 85-50-101

WASHINGTON

(1) A certified physician assistant may perform only those services as outlined in the standardized procedures reference and guidelines established by the commission. If said assistant is being trained to

perform additional procedures beyond those established by the commission, the training must be carried out under the direct, personal supervision of the sponsoring physician or a qualified person mutually agreed upon by the sponsoring physician and the certified physician assistant. Requests for approval of newly acquired skills shall be submitted to the commission and may be granted by a reviewing commission member or at any regular meeting of the commission.

(2) A certified physician assistant may sign and attest to any document that might ordinarily be signed by a licensed physician, to include, but not limited to such things as birth and death certificates.

(3) It shall be the responsibility of the certified physician assistant and the sponsoring physician to ensure that appropriate consultation and review of work are provided.

(4) In the temporary absence of the sponsoring physician, the consultation and review of work shall be provided by a designated alternate sponsor(s).

(5) The certified physician assistant must, at all times when meeting or treating patients, wear a badge identifying him or her as a certified physician assistant.

(6) No certified physician assistant may be presented in any manner which would tend to mislead the public as to his or her title.

WASHINGTON ANN. CODE SEC. 246-918-140

Basic physician assistant-surgical assistant duties. The physician assistant-surgical assistant who is not eligible to take the NCCPA certifying exam shall:

(1) Function only in the operating room as approved by the commission;

(2) Only be allowed to close skin and subcutaneous tissue, placing suture ligatures, clamping, tying and clipping of blood vessels, use of cautery for hemostasis under direct supervision;

(3) Not be allowed to perform any independent surgical procedures, even under direct supervision, and will be allowed to only assist the operating surgeon;

(4) Have no prescriptive authority; and

(5) Not write any progress notes or order(s) on hospitalized patients, except operative notes.

WASHINGTON ANN. CODE SEC. 246-918-250

Physician assistant-surgical assistant—utilization and supervision.

(1) Responsibility of physician assistant-surgical assistant. The physician assistant-surgical assistant is responsible for performing

only those tasks authorized by the supervising physician(s) and within the scope of physician assistant-surgical assistant practice described in WAC 246-918-250. The physician assistant-surgical assistant is responsible for ensuring his or her compliance with the rules regulating physician assistant-surgical assistant practice and failure to comply may constitute grounds for disciplinary action.

(2) Limitations, geographic. No physician assistant-surgical assistant shall be utilized in a place geographically separated from the institution in which the assistant and the supervising physician are authorized to practice.

(3) Responsibility of supervising physician(s). Each physician assistant-surgical assistant shall perform those tasks he or she is authorized to perform only under the supervision and control of the supervising physician(s), but such supervision and control shall not be construed to necessarily require the personal presence of the supervising physician at the place where the services are rendered. It shall be the responsibility of the supervising physician(s) to insure that:

(a) The operating surgeon in each case directly supervises and reviews the work of the physician assistant-surgical assistant. Such supervision and review shall include remaining in the surgical suite until the surgical procedure is complete;

(b) The physician assistant-surgical assistant shall wear a badge identifying him or her as a "physician assistant-surgical assistant" or "P.A.S.A." In all written documents and other communication modalities pertaining to his or her professional activities as a physician assistant-surgical assistant, the physician assistant-surgical assistant shall clearly denominate his or her profession as a "physician assistant-surgical assistant"; or

(c) The physician assistant-surgical assistant is not presented in any manner which would tend to mislead the public as to his or her title.

WASHINGTON ANN. CODE SEC. 246-918-260

WEST VIRGINIA

The tasks a physician assistant may perform are those which require technical skill, execution of standing orders, routine patient care tasks and those diagnostic and therapeutic procedures which the supervising physician may wish to delegate to the physician assistant after the supervising physician has satisfied himself or herself as to the ability and competence of the physician assistant. The supervising physician may, with due regard for the safety of the patient and in keeping with sound medical practice, delegate to the physician assistant those medical procedures and other tasks that are usually performed within the normal scope of the supervising physician's practice, subject to the limitations set forth in this section and the West Virginia Medical Practice Act, W. Va. Code §§30-3-1 et seq., and the training and expertise of the physician assistant.

The physician assistant shall, under appropriate direction and supervision by a physician, augment the physician's data gathering abilities in order to assist the supervising physician in reaching decisions and instituting care plans for the physician's patients. A physician assistant shall have, as a minimum, the knowledge and competency to perform the following functions and may under appropriate supervision perform them; this standard job description is not intended to be specific or all-inclusive:

a. Screen patients to determine the need for medical attention;
b. Review patient records to determine health status;
c. Take a patient history;
d. Perform a physical examination;
e. Perform development screening examinations on children;
f. Record pertinent patient data;
g. Make decisions regarding data gathering and appropriate management and treatment of patients being seen for the initial evaluation of a problem or the follow-up evaluation of a previously diagnosed and stabilized condition;
h. Prepare patient summaries;
i. Initiate requests for commonly performed initial laboratory studies;
j. Collect specimens for and carry out commonly performed blood, urine and stool analyses and cultures;
k. Identify normal and abnormal findings in history, physical examination and commonly performed laboratory studies;
l. Initiate appropriate evaluation and emergency management for emergency situations; for example, cardiac arrest, respiratory distress, injuries, burns and hemorrhage;
m. Perform clinical procedures such as:
   (A) Venipuncture;
   B. Electrocardiogram;
   C. Care and suturing of minor lacerations;
   D. Casting and splinting;
   E. Control of external hemorrhage;
   F. Application of dressings and bandages;
   G. Removal of superficial foreign bodies;

H. Cardiopulmonary resuscitation;

I. Audiometry screening;

J. Visual screening; and

K. Carry out aseptic and isolation techniques;

n. Provide counseling and instruction regarding common patient problems; and

o. Execute documents at the direction of and for the supervising physician.

A physician assistant making application to the Board for job description changes or additions shall document that his or her training and competency supports the request.

A physician assistant may pronounce death provided that:

a. It is contained in his or her job description;

b. The physician assistant has a need to do so within his or her scope of practice; and

c. That the pronouncement is in accordance with applicable West Virginia law and rules.

The supervising physician shall monitor and supervise the activities of the physician assistant and require appropriate documentation, including organized medical records with symptoms, pertinent physical findings, impressions and treatment plans indicated. The supervising physician may also provide written protocols for the use of the physician assistant in the performance of delegated tasks. The established protocols shall be available for public inspection upon request and may be reviewed by the Board as required.

If the supervising physician absents himself or herself in such a manner or to such an extent that he or she is unavailable to aid the physician assistant when required, the supervising physician shall not delegate patient care to his or her physician assistant unless he or she has made appropriate arrangements for an alternate supervising physician. The legal responsibility for the acts and omissions of the physician assistant remains with the supervising physician at all times.

It is the responsibility of the supervising physician to ensure that supervision is maintained in his or her absence.

No physician assistant may be utilized in an office or clinic separate and apart from the supervising physician's primary place for meeting patients unless the supervising physician has obtained specific approval from the Board. A supervising physician may supervise only two (2) satellite operations. The criteria for granting the approval is that the supervising physician demonstrate the following to the satisfaction of the Board:

a. That the physician assistant will be utilized in a designated manpower shortage area or an area of medical need as defined by the Board;

b.   That there is adequate provision for direct communication between the physician assistant and the supervising physician and that the distance between the main office and the satellite operation is not so great as to prohibit or impede appropriate emergency services;

c.   That provision is made for the supervising physician to see each regular patient periodically; for example, every third visit; and

d.   That the supervising physician visits the remote office at least once every fourteen (14) days and demonstrate that he or she spends enough time on site to provide supervision and personal and regular review of the selected records upon which entries are made by the physician assistant. Patient records shall be selected on the basis of written criteria established by the supervising physician and the physician assistant and shall be of sufficient number to assure adequate review of the physician assistant's scope of practice.

The supervising physician shall maintain appropriate records of supervisory contact and shall make them available for Board review if required. A supervising physician who fails to maintain the standards required for a satellite operation may lose the privilege to maintain a satellite operation.

Designated representatives of the Board are authorized to make on-site visits to the offices of supervising physicians and medical care facilities utilizing physician assistants to review the following:

a.   The supervision of physician assistants;

b.   The maintenance of and compliance with, any protocols;

c.   Utilization of physician assistants in conformity with the provisions of this section;

d.   Identification of physician assistants; and

e.   Compliance with licensure and registration requirements.

The Board reserves the right to review physician assistant utilization without prior notice to either the physician assistant or the supervising physician. It is a violation of this rule for a supervising physician or a physician assistant to refuse to undergo a review by the Board.

The provisions of this section shall not be construed to require medical care facilities to accept physician assistants or to use them within their premises. It is appropriate for the physician assistant to provide services to the hospitalized patients of his or her supervising physician under the supervision of the physician, if the medical care facility permits it.

Physician assistants employed directly by medical care facilities shall perform services only under the supervision of a clearly identified supervising physician, and the physician shall supervise no more than three (3) physician assistants or their equivalent, except that a supervising physician may supervise up to four (4) hospital employed physician assistants. Medical facility staff and attending physicians who provide medical direction to or utilize the services of physician assistants employed by a health care facility shall be considered to be alternate supervising physicians.

So long as the facility permits, a physician assistant may:

a. Assess and record the patient's progress within the parameters of an approved job description and report the patient's progress to the supervising physician; and

b. Make entries in medical records and patient charts so long as an appropriate mechanism is established for authentication by the supervising physician through countersignature.

A physician assistant may provide medical care or services in an emergency department so long as he or she has training in emergency medicine, is subject to standard emergency protocols, functions within the parameters of an approved job description which govern his or her performance and is under the supervision of a physician with whom he or she has ready contact and who is willing to assume full responsibility for the physician assistant's performance.

No physician assistant shall render nonemergency outpatient medical services until the patient has been informed that the individual providing care is a physician assistant.

It is the supervising physician's responsibility to be alert to patient complaints concerning the type or quality of services provided by the physician assistant.

In the supervising physician's office and any satellite operation, a notice plainly visible to all patients shall be posted in a prominent place explaining the meaning of the term "Physician Assistant". The physician assistant's license must be prominently displayed in the office and any satellite operation in which he or she may function. A physician assistant may obtain a duplicate license from the Board if required.

The physician assistant is required to notify the Board of changes in his or her employment within thirty (30) days. The physician assistant must provide the Board with his or her new address and telephone number of his or her residence, address and telephone number of employment and name of his or her supervising physician.

The supervising physician is required to notify the Board of any changes in his or her supervision of a physician assistant within ten (10) days.

WEST VIRGINIA RULES SEC. 11-1B-13

WISCONSIN

In providing medical care, the entire practice of any physician assistant shall be under the supervision of a licensed physician. The scope of practice is limited to providing medical care specified in sub.

(2) A physician assistant's practice may not exceed his or her educational training or experience and may not exceed the scope of practice of the supervising physician. A medical care task assigned by the supervising physician to a physician assistant may not be delegated by the physician assistant to another person.

(2) MEDICAL CARE. Medical care a physician assistant may provide include:

(a) Attending initially a patient of any age in any setting to obtain a personal medical history, perform an appropriate physical examination, and record and present pertinent data concerning the patient in a manner meaningful to the supervising physician.

(b) Performing, or assisting in performing, routine diagnostic studies as appropriate for a specific practice setting.

(c) Performing routine therapeutic procedures, including, but not limited to, injections, immunizations, and the suturing and care of wounds.

(d) Instructing and counseling a patient on physical and mental health, including diet, disease, treatment and normal growth and development.

(e) Assisting the supervising physician in a hospital or facility, as defined in s. 50.01 (1m), Stats., by assisting in surgery, making patient rounds, recording patient progress notes, compiling and recording detailed narrative case summaries and accurately writing or executing orders under the supervision of a licensed physician.

(f) Assisting in the delivery of medical care to a patient by reviewing and monitoring treatment and therapy plans.

(g) Performing independently evaluative and treatment procedures necessary to provide an appropriate response to life–threatening emergency situations.

(h) Facilitating referral of patients to other appropriate community health–care facilities, agencies and resources.

(i) Issuing written prescription orders for drugs under the supervision of a licensed physician and in accordance with procedures specified in s. Med 8.08 (2).

WISCONSIN ADMIN. CODE SEC. 8.07

WYOMING

A physician assistant assists in the practice of medicine under the supervision of a licensed physician. Within the physician/physician assistant relationship, physician assistants exercise autonomy in medical decision making and provide a broad range of diagnostic, therapeutic and health promotion and disease prevention services. The physician assistant may perform those duties and responsibilities delegated to him by the supervising physician when the duties and responsibilities are provided under the supervision of a licensed physician approved by the board, within the scope of the physician's practice and expertise and within the skills of the physician assistant.

WYOMING STAT. ANN. SEC. 33-26-502

Supervision Requirements State-by-State

ALABAMA

PHYSICIAN SUPERVISION. A formal relationship between a licensed assistant to a physician and a licensed physician under which the assistant to the physician is authorized to practice as evidenced by a written job description approved by the Board. Physician supervision requires that there shall be at all times a direct, continuing and close supervisory relationship between the assistant to the physician and the physician to whom that assistant is registered. The term supervision does not require direct on-site supervision of the assistant to the physician; however, supervision does include the professional oversight and direction required by these rules and by the written guidelines established by the Board concerning prescribing practices.

ALABAMA ADMIN. CODE R. 540-X-7-.01(6)

Requirements for supervised practice—physician assistants (P.A.).

(1) Physician supervision requires, at all times, a direct, continuing and close supervisory relationship between a physician assistant and the physician to whom the assistant is registered.

(2) There shall be no independent, unsupervised practice by physician assistants.

(3) The supervising physician shall be available for direct communication or by radio, telephone or telecommunication.

(4) The supervising physician shall be available for consultation or referrals of patients from the physician assistant.

(5) In the event the physician to whom the physician assistant is registered is not available, provisions must be made for medical coverage by a physician pursuant to Rule 540-X-7-.24.

(6) If the physician assistant is to perform duties at a site away from the supervising physician, the application for registration must clearly specify the circumstances and provide written verification of physician availability for consultation and/or referral, and direct medical intervention in emergencies and after hours, if indicated. The Board, at its discretion, may waive the requirement of written verification upon documentation of exceptional circumstances. Employees of state and county health departments are exempt from the requirement of written verification of physician availability.

(7) The supervising physician and the physician assistant shall adhere to any written guidelines established by the Board to govern the prescription practices of physician assistants.

(8) If the physician assistant is to perform duties at a site away from the supervising physician, physician supervision requires the following:

(a) Supervising physician receives a daily status report to be made in person, by telephone, or by telecommunications from the assistant on any complications or unusual problems encountered;

(b) Supervising physician visits the clinic, in person, at least once a week during regular business hours to observe and to provide medical direction and consultation;

(c) Supervising physician, during weekly office visits, reviews with the assistant case histories of patients with unusual problems or complications;

(d) An appropriate physician personally diagnoses or treats patients requiring physician follow-up.

(9) The mechanism for quality analysis shall be as follows:

(a) A written plan for review of medical records and patient outcomes shall be submitted with the application for registration, with documentation of the reviews maintained.

(b) Countersignature by supervising physician must be pursuant to established policy and/or applicable legal regulations and accreditation standards.

ALABAMA ADMIN. CODE R. 540-X-7-.23

ALASKA

COLLABORATIVE RELATIONSHIP. (a) A licensed physician assistant may not practice without at least one collaborative relationship established under this chapter.

(b) Documented evidence of an established collaborative relationship consists of a copy of the plan of collaboration approved under 12 AAC 40.980.

(c) A person authorized to practice as a licensed physician assistant shall immediately report to the board, in writing, any change in the physician assistant's collaborative relationship.

(d) A change in a collaborative relationship automatically suspends a licensed physician assistant's authority to practice under that collaborative relationship unless the change is only to replace the primary collaborating physician with an existing alternate collaborating physician and at least one alternate collaborating physician remains in place.

(e) The first time a physician assistant with less than two years of full-time clinical experience practices in a remote location, the physician assistant shall work 160 hours in direct patient care under the direct and immediate supervision of the collaborating physician or alternate collaborating physician. The first 40 hours must be completed before the physician assistant begins practice in the remote location, and the remaining 120 hours must be completed within 90 days of starting practice in the remote location.

(f) A physician assistant with less than two years of full-time clinical experience who practices in a remote location and who has a change of collaborating physician must work 40 hours under the direct and immediate supervision of the new collaborating physician within 60 days of establishing the new collaborative relationship unless the change is only to replace the primary collaborating physician with an existing alternate collaborating physician.

(g) A physician assistant with two or more years of full-time clinical experience who applies for authorization to practice in a remote location shall submit a plan of collaboration that includes the following information or materials:

(1) the location of practice;

(2) a detailed curriculum vitae documenting that the physician assistant's previous experience as a physician assistant is sufficient to meet the requirements of the location assignment; and

(3) a written recommendation and approval from the collaborating physician.

(h) In this section, "remote location" means a location in which a physician assistant practices that is 30 or more miles by road from the collaborating physician's primary office.

12 ALASKA ADMIN. CODE 40.410

ARIZONA

(A) The supervising physician is responsible for all aspects of the performance of a physician assistant, whether or not the supervising physician actually pays the physician assistant a salary. The supervising physician is responsible for supervising the physician assistant and ensuring that the health care tasks performed by a physician assistant are within the physician assistant's scope of training and experience and have been properly delegated by the supervising physician.

B. A supervising physician shall not supervise more than two physician assistants who work the same hours at the same employment location.

C. A supervising physician may designate a supervising physician's agent to provide consultation and supervise a physician assistant when the supervising physician is not immediately available. The supervising physician remains responsible for the acts of a physician assistant when the physician assistant is supervised by a supervising physician's agent.

D. A supervising physician shall develop a system for recordation and review of all instances in which the physician assistant prescribes fourteen day prescriptions of schedule II or schedule III controlled substances. The board shall approve the system.

E. In order to act as a supervising physician or a supervising physician's agent, a physician shall:
   1. Complete an application as prescribed by the board.
   2. Hold a license pursuant to chapter 13 or 17 of this title and not hold a license under probation, restriction or suspension unrelated to rehabilitation.
   3. Submit a statement that the supervising physician or supervising physician's agent is familiar with the statutes and rules regarding the performance of health care tasks of physician assistants and accepts responsibility for supervising the physician assistant.

F. A physician who violates the provisions of this chapter shall not serve as a supervising physician or supervising physician's agent.

G. The supervising physician's agent is responsible for the acts of a physician assistant in the absence of the supervising physician if the board approves. The board considers the supervising physician's agent's signature on a physician assistant's current notification of supervision to be acknowledgment by the supervising physician's agent that the agent understands and is familiar with the physician assistant's approved health care tasks.

H. A supervising physician or supervising physician's agent shall not delegate to the physician assistant any health care task that the supervising physician or supervising physician's agent does not have training or experience in and does not perform.

ARIZONA REV. STAT. ANN. SEC. 32-2533

ARKANSAS

(a) Supervision of physician assistants shall be continuous but shall not be construed as necessarily requiring the physical presence of the supervising physician at the time and place that the services are rendered.
(b) It is the obligation of each team of physicians and physician assistants to ensure that:
    (1) The physician assistant's scope of practice is identified;
    (2) The delegation of medical task is appropriate to the physician assistant's level of competence;
    (3) The relationship and access to the supervising physician is defined; and
    (4) A process of evaluation of the physician assistant's performance is established.
(c) The physician assistant and supervising physician may designate back-up physicians who are agreeable to supervise the physician assistant during the absence of the supervising physician.

ARKANSAS CODE 17-105-109

CALIFORNIA

(a) A supervising physician shall be available in person or by electronic communication at all times when the physician assistant is caring for patients.
(b) A supervising physician shall delegate to a physician assistant only those tasks and procedures consistent with the supervising physician's specialty or usual and customary practice and with the patient's health and condition.
(c) A supervising physician shall observe or review evidence of the physician assistant's performance of all tasks and procedures to be delegated to the physician assistant until assured of competency.
(d) The physician assistant and the supervising physician shall establish in writing transport and back-up procedures for the immediate care of patients who are in need of emergency care beyond the physician assistant's scope of practice for such times when a supervising physician is not on the premises.

e) A physician assistant and his or her supervising physician shall establish in writing guidelines for the adequate supervision of the physician assistant which shall include one or more of the following mechanisms:

   (1) Examination of the patient by a supervising physician the same day as care is given by the physician assistant;

   (2) Countersignature and dating of all medical records written by the physician assistant within thirty (30) days that the care was given by the physician assistant;

   (3) The supervising physician may adopt protocols to govern the performance of a physician assistant for some or all tasks. The minimum content for a protocol governing diagnosis and management as referred to in this section shall include the presence or absence of symptoms, signs, and other data necessary to establish a diagnosis or assessment, any appropriate tests or studies to order, drugs to recommend to the patient, and education to be given the patient. For protocols governing procedures, the protocol shall state the information to be given the patient, the nature of the consent to be obtained from the patient, the preparation and technique of the procedure, and the follow-up care. Protocols shall be developed by the physician, adopted from, or referenced to, texts or other sources. Protocols shall be signed and dated by the supervising physician and the physician assistant. The supervising physician shall review, countersign, and date a minimum of 10% sample of medical records of patients treated by the physician assistant functioning under these protocols within thirty (30) days. The physician shall select for review those cases which by diagnosis, problem, treatment or procedure represent, in his or her judgment, the most significant risk to the patient;

   (4) Other mechanisms approved in advance by the committee.

(f) In the case of a physician assistant operating under interim approval, the supervising physician shall review, sign and date the medical record of all patients cared for by that physician assistant within seven (7) days if the physician was on the premises when the physician assistant diagnosed or treated the patient. If the physician was not on the premises at that time, he or she shall review, sign and date such medical records within 48 hours of the time the medical services were provided.

(g) The supervising physician has continuing responsibility to follow the progress of the patient and to make sure that the physician assistant does not function autonomously. The supervising physician shall be responsible for all medical services provided by a physician assistant under his or her supervision.

CALIFORNIA CODE REGS. SEC. 1399.545

COLORADO

Responsibilities of All Physician Supervisors

(A) Two Physician Assistant Limit. A physician may not supervise more than two physician assistants at any one particular moment in time.

B. Charts to be Reviewed Every Seven Working Days. A physician supervisor shall review the chart for every patient seen by a supervised physician assistant no later than seven working days after the physician assistant has performed an act defined as the practice of medicine. The physician supervisor shall document the performance of such review by signing the chart in a legible manner. In lieu of signing the chart, the physician supervisor may document the performance of such review by the use of an electronically generated signature provided that reasonable measures have been taken to prevent the unauthorized use of the electronically generated signature. Physician assistants performing delegated medical functions in an acute care hospital setting must comply with the requirements of Section 12-36-106(5)(b)(II)(A), (B) and (C), C.R.S.

III. Responsibilities of the Primary Physician Supervisor

(A) Primary Physician Supervisor. Except as set forth in subsection IV below, a physician licensed to practice medicine by the Board may delegate to a physician assistant licensed by the Board the authority to perform acts which constitute the practice of medicine only if a form in compliance with Section 4 of this rule is on record with the Board. The physician whose name appears on the form in compliance with Section 4 of this rule shall be deemed the "primary physician supervisor". The supervisory relationship shall be deemed to be effective for all time periods in which a form in compliance with Section 4 of this rule is on file with the Board.

B. Liability for Actions of a Physician Assistant. A primary physician supervisor may supervise and delegate responsibilities to a physician assistant in the manner the primary physician supervisor deems fit. Except as provided in subsection IV - B below, the primary physician supervisor shall be deemed to have violated this rule if a supervised physician assistant commits unprofessional conduct as defined in Section 12-36-117(1)(p), C.R.S., or if such physician assistant otherwise violates these rules. The primary physician supervisor shall not be responsible for the conduct of a physician assistant where that physician assistant was acting under the supervision of another primary physician supervisor and there is a form in compliance with Section 4 of these rules signed by that other primary physician supervisor.

C. Limitation to Two Supervised Physician Assistants. A primary physician supervisor shall be the primary physician supervisor for no more than two specific, individual physician assistants. The names of such physician assistants shall appear on the form in compliance with Section 4 of this rule. The primary physician supervisor may supervise additional physician assistants other than those who appear on the form in compliance with Section 4 of this rule. In other words, a primary physician supervisor may also be a secondary physician supervisor, as set forth below, for additional physician assistants. However, the primary physician supervisor may do so only in compliance with the limitations set forth in subsection II A above.

D. One Primary Physician Supervisor Per Employer. A physician assistant shall not have more than one primary physician supervisor for each employer. For purposes of this rule, any hospital system or health maintenance organization shall constitute a single employer.

IV. Responsibilities of the Secondary Physician Supervisor

(A) Secondary Physician Supervisor. A physician licensed to practice medicine by the Board other than the supervisor whose name appears on the form in compliance with Section 4 of this rule, may delegate to a physician assistant licensed by the Board, the authority to perform acts which constitute the practice of medicine only as permitted by this subsection IV. Such physician shall be termed the "secondary physician supervisor."

B. Liability on the Part of a Secondary Physician Supervisor for the Actions of a Physician Assistant. If a physician signs the chart for a patient seen by a physician assistant as a secondary physician supervisor, such physician shall be deemed to be responsible for any act defined as the practice of medicine performed by such physician assistant while supervised by the secondary physician supervisor. If, from the signature on the chart and all the surrounding facts and circumstances, a physician has assumed the role of secondary physician supervisor, that physician shall have assumed the responsibility for supervision of the physician assistant and shall be deemed to have relieved the primary physician supervisor of the supervisory responsibilities set forth in subsection III - B above. Such assumption of responsibility shall relate only to those particular actions of the physician assistant supervised by the secondary physician supervisor. The secondary physician supervisor shall be deemed to have violated this rule if such supervised physician assistant commits unprofessional conduct as defined in Section 12-36-117(1)(p), C.R.S., or if such physician assistant otherwise violates these rules.

C. Other Responsibilities of the Secondary Physician Supervisor. In the event that a physician undertakes the supervision of a physician assistant who does not have a primary physician supervisor, or who does not have a form in compliance with Section 4 of this rule on file with the Board, such physician shall be deemed to be the primary physician supervisor and shall be subject to all responsibilities of the primary physician supervisor including the two physician assistant limit. The Board recommends but does not require that any physician acting as a secondary physician supervisor sign every chart with the words "secondary physician supervisor" and identify the primary physician supervisor.

D. Effect of the Failure of the Secondary Physician Supervisor to Supervise. Absent a review and signing of the chart by the secondary physician supervisor, the primary physician supervisor for that employer shall be deemed to have been the supervisor rather than the secondary supervisor. In such event, the primary physician supervisor shall be responsible for the practice of medicine of the physician assistant as set forth above.

COLORADO CODE REGS. SEC. 400-2 (II)

CONNECTICUT

"Supervision" means the exercise by the supervising physician of oversight, control and direction of the services of a physician assistant. Supervision includes but is not limited to:

(A) Continuous availability of direct communication either in person or by radio, telephone or telecommunications between the physician assistant and the supervising physician;

(B) active and continuing overview of the physician assistant's activities to ensure that the supervising physician's directions are being implemented and to support the physician assistant in the performance of his services;

(C) personal review by the supervising physician of the physician assistant's practice at least weekly or more frequently as necessary to ensure quality patient care;

(D) review of the charts and records of the physician assistant on a regular basis as necessary to ensure quality patient care;

(E) delineation of a predetermined plan for emergency situations; and

(F) designation of an alternate licensed physician in the absence of the supervising physician.

CONNECTICUT GEN. STATUTE SEC. 20-12A(7)

DELAWARE

"Supervision of physician's assistants" means the ability of the supervising physician to provide or exercise control and direction over the services of physician's assistants. The constant physical presence of the supervising physician is not required, provided that the supervising physician is readily accessible by some form of electronic communication and that the supervising physician can be physically present within 30 minutes if necessary.

a. Any physician who delegates medical responsibility to a physician's assistant is responsible for that individual's medical activities and must provide adequate supervision. No function may be delegated to a physician's assistant who by statute or professional regulation is prohibited from performing that function. The delegating physician cannot be involved in patient care in name only. A physician's assistant shall not maintain or manage an office separate and apart from the supervision physician. No regulation of the Board shall purport to authorize physician's assistants to engage in diagnosis, to prescribe or dispense legend drugs or therapeutics, to practice medicine or surgery or refractions or to pronounce a patient dead in any setting independent of the supervision of a physician who is licensed to practice medicine and surgery. Such licensed physician's assistants shall not delegate an assigned task to any other individual, nor shall they independently bill a patient for services rendered at the request of the physician.

b. For the purpose of clarification, the terms "guidelines," "standing orders," "protocols" and "algorithms" are synonymous in their application under these regulations. Hereafter, the term "standing orders" will be used. Prescription and nonprescription medications may be initiated by standing orders if these standing orders have been approved by the responsible delegating physician and by the Physician's Assistant Regulatory Council. Emergency care as defined in the Medical Practices Act is exempted from these regulations.

c. It is appropriate and good medical procedure for all responsible physicians who choose to have their patients followed by physician's assistants to personally reevaluate at least every 3 months any patient receiving controlled substances or at least every 6 months any patient receiving other prescription medications or therapeutics.

d. A supervising physician may not delegate responsibilities in assisting the physician to a physician's assistant that exceed the physician's specialty.

e. A supervising physician who fails to adhere to these regulations would be considered to be permitting the unauthorized practice of medicine (as defined under § 1703(c) of this chapter (the Medical Practices Act)) and would be subject to disciplinary action by the Board of Medical Practice.

A physician's assistant will at all times be under the control of a licensed physician, as defined in this chapter.

Tit. 24 Delaware Code sec. 1770A-2

DISTRICT OF COLUMBIA

A supervising physician has ultimate responsibility for the medical care and treatment given to a patient by a physician assistant to whom the supervising physician has delegated authority to perform health care tasks.

Subject to the limitations of the Act and this chapter, a physician who is registered as a supervising physician by the Board may delegate to a physician assistant medical procedures and other tasks that are usually performed within the normal scope of the supervising physician's practice.

A supervising physician shall not permit a physician assistant to practice medicine independently, and shall ensure that all actions undertaken by a physician assistant are as follows:
(a) Governed by a standard or advanced job description registered by the Board;
(b) Performed in immediate collaboration with the supervising physician; or
(c) Performed pursuant to § 4911.5.

A supervising physician may delegate to a physician assistant only those tasks and duties that are consistent with sound medical practice, taking into account the following:
(a) The physician assistant's education, skill, training, and experience;
(b) The patient's health and safety;
(c) The degree of supervision provided by the supervising physician;
(d) The qualifications of the supervising physician; and
(e) The nature of the supervising physician's practice.

A supervising physician shall be responsible for supervising a physician assistant at all times that a physician assistant performs health care tasks delegated by a supervising physician. Unless a job description registered by the Board expressly requires a greater level of supervision, a supervising physician shall do the following:

(a) Be present within a fifteen (15) mile radius of the District;

(b) Be available for consultation by voice communication;

(c) Countersign all medical orders and progress notes within forty-eight (48) hours; and

(d) Provide immediate collaboration for health care tasks that are not governed by a job description registered by the Board.

A supervising physician who is temporarily unavailable to supervise a physician assistant shall designate a back-up supervising physician to provide substitute supervision during the supervising physician's absence.

A physician who is designated to provide substitute supervision of a physician assistant pursuant to a § 4914.6 shall be registered in a job description as a back-up supervising physician before providing supervision.

A back-up supervising physician shall have ultimate responsibility for the medical care and treatment given to a patient by a physician assistant acting under the supervision of the back-up supervising physician.

The Director may amend a registered job description to name additional back-up supervising physicians; provided, that each named physician is licensed in good standing in the District and, on a form approved by the Board, certifies as follows:

(a) That the physician has read and understood the contents of the job description, this chapter, and the Act; and

(b) That the physician agrees to observe the requirements for supervising the practice of a physician assistant set forth in those documents.

A supervising physician shall not delegate patient care responsibility to a physician assistant during the absence of the supervising physician unless substitute supervision has been arranged.

A health care facility, organization, association, institution, or group practice which employs a physician assistant shall designate one physician to supervise the physician assistant. The physician who is designated has ultimate responsibility for the care and treatment of a patient attended by the physician assistant regardless of whether the designated supervising physician actually pays the salary of the physician assistant.

Except as provided in § 4914.13, a physician shall not supervise more than two (2) physician assistants at one time.

A supervising physician employed by a health care facility that provides inpatient treatment may supervise four (4) physician assistants; Provided, that the health care tasks delegated to the physician assistants are restricted to the case and treatment of the facility's in-patient population.

Tit. 17 District of Columbia Mun. Regs. sec. 4914

FLORIDA

"Supervision" means responsible supervision and control. Except in cases of emergency, supervision requires the easy availability or physical presence of the licensed physician for consultation and direction of the actions of the physician assistant. For the purposes of this definition, the term "easy availability" includes the ability to communicate by way of telecommunication. The boards shall establish rules as to what constitutes responsible supervision of the physician assistant.

FLORIDA STAT. ANN. SEC. 458.347 (2)(F)

GEORGIA

No physician shall have more than four Physician assistants licensed to him or her at any one time. Additionally, no physician may supervise more than two physician assistants at one time, except that a physician may supervise more than two physician assistants while on call for a solo practioner or as a member of a group in a practice setting including, but not limited to, clinics, hospitals and other institutions. The physician taking call must be approved to supervise the physician assistant of the physician for whom he or she is taking call.

RULES AND REGS. OF THE STATE OF GEORGIA SEC. 360-5-.07

HAWAII

The supervising physician shall:
(1) Possess a current unrestricted Hawaii license to practice medicine and surgery that is in good standing with the board;
(2) Submit a statement that the supervising physician will direct and exercise supervision over any subordinate physician assistant in accordance with this subchapter and recognizes that the supervising physician retains full professional and legal responsibility for the performance of the physician assistant and the care and treatment of the patient;
(3) Permit the physician assistant to be utilized in any setting authorized by the supervising physician including, but not limited to, clinics, hospitals, ambulatory centers, patient homes, nursing homes, other lodging, and other institutional settings;
(4) Provide adequate means for direct communication between the physician assistant and the supervising physician; provided that where the physical presence of the supervising physician is not required, the direct communication may occur through the use of technology which may include but is not limited to, two way

radio, telephone, fax machine, modem, or other telecommunication device;

(5) Personally review the records of each patient seen by the physician assistant within seven working days;

(6) Designate an alternate supervising physician in the physician's absence;

(7) Supervise no more than two physician assistants at any one time; and

(8) Be authorized to allow the physician assistant to prescribe, dispense, and administer medications and medical devices to the extent delegated by the supervising physician and subject to the following requirements:

(A) Prescribing and dispensing of medications may include Schedule III through V and all legend medications. No physician assistant may prescribe Schedule II medications;

(B) A physician assistant who has been delegated the authority to prescribe Schedule III through V medications shall register with the Drug Enforcement Administration (DEA);

(C) Each prescription written by a physician assistant shall include the name, address, and phone number of the supervising physician and physician assistant. The printed name of the supervising physician shall be on one side of the form and the printed name of the physician assistant shall be on the other side. A physician assistant who has been delegated the authority to prescribe shall sign the prescription next to the printed name of the physician assistant;

(D) A physician assistant employed or extended privileges by a hospital or extended care facility may, if allowed under the bylaws, rules, and regulations of the hospital or extended care facility, write orders for medications Schedule II through V, for inpatients under the care of the supervising physician;

(E) The board of medical examiners shall notify the pharmacy board in writing, at least annually or more frequently if required by changes, of each physician assistant authorized to prescribe;

(F) A physician assistant may request, receive, and sign for professional samples and may distribute professional samples to patients; and

(G) All dispensing activities shall comply with appropriate federal and state regulations.

(b) The supervising physician or physicians and the physician assistant shall notify the board within ten days of severance of supervision or employment of the physician assistant.

HAWAII ADMIN. R. SEC. 16-85-49

IDAHO

The supervising physician accepts full responsibility for the medical acts of and patient services provided by physician assistants, graduate physician assistants, nurse practitioners, certified nurse-midwives, and clinical nurse specialists and for the supervision of such acts which shall include, but are not limited to: (3-16-04)

a. An on-site visit at least monthly to personally observe the quality of care provided; (3-16-04)

b. A periodic review of a representative sample of medical records to evaluate the medical services that are provided. When applicable, this review shall also include an evaluation of adherence to the delegation of services agreement between the physician and physician assistant or graduate physician assistant; and (3-16-04)

c. Regularly scheduled conferences between the supervising physician and such licensees. (3-16-04)

02. Patient Complaints. The supervising physician shall report to the Board of Medicine all patient complaints received against the physician assistant or graduate physician assistant which relate to the quality and nature of medical care or patient services rendered. The supervising physician shall report to the Board of Nursing all patient complaints received against the nurse practitioner, certified nurse-midwife, or clinical nurse specialist, that relate to the quality and nature of medical care rendered. (3-16-04)

03. Pre-Signed Prescriptions. The supervising physician shall not utilize or authorize the physician assistant, nurse practitioner, certified nurse-midwife, or clinical nurse specialist to use any pre-signed prescriptions. (3-16-04)

04. Supervisory Responsibility. A supervising physician or alternate supervising physician shall not supervise more than three (3) physician assistants, graduate physician assistants, nurse practitioners, certified nurse-midwives, or clinical nurse specialists contemporaneously. The Board, however, may authorize a supervising physician or alternate supervising physician to supervise a total of six (6) such licensees contemporaneously if necessary to provide adequate medical care and upon prior petition documenting adequate safeguards to protect the public health and safety. The responsibilities and duties of a supervising physician may not be transferred to a business entity, professional corporation or partnership, nor may they be assigned to another physician without prior notification and Board approval. (3-16-04)

05. Available Supervision. The supervising physician shall oversee the activities of the nurse practitioner, physician assistant, graduate physician assistant, certified nurse-midwife, or clinical nurse special-ist, and must always be available either in person or by telephone to supervise, direct and counsel such licensees. The scope and nature of the supervision of the physician assistant and graduate physician assistant shall be outlined in a delegation of services agreement, as set forth in IDAPA 22.01.03, "Rules for the Licensure of Physician Assistants," Subsection 030.03. (3-16-04)

06. Disclosure. It shall be the responsibility of each supervising physician to ensure that each patient who receives the services of a physician assistant, graduate physician assistant, nurse practitio-ner, certified nurse-midwife, or clinical nurse specialist is aware of the fact that said person is not a licensed physician. This disclosure requirement can be fulfilled by the use of nametags, correspondence, oral statements, office signs or such other procedures that under the involved circumstances adequately advise the patient of the education and training of the person rendering medical services. (3-16-04)

The Board, by and through its designated agents, is authorized to conduct on-site reviews of the activities of the supervising physicians at the locations and facilities in which the physician assistant, gradu-ate physician assistant, nurse practitioner, certified nurse-midwife, or clinical nurse specialist practices at such times as the Board deems necessary.

IDAHO ADMIN. CODE SEC. 22.01.04.02

ILLINOIS

a) The supervising physician/alternate supervising physician shall maintain the final responsibility for the care of the patient and the performance of the physician assistant.

b) Delegated procedures and tasks performed by the physician assis-tant shall be within the current scope of practice of the supervis-ing physician or designated alternate supervising physician with whom the physician assistant is working at the time.

c) The supervising physician may supervise no more than two phy-sician assistants. However, a physician assistant shall be able to hold more than one professional position.

d) Any time the supervising physician is unable to provide the appropriate supervision to the physician assistant, he/she shall designate an alternate supervising physician to provide such supervision. The name(s) of the alternate supervising physician(s) shall be identified in the guidelines established by the supervising physician. If the supervising physician will be unable to supervise the physician assistant for more than 30 days, he/she shall notify the Department, on forms prescribed by the Department. Failure of the supervising physician to notify the Department shall be grounds for discipline of the physician's license.

e) When under supervision of an alternate supervising physician, the physician assistant may carry out those duties that are contained within the established guidelines of the physician/physician assistant team. An alternate supervising physician shall be subject to the same supervision responsibilities as the supervising physician.

f) It is the responsibility of the supervising physician to direct and review the work, records and practice of the physician assistant on a timely basis to ensure that appropriate directions are given and understood and that appropriate treatment is being rendered.

g) In the event that the supervising physician is not present in the same facility as the physician assistant, the supervising physician should be within reasonable travel distance from the facility so that the supervising physician can personally assure the proper care of his/her patients.

h) The supervising physician shall have full authority and responsibility to direct, supervise and limit the role of a physician assistant. Nothing contained herein shall be deemed to alter the fact that a physician assistant shall continue to bear responsibility for his/her actions to the extent that the physician assistant fails to comply with physician directives or is not carrying out those directives in a professional and appropriate manner in conformance with his/her training.

i) The physician assistant shall only work under the direction of the current supervising physician or alternate supervising physician and may undertake patient care responsibilities only for the patients of the supervising physician or alternate supervising physician.

ILLINOIS ADMIN. CODE TIT. 68 SEC. 1350.80

INDIANA

(a) A physician licensed under IC 25-22.5 who intends to supervise a physician assistant shall register his or her intent to do so with the board on a form approved by the board prior to commencing supervision of a physician assistant. The supervising physician shall include the following information on the form supplied by the board:

   (1) The name, business address, and telephone number of the supervising physician.

(2) The name, business address, telephone number, and certification number of the physician assistant.

(3) The current license number of the physician.

(4) A statement that the physician will be supervising no more than two (2) physician assistants, and the name and certificate numbers of the physician assistants he or she is currently supervising.

(5) A description of the setting in which the physician assistant will practice under the supervising physician, including the specialty, if any, of the supervising physician.

(6) A statement that the supervising physician:

    (A) will exercise continuous supervision over the physician assistant in accordance with IC 25-27.5-6 and this article;

    (B) shall review all patient encounters maintained by the physician assistant within twenty-four (24) hours after the physician assistant has seen a patient; and

    (C) at all times, retain professional and legal responsibility for the care rendered by the physician assistant.

(7) Detailed description of the process maintained by the physician for evaluation of the physician assistant's performance.

(b) The supervising physician may not be the designated supervising physician for more than two (2) physician assistants and may not supervise more than two (2) physician assistants at one (1) time as the primary or designated supervising physician.

(c) The designated supervising physician is to accept responsibility of supervising the physician assistant in the absence of the primary supervising physician of record. Protocol is to be established by the physician practice.

(d) The supervising physician shall, within fifteen (15) days, notify the board when the supervising relationship with the physician assistant is terminated, and the reason for such termination. In addition, notification shall be submitted to the committee.

INDIANA ADMIN. CODE TIT. 844 R. 2.2-2-2

IOWA

Physician assistants shall use the board-approved forms to notify the board of the identity of their supervising physicians at the following times:

a. Prior to beginning practice in Iowa.

b. Within 90 days of any change in supervisory relationship or change in supervisory physicians.

c. At the time of license renewal. The physician assistant shall provide the identity of the current supervising physician(s) and of the supervising physician(s) who has provided supervision during the physician assistant's current biennium.

The physician assistant shall maintain documentation of current supervising physicians, which shall be made available to the board upon request.

A physician assistant who provides medical services shall be supervised by one or more physicians; but a physician shall not supervise more than two physician assistants at the same time.

It shall be the responsibility of the physician assistant with a supervising physician to ensure that the physician assistant is adequately supervised.

a. Patient care provided by the physician assistant shall be reviewed with a supervising physician on an ongoing basis as indicated by the clinical condition of the patient. Although every chart need not be signed nor every visit reviewed, nor does the supervising physician need to be physically present at each activity of the physician assistant, it is the responsibility of the supervising physician and physician assistant to ensure that each patient has received the appropriate medical care.

b. Patient care provided by the physician assistant may be reviewed with a supervising physician in person, by telephone or by other telecommunicative means.

c. When signatures are required, electronic signatures are allowed if:
    (1) The signature is transcribed by the signer into an electronic record and is not the result of electronic regeneration; and
    (2) A mechanism exists allowing confirmation of the signature and protection from unauthorized reproduction.

d. If the physician assistant is being trained to perform new medical procedures, the training may be carried out only under the direct, personal supervision of a supervising physician or another qualified individual.

Iowa Admin. Code r. 645-326.8

KANSAS

Direction and supervision of the physician assistant shall be considered to be adequate if the responsible physician meets all of the following requirements:

(a) At least annually, reviews and evaluates the professional competency of the physician assistant;

(b) at least annually, reviews any drug prescription protocol and determines if any modifications, restrictions, or terminations are required. Any of these changes shall be conveyed to the physician assistant and set forth in all copies of the protocol required by K.A.R. 100-28a-9 to be maintained and provided;

(c) engages in the practice of medicine and surgery in this state;

(d) insures that the physician assistant has a current license issued by the board;

(e) within 10 days, reports to the board any knowledge of disciplinary hearings, formal hearings, public or private censure, or other disciplinary action taken against the physician assistant by any state's licensure or registration authority or any professional association;

(f) within 10 days, reports to the board any litigation, threatened litigation, or claim alleging professional incompetency or professional negligence on the part of the physician assistant;

(g) at least every 14 days, reviews all records of patients treated by the physician assistant and authenticates this review in the patient record;

(h) reviews patient records and authenticates the review in each patient record within 48 hours of treatment provided by the physician assistant if the treatment provided in an emergency exceeded the authority granted to the physician assistant by the responsible physician request form required by K.A.R.100-28a-9;

(i) provides for a designated physician to provide supervision and direction on each occasion when the responsible physician is temporarily absent, is unable to be immediately contacted by telecommunication, or is otherwise unavailable at a time the physician assistant could reasonably be expected to provide professional services; and

(j) delegates to the physician assistant only those acts that constitute the practice of medicine and surgery that the responsible physician believes or has reason to believe can be competently performed by the physician assistant, based upon the physician assistant's background, training, capabilities, skill, and experience.

KANSAS ADMIN. REGS. 100-28A-10

KENTUCKY

"Supervision" means overseeing the activities of and accepting of responsibility for the medical services rendered by a physician assistant. Each team of physicians and physician assistants shall ensure that the delegation of medical tasks is appropriate to the physician assistant's level of training and experience, that the identifications of and access to the supervising physician are clearly defined, and that a process for evaluation of the physician assistant's performance is established.

KENTUCKY REV. STAT. SEC. 311.840(6)

A supervising physician shall:

(1) Restrict the services of a physician assistant to services within the physician assistant's scope of practice and to the provisions of KRS 311.840 to 311.862;

(2) Prohibit a physician assistant from prescribing or dispensing controlled substances;

(3) Inform all patients in contact with a physician assistant of the status of the physician assistant;

(4) Post a notice stating that a physician assistant practices medicine or osteopathy in all locations where the physician assistant may practice;

(5) Require a physician assistant to wear identification that clearly states that he or she is a physician assistant;

(6) Prohibit a physician assistant from independently billing any patient or other payor for services rendered by the physician assistant;

(7) If necessary, participate with the governing body of any hospital or other licensed health care facility in a credentialing process established by the facility;

(8) Not require a physician assistant to perform services or other acts that the physician assistant feels incapable of carrying out safely and properly;

(9) Maintain adequate, active, and continuous supervision of a physician assistant's activities to assure that the physician assistant is performing as directed and complying with the requirements of KRS 311.840 to 311.862 and all related administrative regulations;

(10) Sign all records of service rendered by a physician assistant in a timely manner as certification that the physician assistant performed the services as delegated;

(11) (a) Reevaluate the reliability, accountability, and professional knowledge of a physician assistant two (2) years after the physician assistant's original certification in this Commonwealth and every two (2) years thereafter; and

(b) Based on the reevaluation, recommend approval or disapproval of certification or recertification to the board; and

(12) Notify the board within three (3) business days if the supervising physician:

(a) Ceases to supervise or employ the physician assistant; or

(b) Believes in good faith that a physician assistant violated any disciplinary rule of KRS 311.840 to 311.862 or related administrative regulations.

KENTUCKY REV. STAT. SEC. 311.856

LOUISIANA

Supervising Physician is a physician approved by and registered with the board under this Chapter to supervise a physician assistant.

Supervision, responsible direction and control, with the supervising physician assuming legal liability for the services rendered by the physician assistant in the course and scope of the physician assistant's employment.

Such supervision shall not be construed in every case to require the physical presence of the supervising physician.

However, the supervising physician and physician assistant must have the capability to be in contact with each other by either telephone or other telecommunications device. Supervision shall exist when the supervising physician responsible for the patient gives informed concurrence of the actions of the physician assistant, whether given prior to or after the action, and when a medical treatment plan or action is made in accordance with written clinical practice guidelines or protocols set forth by the supervising physician.

LOUISIANA ADMIN. CODE SEC. 1503

MAINE

Supervision shall be continuous but shall not be construed as necessarily requiring the physical presence of the supervising physician at the time and place that the services are rendered.

(A) SUPERVISORS

Physician assistants may practice medicine and perform medical activities only when provided supervision by the following:

1. a primary or secondary supervising physician; or
2. a physician in an organized health care delivery system in which there is a primary supervising physician, or
3. a physician licensed by the Board of Osteopathic Licensure who is permitted under rules promulgated by that Board to be a secondary supervisor of physician assistants.

B. QUALIFICATION FOR APPROVAL AS PRIMARY SUPERVISING PHYSICIAN

1. Except as otherwise provided in this chapter, any physician must be approved by the Board, before the physician may become a Primary Supervising Physician, for each individual wishing to be supervised. The Board may grant approval to a physician to become a Primary Supervising Physician who:

a. has an active, unrestricted, permanent license to practice medicine in this state;

b. submits a statement to the Board that the licensee will oversee and accept responsibility and liability for the medical activities delegated to the physician assistant. If the physician is to serve as the Primary Supervising Physician for an Organized Health Care Delivery System or Group Practice, the statement must so indicate;

c. submits an affidavit that a written Plan of Supervision addressing the technical requirements of supervision (as set forth in Section 5 of this Chapter) is on file in the practice setting; and

d. pays the appropriate fee as determined by the Board.

2. Prohibited Physician Conduct

a. No physician shall delegate to any person other than another physician licensed by the Board of Licensure in Medicine or the Board of Osteopathic Licensure the performance of duties which constitute the practice of medicine or surgery, except in full compliance with this chapter or pursuant to 32 M.R.S.A. §3270 B.

b. No physician shall supervise an unlicensed physician assistant.

c. No physician shall supervise a physician assistant unless:

1. the physician has been approved by the Board to become a Primary Supervising Physician and has completed a statement that the physician agrees to provide supervision to a particular physician assistant (as required by section 2 or 9) and has ensured that the statement has been provided to the Board; or

2. the physician has ensured that the physician assistant has a primary supervising physician, or is supervised by a physician licensed by the Board of Osteopathic Licensure who is permitted to exercise primary supervision of physician assistants by that board, and provides supervision only in an Organized Health Care Delivery System; or

3. the physician assistant has a Primary Supervising Physician or is supervised by a physician licensed by the Board of Osteopathic Licensure who is permitted to exercise primary supervision of physician assistants by that board, and agrees in writing to accept delegated responsibility as a secondary supervising physician from the Primary Supervising Physician under the Plan Of Supervision.

3. Sanctions

Any physician licensed by the Board who is determined to have violated this section shall be deemed to have violated 32

M.R.S.A. §3282-A.2 and shall be subject to disciplinary action by the Board.

The Board may terminate a physician from acting as a secondary or Primary Supervising Physician or teaching-supervising physician in accordance with due process.

C. ELEMENTS AND TECHNICAL REQUIREMENTS OF SUPERVISION

As a part of the supervising physician/physician assistant team, a physician assistant is responsible for ensuring that:

1. the physician assistant's basic scope of practice and practice setting is identified;
2. the delegation of medical tasks is appropriate to the physician assistant's level of competence;
3. the relationship of, and access to, a supervising physician is defined; and
4. a process for evaluation of the physician assistant's performance is established.

D. WRITTEN PLAN OF SUPERVISION

Physician assistants licensed to practice in accordance with these rules and their primary supervising physician must prepare and have on file in the practice setting a written, dated plan of supervision containing specified practice descriptions of the elements of supervision as outlined in subparagraph C. This plan of supervision must be reviewed and updated as necessary, but in any event, whenever the physician assistant's license is renewed a copy of the updated plan must be submitted with the renewal application. A statement shall be attached to the plan stating the date the plan was reviewed and any changes to the plan, and shall be signed by the physician assistant and primary supervising physician. If a physician assistant is to be supervised by a secondary supervising physician(s), the secondary supervising physician(s) must accept delegation of supervision in writing as part of the plan of supervision. Appendix 1 of these Rules provides one sample format for a written plan of supervision.

E. PLAN TO BE AVAILABLE ON DEMAND

A physician assistant shall provide, at the request of any Board member or authorized person, a copy of the plan of supervision and, if applicable, the document showing the delegation of that plan to a secondary supervising physician. Such request may be made in writing or by appearing at the practice setting in which case the plan shall be provided immediately. The Board may require the plan to be amended for purposes of ensuring public safety as required by state law.

Assumption of Responsibility

If a physician assistant is employed by a physician or group of physicians, the physician assistant must still be provided supervision by an approved primary or secondary supervising physician. Liability under these rules for the physician assistant's medical activities shall remain that of the approved primary or secondary supervising physician, including when the physician assistant provides care and treatment for patients in an organized health care delivery system facility. If a physician assistant is employed by or a principal in an organized health care delivery system facility, nothing in these rules shall be construed to limit the liability of the organized health care delivery system facility for the physician assistant's actions or omissions. A physician assistant who is employed by or who is a principal in such facilities must still be provided supervision by an approved primary or secondary supervising physician.

Notification of Change in or Addition of Supervising Physician

A physician assistant licensed by this Board, upon changing primary supervising physicians or adding an additional primary supervising physician or multiple work site, must notify the Board. Such notification shall include:

(A) the name, business address, and telephone number of the new or additional primary supervising physician(s); the name, business address, and telephone number of the physician assistant; and at least one of the following:
  1. a signed statement (as required in Section 2 and/or 9) from each new or additional primary supervising physician;
  2. if a physician assistant is to be employed by or a principal in an organized health care delivery system facility, a statement (as required in Section 2 and/or 9) from the organized health care delivery system facility certifying employment and signed by the physician in the organized health care delivery system facility who has been approved as a primary supervising physician; or
  3. if a physician assistant is to be employed by or practice in a group practice, a statement (as required in Section 2 and/or 9) from the primary supervising physician in the group practice agreeing to provide supervision as defined in Section 2 and/or 9.
(B) A physician assistant will notify the Board of any changes, additions, or deletions in supervising physicians no later than 14 days after the effective date of the change or addition.
(C) The statement of the primary supervising physician or the certification of employment by the organized health care delivery

system facility must be executed by the physician or an organized health care delivery system prior to the physician assistant's initiation of practice under the new supervising physician.

(D) Notifications not submitted in writing within 14 days will be subject to a late fee of not more than $100.

CODE MAINE R. SEC. 02 373 7-9

MARYLAND

(A) The physician assistant and supervising physician shall submit the delegation agreement with original signatures on a form approved by the Board.

(B) The applicant shall submit a fee of $200 for the first delegation agreement and $100 for each additional delegation agreement.

(C) In order for a physician to use a physician assistant for the performance of delegated medical duties, the supervising physician shall:

(1) Give the physician's license number or registration number;

(2) Give the State certification number of the physician assistant;

(3) Give the location where the physician assistant will perform duties delegated by the physician;

(4) Give the scope of the physician's practice;

(5) Describe the job duties and delegated medical acts which the physician assistant will perform and the conditions under which they will be performed;

(6) Describe the qualifications of the supervising physician and physician assistant;

(7) Describe the setting in which the physician assistant will practice;

(8) Describe the continuous supervision mechanisms that the supervising physician or physicians shall utilize;

(9) Include an attestation that all medical acts to be delegated to the physician assistant are within the scope of practice of the supervising physician and appropriate to the physician assistant's education, training, and level of competence;

(10) Include an attestation that the supervising physician will utilize the mechanisms of continuous supervision as described in the delegation agreement;

(11) Include an attestation that the supervising physician accepts responsibility for any care given by the physician assistant;

(12) Include an attestation that the supervising physician will respond in a timely manner when contacted by the physician assistant; and

(13) Describe the method of evaluating the physician assistant's performance.

(D) In a hospital, the supervising physician shall meet the requirements under §C(1)(13) of this regulation, and may act as the primary supervision physician by:

(1) Preparing a statement describing the supervisory arrangements, which includes an ongoing list of all approved alternating supervising physicians, with the alternating supervising physicians' scope of practice, signed and dated by each alternating supervising physician;

(2) Keeping the list described in §D(1) of this regulation on file at all practice sites; and

(3) Providing the list on request in writing, during all business hours, to representatives of the Board or the Licensing and Certification Administration.

(E) In a hospital, the requirements of Health Occupations Article, §15-302(b)(4), Annotated Code of Maryland, and §C(9) of this regulation are met if the primary supervising physician attests that the:

(1) Physician assistant will practice only within the scope of practice of any assigned alternate supervising physician; and

(2) Primary supervising physician assumes the responsibility for maintaining and enforcing mechanisms which assure that this requirement is met on a continual basis.

(F) All supervising physicians shall:

(1) Provide on-site supervision at all times for a physician assistant who has a temporary certificate;

(2) Report to the Board within 10 days any termination of employment of a physician assistant for reasons including, but not limited to:

(a) Voluntary resignation,

(b) Termination for conduct which may be grounds for discipline as listed in Regulation .13 of this chapter, and

(c) Resignation after notice of intent to terminate;

(3) Be familiar with the statute and regulations which govern physician assistants; and

(4) Maintain a system to assure that the physician assistant is not practicing beyond the scope of the delegation agreement.

MARYLAND REGS. CODE TIT. 10 SEC. 32.03.06

MASSACHUSETTS

(1) All professional activities of a physician assistant must be supervised by a supervising physician approved by the Massachusetts

Board of Registration in Medicine pursuant to 243 CMR 2.08(7). A "supervising physician," for purposes of this subchapter, shall mean a physician who is a "full licensee" of the Massachusetts Board of Registration in Medicine.

(2) A supervising physician shall not supervise more than two physician assistants at any one time.

(3) A supervising physician may use a physician assistant to assist him or her in the process of gathering data necessary to make decisions and institute patient care plans. A physician assistant shall not, however, supplant a licensed physician as the principal medical decision-maker.

(4) A supervising physician shall afford supervision adequate to ensure all of the following:

(a) The physician assistant practices medicine in accordance with accepted standards of medical practice. 263 CMR 5.05(4)(a) does not require the physical presence of the supervising physician in every situation in which a physician assistant renders medical services.

(b) The physician assistant, except in life-threatening emergencies where no licensed physician is available, informs each patient that he or she is a physician assistant and that he or she renders medical services only under the supervision of a licensed physician.

(c) The physician assistant wears a name tag which identifies him or her as a physician assistant.

(d) The supervising physician reviews diagnostic and treatment information, as agreed upon by the supervising physician and the physician assistant, in a timely manner consistent with the patient's medical condition.

(e) On follow-up care, hospital visits, nursing home visits, attending the chronically ill at home, and in similar circumstances in which the supervising physician has established a therapeutic regimen or other written protocol, the physician assistant checks and records a patient's progress and reports the patient's progress to the supervising physician. Supervision is adequate under this subparagraph if it permits a physician assistant who encounters a new problem not covered by a written protocol or which exceeds established parameters to initiate a new patient care plan and consult with the supervising physician.

(f) In an emergency, the physician assistant renders emergency medical services necessary to avoid disability or death of an injured person until a licensed physician arrives.

(g) When a supervising physician is unable or unavailable to be the principal medical decision-maker, another licensed physician must be designated to assume temporary supervisory responsibilities with respect to the physician assistant. The name and scope of responsibility of the physician providing such temporary supervision must be readily ascertainable from records kept in the ordinary course of business which are available to patients. The supervising physician(s) of record is ultimately responsible for ensuring that each task performed by a physician assistant is properly supervised.

CODE MASSACHUSETTS REGS. TIT. 263 SEC. 5.05

MICHIGAN

(1) Except as otherwise provided in this subsection and section 17049(5), a physician who is a sole practitioner or who practices in a group of physicians and treats patients on an outpatient basis shall not supervise more than 4 physician's assistants. If a physician described in this subsection supervises physician's assistants at more than 1 practice site, the physician shall not supervise more than 2 physician's assistants by a method other than the physician's actual physical presence at the practice site.

(2) A physician who is employed by, under contract or subcontract to, or has privileges at a health facility or agency licensed under article 17 or a state correctional facility may supervise more than 4 physician's assistants at the health facility or agency or state correctional facility.

(3) To the extent that a particular selected medical care service requires extensive medical training, education, or ability or pose serious risks to the health and safety of patients, the board may prohibit or otherwise restrict the delegation of that medical care service or may require higher levels of supervision.

(4) A physician shall not delegate ultimate responsibility for the quality of medical care services, even if the medical care services are provided by a physician's assistant.

(5) The board may promulgate rules for the delegation by a supervising physician to a physician's assistant of the function of prescription of drugs. The rules may define the drugs or classes of drugs the prescription of which shall not be delegated and other procedures and protocols necessary to promote consistency with federal and state drug control and enforcement laws. Until the rules are promulgated, a supervising physician may delegate the prescription of drugs other than controlled substances as

defined by article 7 or federal law. When delegated prescription occurs, both the physician's assistant's name and the supervising physician's name shall be used, recorded, or otherwise indicated in connection with each individual prescription.

(6) A supervising physician may delegate in writing to a physician assistant the ordering, receipt, and dispensing of complimentary starter dose drugs other than controlled substances as defined by article 7 or federal law. When the delegated ordering, receipt, or dispensing of complimentary starter dose drugs occurs, both the physician assistant's name and the supervising physician's name shall be used, recorded, or otherwise indicated in connection with each order, receipt, or dispensing. As used in this subsection, "complimentary starter dose" means that term as defined in section 17745. It is the intent of the legislature in enacting this subsection to allow a pharmaceutical manufacturer or wholesale distributor, as those terms are defined in part 177, to distribute complimentary starter dose drugs to a physician assistant, as described in this subsection, in compliance with section 503(d) of the federal food, drug, and cosmetic act, chapter 675, 52 Stat. 1051, 21 U.S.C. 353.

MICHIGAN COMPLIED LAWS SEC. 333.17048

Responsibilities of physician supervising physician's assistant.

(1) In addition to the other requirements of this section and subject to subsection (5), a physician who supervises a physician assistant is responsible for all of the following:
 (a) Verification of the physician assistant's credentials.
 (b) Evaluation of the physician assistant's performance.
 (c) Monitoring the physician assistant's practice and provision of medical care services.

(2) Subject to section 17048, a physician who supervises a physician assistant may delegate to the physician assistant the performance of medical care services for a patient who is under the case management responsibility of the physician, if the delegation is consistent with the physician assistant's training.

(3) A physician who supervises a physician assistant is responsible for the clinical supervision of each physician assistant to whom the physician delegates the performance of medical care service under subsection (2).

(4) Subject to subsection (5), a physician who supervises a physician assistant shall keep on file in the physician's office or in the health facility or agency or correctional facility in which the physician

supervises the physician assistant a permanent, written record that includes the physician's name and license number and the name and license number of each physician assistant supervised by the physician.

(5) A group of physicians practicing other than as sole practitioners may designate 1 or more physicians in the group to fulfill the requirements of subsections (1) and (4).

MICHIGAN COMPLIED LAWS SEC. 333.17049

MINNESOTA

"Supervising physician" means a Minnesota licensed physician who accepts full medical responsibility for the performance, practice, and activities of a physician assistant under an agreement as described in section 147A.20. A supervising physician shall not supervise more than two full-time equivalent physician assistants simultaneously.

"Supervision" means overseeing the activities of, and accepting responsibility for, the medical services rendered by a physician assistant. The constant physical presence of the supervising physician is not required so long as the supervising physician and physician assistant are or can be easily in contact with one another by radio, telephone, or other telecommunication device. The scope and nature of the supervision shall be defined by the individual physician-physician assistant agreement.

MINNESOTA STAT. ANN. SEC. 147A.01(23-24)

MISSISSIPPI

1. Before any physician shall supervise a Physician Assistant, the physician must first
   (a) present to the Board's Executive Director, a duly executed protocol,
   (b) appear personally before the Board or its Executive Director, and
   (c) obtain written approval to act as a supervising physician. The facts and matters to be considered by the Board when approving or disapproving a protocol or supervision arrangement, shall include, but are not limited to, how the supervising physician and Physician Assistant plan to implement the protocol, the method and manner of supervision, consultation, referral and liability.
2. Where two or more physicians anticipate executing a protocol to supervise a Physician Assistant, it shall not be necessary that all

of the physicians personally appear before the Board or Executive Director as required in Subsection 1 above. In this situation, the physician who will bear the primary responsibility for the supervision of the Physician Assistant shall make the required personal appearance.

Supervising Physician Limited

1. No physician shall be authorized to supervise a Physician Assistant unless that physician holds an unrestricted license to practice medicine in the State of Mississippi.

2. Supervision means overseeing activities of, and accepting responsibility for, all medical services rendered by the Physician Assistant. Except as described in Subsection 3, supervision must be continuous, but shall not be construed as necessarily requiring the physical presence of the supervising physician.

3. New graduate Physician Assistants and all Physician Assistants newly practicing in Mississippi, except those licensed under provision C1, require the on-site presence of a supervising physician for one hundred twenty (120) days.

4. The Physician Assistant's practice shall be confined to the primary office or clinic of the supervising physician or any hospital(s) or clinic or other health care facility within the same community where the primary office is located, wherein the supervising physician holds medical staff privileges. Exceptions to this requirement may be granted on an individual basis, provided the location(s) of practice are thereafter set forth in the protocol.

5. The supervising physician must provide adequate means for communication with the Physician Assistant. Communication may occur through the use of technology which may include, but is not limited to, radio, telephone, fax, modem, or other telecommunication device.

6. The supervising physician shall, on at least a monthly basis, conduct a review of the records/charts of at least ten percent (10%) of the patients treated by the Physician Assistant, said records/charts selected on a random basis. During said review, the supervising physician shall note the medical and family histories taken, results of any and all examinations and tests, all diagnoses, orders given, medications prescribed, and treatments rendered. The review shall be evidenced by the supervising physician placing his signature or initials next to each of the above areas of review, and shall submit proof of said review to the Board upon request.

Number of Physician Assistants Supervised

No physician shall supervise more than two (2) Physician Assistants at any one time. A physician supervising two (2) nurse practitioners may not supervise a Physician Assistant.

Termination

The Physician Assistant and supervising physician shall notify the Board in writing immediately upon the Physician Assistant's termination; physician retirement; withdrawal from active practice; or any other change in employment, functions or activities. Failure to notify can result in disciplinary action.

MISSISSIPPI RULES CH. XXII SEC. 4 (E-H)

MISSOURI

(1) As used in this rule, unless specifically provided otherwise, the term:
    (A) Supervising physician shall mean a physician so designated pursuant to 4 CSR 150-7.100(4) who holds a permanent license to practice medicine in the state of Missouri and who is actively engaged in the practice of medicine, except that this shall not include physicians who hold a limited license pursuant to section 334.112, RSMo, or a temporary license pursuant to section 334.045 or 334.046, RSMo, or physicians who have retired from the practice of medicine. A physician meeting these requirements but not so designated may serve as a supervising physician, upon signing a physician assistant supervision agreement for times not to exceed fifteen (15) days, when the supervising physician is unavailable if so specified in the physician assistant supervision agreement;
    (B) Physician assistant supervision agreements refers to written agreements, jointly agreed upon protocols, or standing orders between a supervising physician and a licensed physician assistant which provide for the delegation of health care services from a supervising physician to a licensed physician assistant and the review of such services;
    (C) Consultation shall mean the process of seeking a supervising physician's input and guidance regarding patient care including, but not limited to, the methods specified in the physician assistant supervision agreement;
    (D) Assistance shall mean participation by a supervising physician in patient care;
    and

(E) Intervention refers to the direct management of a patient's care by a supervising physician.

(2) No physician assistant shall practice pursuant to the provisions of sections 334.735 through 334.748, RSMo, or to the provisions of this rule unless licensed and pursuant to a written physician assistant supervision agreement.

(3) A supervising physician as designated pursuant to 4 CSR 150-7.100(4) or otherwise in the physician assistant supervision agreement shall at all times be immediately available to the licensed physician assistant for consultation, assistance, and intervention within the same office facility unless making follow-up patient examinations in hospitals, nursing homes and correctional facilities pursuant to section 334.735.9, RSMo, or unless practicing under federal law. No physician assistant shall practice without physician supervision or in any location where a supervising physician is not immediately available for consultation, assistance and intervention, except in an emergency situation, pursuant to federal law, or as provided in section 334.735.9, RSMo.

(4) A physician assistant shall be limited to making follow-up patient examinations in hospitals, nursing homes and correctional facilities where the supervising physician as designated pursuant to 4 CSR 150-7.100(4) or otherwise in the physician assistant supervision agreement, is no further than thirty (30) miles by road, using the most direct route available, or in any other fashion so distanced as to create an impediment to effective intervention, supervision of patient care or adequate review of services. Physician assistants practicing in federally designated health professional shortage areas (HPSAs), shall be limited to practice locations where the supervising physician as designated pursuant to 4 CSR 150-7.100(4) or otherwise in the physician assistant supervision agreement, is no further than fifty (50) miles by road, using the most direct route available.

(5) No physician may be designated to serve as supervising physician for more than three (3) full-time equivalent licensed physician assistants. This limitation shall not apply to physician assistant supervision agreements of hospital employees providing in-patient care services in hospitals as defined in Chapter 197, RSMo.

(6) Upon entering into a physician assistant supervision agreement, the supervising physician shall be familiar with the level of skill, training and the competence of the licensed physician assistant whom the physician will be supervising. The provisions contained in the physician assistant supervision agreement between

the licensed physician assistant and the supervising physician shall be within the scope of practice of the licensed physician assistant and consistent with the licensed physician assistant's skill, training and competence.

(7) A licensed physician assistant practicing pursuant to a physician assistant supervision agreement shall work in the same office facility as the supervising physician except as provided in section 334.735(9), RSMo.

(8) The delegated health care services provided for in the physician assistant supervision agreement shall be consistent with the scopes of practice of both the supervising physician and licensed physician assistant including, but not limited to, any restrictions placed upon the supervising physician's practice or license.

(9) The physician assistant supervision agreement between a supervising physician and a licensed physician assistant shall:

   (A) Include consultation, transportation and referral procedures for patients needing emergency care or care beyond the scope of practice of the licensed physician assistant if the licensed physician assistant practices in a setting where a supervising physician is not continuously present;

   (B) Include the method and frequency of review of the licensed physician assistant's practice activities;

   (C) Be reviewed at least annually and revised as the supervising physician and licensed physician assistant deem necessary;

   (D) Be maintained by the supervising physician and licensed physician assistant for a minimum of eight (8) years after the termination of the agreement;

   (E) Be signed and dated by the supervising physician and licensed physician assistant prior to its implementation; and

   (F) Contain the mechanisms for input for serious or significant changes to a patient.

(10) It is the responsibility of the supervising physician to determine and document the completion of at least a one (1)-month period of time during which the licensed physician assistant shall practice with a supervising physician continuously present before making follow-up visits in hospitals, nursing homes and correctional facilities.

(11) It is the responsibility of the supervising physician and licensed physician assistant to jointly review and document the work, records, and practice activities of the licensed physician assistant at least once every two (2) weeks. For nursing home practice, such review shall occur at least once a month. The supervising physician and the licensed physician assistant shall conduct this review at the site of

service except in extraordinary circumstances which shall be documented. The documentation of this review shall be available to the Board of Registration for the Healing Arts for review upon request.

(12) If any provisions of these rules are deemed by the appropriate federal or state authority to be inconsistent with guidelines for federally funded clinics, individual provisions of these rules shall be considered severable and supervising physicians and licensed physician assistants practicing in such clinics shall follow the provisions of such federal guidelines in these instances. However, the remainder of the provisions of these rules not so affected shall remain in full force and effect for such practitioners.

MISSOURI CODE OF REGS. TIT. 4 SEC. 150-7.135

MONTANA

(1) Each supervising physician named in the utilization plan required by 37-20-301 shall:

   (a) possess a current, unrestricted license to practice medicine in this state;

   (b) submit a statement to the Montana state board of medical examiners that, in his opinion, the physician assistant-certified to be employed is of good character and is both mentally and physically able to perform the duties of a physician assistant-certified described in the utilization plan;

   (c) submit a statement to the board that he will exercise supervision over the physician assistant-certified in accordance with any rules adopted by the board and will retain professional and legal responsibility for the care and treatment of his patients; and

   (d) submit detailed information to the board regarding the physician's professional background, medical education, internship and residency, continuing education received, membership in state and national medical associations, hospital and staff privileges, and such other information as the board may require.

(2) Each physician assistant-certified named in the utilization plan required by 37-20-301 shall meet the criteria for approval as a physician assistant-certified as provided in 37-20-402.

MONTANA CODE ANN. SEC. 37-20-101

NEBRASKA

Supervision must be sufficient to provide quality medical care.

The supervising physician and the physician assistant must have a written scope of practice agreement which is kept on file at the primary practice site and available for review by the Department upon request.

1. The scope of practice agreement must delineate:
    (a) The activities of the physician assistant; and
    (b) The limits of the physician assistant.
2. The physician assistant's practice agreement must include only the procedures in which the supervising physician is trained.

When the supervising physician utilizes a backup supervising physician s/he must maintain an agreement at all times with such physician to act as a backup supervising physician for him/her when s/he is not readily available to supervise the physician assistant. Such agreement must be maintained at the supervising physician's primary practice site, and the Department must be allowed access to such agreement at any point in time.

Supervising physician(s) or backup supervising physician(s) must notify the physician assistant of any license limitation or disciplinary action taken on the physician's license.

The supervising physician and the physician assistant must be together at any practice site 20% of the time when a physician assistant is providing medical services.

1. Calls outside the offices of the primary and secondary sites may be included in the calculation of the 20% of the time that the physician assistant and supervising physician must be together. Such calls must include but are not limited to: family planning clinics, school health, home visits, on-call time, sporting events, public health agencies, skilled nursing facilities, migrant health centers, nursing homes, and sexually transmitted disease clinics.

The time the supervising physician and physician assistant are together may not be less than 20% unless approved by the Board upon showing of good cause by the supervising physician. In determining good cause, the factors to consider include but are not limited to: the proposed practice site; percentage of time together to include time together on calls outside the offices as referenced in 172 NAC 90-006.01E; number of years of experience of physician assistant; number of years supervising physician has supervised physician assistants; any previous knowledge the supervising physician has had with the physician assistant's patient care in the community; if the site serves a state or federally designated shortage or underserved areas; and general level of patient problem complexity.

The supervising physician must obtain a physician to accept responsibility for supervision of the physician assistant whenever the supervising physician will not be readily available to the practice. A physician wishing to serve as a back-up physician must be licensed to practice medicine or osteopathic medicine and surgery in the State of Nebraska, not be prohibited by the Board from supervising a physician assistant, and be approved by the supervising physician as a person willing and qualified to assume responsibility for the care rendered by the physician assistant in the absence of the supervising physician.

A physician assistant may not practice at a secondary site without the personal presence of the supervising physician unless approval has been granted on an individual basis by the Board. Such approval must be granted when the following conditions are met:

1. The physician assistant holds a permanent license.
2. The physician assistant has practiced in Nebraska for at least 25 hours a week for a period of six weeks under the supervision of the physician who is currently approved to supervise the physician assistant and is requesting approval for such physician assistant to practice at the secondary site.
   a. The six-week time period that the supervising physician and the physician assistant must be together may be shortened if approved by the Board upon a showing of good cause by the supervising physician. In determining such good cause, the factors to consider include but are not limited to: the number of years of experience the physician assistant has practiced, the number of years of experience the supervising physician has had supervising physician assistants, type of practice setting, and the familiarity the supervising physician has with the physician assistant's patient care in the community.
3. The supervising physician makes site visits to the secondary site. Such site visits must occur at a minimum of one-half day per month. Site visits may be less if approved by the Board upon showing of good cause.
   a. In determining good cause, the factors to consider include but are not limited to; practice site hours, general level of patient problem complexity, number of years of experience by the physician assistant, number of years of experience the supervising physician has supervised physician assistants and type of practice setting. A systematic documentation of these visits must be established and maintained by the supervising physician.
4. The supervising physician, as a method of regular reporting, must review 100% of the charts of the patients seen by the physician assistant. A systematic documentation of these reviews must be established and maintained by the supervising physician.
5. The supervising physician must maintain and make available to the Department, upon request, all documentation of supervision of physician assistant activities.

The supervising physician who wishes to supervise a physician assistant in a secondary site without being physically present must submit an application to the Department, on a form provided by the Department or on an alternate format. The secondary site application may be submitted at the time of the initial application or at a later date as an addendum. The application must include the following information:

1. Name of supervising physician.
2. Name of physician assistant.
3. Name and address of medical practice.
4. Secondary site address.
   a. Street address.
   b. City/State/Zip/County.
   c. Phone number (optional).
5. Weekly practice schedule.
   a. Office hours (primary/secondary sites).
   b. Physician hours, when physician is present (primary/secondary sites).
   c. Physician assistant hours, when physician assistant is present (primary/secondary sites).
   d. Total hours of each provider at each site.
6. Will the supervising physician/designated backup physician, when acting as the supervising physician, be present at the secondary site one-half day per month during the time that the practice is open?
   a. If the supervising physician is proposing to be present at the secondary site less than one half day per month during the time the practice is open, describe:
      (1) Practice site hours.
      (2) General level of patient complexity.
      (3) Number of years of experience of the physician assistant.
      (4) Number of years of experience the supervising physician has supervising physician assistants.
      (5) Type of practice setting.
      (6) Other pertinent information.
7. Will the supervising physician/designated backup physician, when acting as the supervising physician, and the physician assistant be together 20% of the time at any site that the physician assistant is performing medical services?
   a. If the supervising physician is proposing to be present at any site less than 20% of the time when the physician assistant is performing medical services, describe:
      (1) Proposed practice site.

(2) Percentage of time together.

(3) Number of years of experience of the physician.

(4) Number of years of experience of the physician assistant.

(5) Any previous knowledge of the supervising physician has had with the physician assistant's patient care in the community.

(6) If the site serves a state or federally designated shortage or underserved area.

(7) General level of patient problem complexity.

(8) Other pertinent/relative information.

8. Will the supervising physician/designated backup physician, when acting as the supervising physician, review 100% of the patient charts?

9. Include a notarized statement by the supervising physician and the physician assistant that states that the statements on the application are true and complete.

The supervising physician may be certified to supervise only two physician assistants unless there is showing of good cause by the supervising physician. In determining such good cause, the factors to consider include, but are not limited to:

1. Group practices;

2. Temporary loss of a supervising physician;

3. Part-time employment of the physician assistant; and

4. Practicing in facilities that serve state or federally designated shortage areas or under-served areas.

If the supervision of a physician assistant is terminated by the physician or physician assistant, the supervising physician must notify the Department of such termination. A physician assistant must cease providing any medical services when the supervising physician terminates supervision unless the physician assistant is acting pursuant to another active scope of practice agreement with another supervising physician.

A physician assistant may not provide medical services when a supervising physician:

1. Is not readily available and there is no backup physician; or

2. The Certificate of Approval to Supervise has been revoked or suspended.

172 NEBRASKA CODE ANN. SEC. 90-006

NEVADA

1. The supervising physician is responsible for all the medical activities of his physician assistant. The supervising physician shall ensure that:

(a) The physician assistant is clearly identified to the patients as a physician assistant;

(b) The physician assistant performs only those medical services which have been approved by his supervising physician;

(c) The physician assistant does not represent himself in any manner which would tend to mislead the general public, the patients of the supervising physician or any other health professional; and

(d) There is strict compliance with:

    (1) The provisions of the license issued by the board to his physician assistant regarding controlled substances, poisons, dangerous drugs or devices;

    (2) The provisions of the certificate of registration issued to his physician assistant by the state board of pharmacy pursuant to NRS 639.1373; and

    (3) The regulations of the state board of pharmacy regarding controlled substances, poisons, dangerous drugs or devices.

2. Except as otherwise required in subsection 3 or 4, the supervising physician shall review and initial selected charts of the patients of the physician assistant. He shall be available at all times that his physician assistant is providing medical services, to consult with his assistant. Those consultations may be indirect, including, without limitation, by telephone.

3. At least once a month, the supervising physician shall spend part of a day at any location where the physician assistant provides medical services to act as a consultant to the physician assistant and to monitor the quality of care provided by the physician assistant.

4. If the supervising physician is unable to supervise the physician assistant as required by this section, he shall designate a qualified substitute physician, who practices medicine in the same specialty as the supervising physician, to supervise the assistant. If the substitute physician's supervision will exceed 72 hours, the supervising physician shall notify the board of the designated substitute for approval by the board.

5. A physician who supervises a physician assistant shall develop and carry out a program to ensure the quality of care provided by a physician assistant. The program must include, without limitation:

(a) An assessment of the medical competency of the physician assistant;

(b) A review and initialing of selected charts;

(c) An assessment of a representative sample of the referrals or consultations made by the physician assistant with other health professionals as required by the condition of the patient;

(d) Direct observation of the ability of the physician assistant to take a medical history from and perform an examination of patients representative of those cared for by the physician assistant; and

(e) Maintenance by the supervising physician of accurate records and documentation regarding the program for each physician assistant supervised.

6. A physician may not supervise a physician assistant unless the physician has been approved by the board and has paid the applicable fee.

NEVADA ADMIN. CODE SEC. 630.370

NEW HAMPSHIRE

Responsibility of the registered supervisory physician.

(a) The RSP or ARSP shall be available for consultation with the physician assistant and shall be responsible for assuring that appropriate directions are given to, and understood and executed by, the physician assistant.

(b) The RSP or ARSP shall not be required to be physically present while the physician assistant is providing care, so long as the RSP or ARSP and the physician assistant are or can easily be in contact with each other by radio, telephone or telecommunication.

(c) The RSP shall establish a regular, ongoing evaluation of a representative sample of patient records as part of a review of the physician assistant's performance.

(d) The RSP shall designate in writing one or more alternate supervising physicians whose scope of practice encompasses the RSP's scope of practice, and such alternates shall assume responsibility for the supervision of the physician assistant when the RSP is unavailable.

NEW HAMPSHIRE CODE ADMIN. R. ANN. (MED) SEC. 602.01

NEW JERSEY

a. A physician assistant and a temporary licensed physician assistant shall be under the direct supervision of a physician at all times during which the physician assistant or temporary licensed physician assistant is working in his official capacity.

b. In an inpatient setting, direct supervision of a physician assistant shall include, but not be limited to:

(1) continuing or intermittent presence with constant availability through electronic communications;

(2) regularly scheduled review of the practice of the physician assistant; and

(3) personal review by a physician of all charts and records of patients and countersignature by a physician of all medical orders, including prescribing and administering medication, within 24 hours of their entry by the physician assistant.

c. In an outpatient setting, direct supervision of a physician assistant shall include, but not be limited to:

(1) constant availability through electronic communications;

(2) regularly scheduled review of the practice of the physician assistant; and

(3) personal review by a physician of the charts and records of patients and countersignature by a physician of all medical orders, within seven days of their entry by the physician assistant, except that in the case of any medical order prescribing or administering medication, a physician shall review and countersign the order within 48 hours of its entry by the physician assistant.

d. In any setting, direct supervision of a temporary licensed physician assistant shall include, but not be limited to:

(1) continuing physical presence of a physician or a licensed physician assistant;

(2) regularly scheduled review by a physician of the practice of the temporary licensed physician assistant; and

(3) personal review by a physician of all charts and records of patients within 24 hours of an entry by the temporary licensed physician assistant.

NEW JERSEY STAT. ANN. SEC. 45: 9-27.18

NEW MEXICO

(A) As a condition of licensure, all physician assistants practicing in New Mexico shall inform the board of the name of the physician under whose supervision they will practice. All supervising physicians shall be licensed under the Medical Practice Act and shall be approved by the board.

B. Every licensed physician supervising a licensed physician assistant shall be individually responsible and liable for the performance of the acts and omissions delegated to the physician assistant.

Nothing in this section shall be construed to relieve the physician assistant of responsibility and liability for the acts and omissions of the physician assistant.

C. A licensed physician shall not supervise more than two physician assistants; except, where a physician is working in a health facility providing health service to the public primarily on a free or reduced fee basis, that is funded in whole or in part out of public funds or the funds of private charitable institutions or for good cause shown, the board may authorize a greater number upon a finding that the program provides adequate supervision of the physician assistants.

NEW MEXICO STAT. ANN. SEC. 61-6-10

NEW YORK

1. Notwithstanding any other provision of law, a physician assistant may perform medical services, but only when under the supervision of a physician and only when such acts and duties as are assigned to him are within the scope of practice of such supervising physician.
2. Notwithstanding any other provision of law, a specialist assistant may perform medical services, but only when under the supervision of a physician and only when such acts and duties as are assigned to him are related to the designated medical specialty for which he is registered and are within the scope of practice of his supervising physician.
3. Supervision shall be continuous but shall not be construed as necessarily requiring the physical presence of the supervising physician at the time and place where such services are performed.
4. No physician shall employ or supervise more than two physician assistants and two specialist assistants in his private practice.
5. Nothing in this article shall prohibit a hospital from employing physician assistants or specialist assistants provided they work under the supervision of a physician designated by the hospital and not beyond the scope of practice of such physician. The numerical limitation of subdivision four of this section shall not apply to services performed in a hospital.
6. Notwithstanding any other provision of this article, nothing shall prohibit a physician employed by or rendering services to the department of correctional services under contract from supervising no more than four physician assistants or specialist assistants in his practice for the department of correctional services.

7. Notwithstanding any other provision of law, a trainee in an approved program may perform medical services when such services are performed within the scope of such program.
8. Nothing in this article, or in article thirty-seven of the public health law, shall be construed to authorize physician assistants or specialist assistants to perform those specific functions and duties specifically delegated by law to those persons licensed as allied health professionals under the public health law or the education law.

NEW YORK STAT. C. L. SEC. 6542

NORTH CAROLINA

(a) A physician assistant may perform medical acts, tasks, or functions only under the supervision of a physician. Supervision shall be continuous but, except as otherwise provided in these Rules, shall not be construed as requiring the physical presence of the supervising physician at the time and place that the services are rendered.

(b) It is the obligation of each team of physician(s) and physician assistant(s) to ensure that the physician assistant's scope of practice is identified; that delegation of medical tasks is appropriate to the skills of the supervising physician(s) as well as the physician assistant's level of competence; that the relationship of, and access to, each supervising physician is defined; and that a process for evaluation of the physician assistant's performance is established. A statement describing these supervisory arrangements in all settings must be signed by each supervising physician and the physician assistant and shall be kept on file at all practice sites. This statement describing supervisory arrangements and instructions for prescriptive authority shall be available upon request by the Board or its representatives.

(c) The time interval between the physician assistant's contact with the patient and the chart review and countersigning by the supervising physician may be a maximum of seven days for outpatient (clinic/office) charts. Entries by a physician assistant into patient charts of inpatients (hospital, long term care institutions) must comply with the rules and regulations of the institution; but, at a minimum, the initial work up and treatment plan and the discharge summary must be countersigned by the supervising physician within seven days of the time of generation of these notes. In the acute inpatient setting, the initial work-up, orders, and treatment plan must be signed and dated within two working days.

21 NORTH CAROLINA ANN. CODE 32 SEC. .0110

NORTH DAKOTA

Upon undertaking the supervision of a physician assistant as contemplated by this chapter, the physician shall file with the board a copy of the contract establishing that relationship. That contract must be approved by the board of medical examiners.

The contract must be confirmed annually by completing and filing with the board such forms as are requested and provided by the board. The board must be notified within seventy-two hours of any contract termination or modification.

Every physician who supervises a physician assistant under this chapter must practice medicine in North Dakota. No physician may act as a supervising physician for any physician assistant who is a member of the physician's immediate family unless specific authorization for such supervision has been approved by the board of medical examiners. For purposes of this section, "immediate family" means a spouse, parent, child, or sibling of the supervising physician.

NORTH DAKOTA ADMIN. CODE SEC. 50-03-01-03

For the purpose of this section, "supervision" means overseeing the activities of, and accepting the responsibility for, the medical services rendered by a physician assistant. Supervision shall be continuous but shall not be construed as necessarily requiring the physical presence of the supervising physician at the time and place that the services are rendered. It is the responsibility of the supervising physician to direct and review the work, records, and practice of the physician assistant on a continuous basis to ensure that appropriate and safe treatment is rendered. The supervising physician must be available continuously for contact personally or by telephone or other electronic means. It is the obligation of each team of physicians and physician assistants to ensure that the physician assistant's scope of practice is identified; that delegation of medical tasks is appropriate to the physician assistant's level of competence; that the relationship of, and access to, the supervising physician is defined; and that a process for evaluation of the physician assistant's performance is established.

NORTH DAKOTA ADMIN. CODE SEC. 50-03-01-04

Under no circumstances shall the supervising physician designate the physician assistant to take over the physician's duties or cover the physician's practice. During any absence or temporary disability of a supervising physician, it is mandatory that the supervising physician designate a substitute physician to assume all duties and responsibilities of the supervising physician. The physician assistant, during this period, will be responsible to the substitute physician. The designation of a substitute supervising physician must be in writing; signed by the supervising physician, the substitute supervising physician, and the physician assistant; and contain the following information:

1. The name of the substitute supervising physician.
2. The period during which the substitute supervising physician will assume the duties and responsibilities of the supervising physician.
3. Any substantive change in the physician assistant's duties or responsibilities. The appointment of a substitute supervising physician does not become effective unless it is first approved by the board of medical examiners.

NORTH DAKOTA ADMIN. CODE SEC. 50-03-01-05

OHIO

(A) A supervising physician shall supervise a physician assistant within the terms, conditions, and limitations set forth in a standard or supplemental physician assistant utilization plan approved by the board, including the degree of supervision specified in that plan.

(B) As used in any standard or supplemental physician assistant utilization plan, the terms direct supervision, on-site supervision, and off-site supervision mean the following:

(1) "Direct supervision" means that the supervising physician is actually in sight of the physician assistant when the physician assistant is performing the function requiring direct supervision. Although the physician may be performing some other task at the same time, he is physically present in the same room, so that he may immediately provide direction or assume the performance of the task if difficulties arise. This does not require that the physician is watching "over the shoulder" of the physician assistant as would be required during the training period to ensure that the physician assistant is competent to perform the task. The term "immediate presence" means that direct supervision is being provided. While direct supervision would not be required for performance of tasks included on a standard utilization plan, it may be required for certain functions carrying high risks that are requested on a supplemental utilization plan.

(2) "On-site supervision" requires the physical presence of the supervising physician in the same location (e.g., the physician's office suite) as the physician assistant, but does not require his physical presence in the same room. This level of

supervision is normally required by statute for all physician assistants when new patients are being seen. It is also required by statute for all physician assistants practicing within a facility's emergency department. This level of supervision may also be appropriately required for the performance of specific functions requested through a supplemental utilization plan. If a physician states in the standard utilization plan that supervision will be on-site at all times, then he and the physician assistant must practice in accordance with that declaration.

(3) "Off-site supervision" means that the supervising physician must be continuously available for direct communication with the physician assistant and must be in a location that under normal conditions is not more than sixty minutes travel time from the physician assistant's location. Off-site supervision is appropriate for some functions included in the standard utilization plan (subject to the additional restraints of division (D) of section 4730.21 of the Revised Code), but would rarely be authorized for functions requested on supplemental utilization plans.

(C) When a supervising physician authorizes a physician assistant to practice in a facility's emergency department, the supervising physician shall provide on-site supervision of the physician assistant, unless certain services requiring direct supervision are specified in a standard or supplemental physician assistant utilization plan and approved by the board.

(D) A patient new to a physician's practice may be seen by a physician assistant only when a supervising physician is on the premises, except in those situations specified in a standard or supplemental utilization plan under which the presence of the physician is not necessary. A patient new to a physician's practice or an established patient of a physician with a new condition shall be seen and personally evaluated by a supervising physician prior to initiation of any treatment plan proposed by a physician assistant for the new patient or the established patient's new condition.

OHIO ADMIN. RULES SEC. 4731-4.03

OKLAHOMA

(A) No health care services may be performed by a physician assistant unless a current application to practice, jointly filed by the supervising physician and physician assistant, is on file with and approved by the State Board of Medical Licensure and Supervision.

The application shall include a description of the physician's practice, methods of supervising and utilizing the physician assistant, and names of alternate supervising physicians who will supervise the physician assistant in the absence of the primary supervising physician.

B. The supervising physician need not be physically present nor be specifically consulted before each delegated patient care service is performed by a physician assistant, so long as the supervising physician and physician assistant are or can be easily in contact with one another by radio, telephone or other means of telecommunication. In all patient care settings, the supervising physician shall provide appropriate methods of supervising the health care services provided by the physician assistant including:

a. being responsible for the formulation or approval of all orders and protocols, whether standing orders, direct orders or any other orders or protocols, which direct the delivery of health care services provided by a physician assistant, and periodically reviewing such orders and protocols,

b. regularly reviewing the health care services provided by the physician assistant and any problems or complications encountered,

c. being available physically or through direct telecommunications for consultation, assistance with medical emergencies or patient referral,

d. being on-site to provide medical care to patients a minimum of one-half (1/2) day per week. Additional on-site supervision may be required at the recommendation of the Physician Assistant Committee and approved by the Board; and

e. that it remains clear that the physician assistant is an agent of the supervising physician; but, in no event shall the supervising physician be an employee of the physician assistant.

C. In patients with newly diagnosed chronic or complex illnesses, the physician assistant shall contact the supervising physician within forty-eight (48) hours of the physician assistant's initial examination or treatment and schedule the patient for appropriate evaluation by the supervising physician as directed by the physician.

D. (1) A physician assistant under the direction of a supervising physician may prescribe written and oral prescriptions and orders. The physician assistant may prescribe drugs, including controlled medications in Schedules II through V pursuant to Section 2-312 of Title 63 of the Oklahoma Statutes, and medical supplies and services as delegated by the supervising physician and as approved by the State Board of Medical Licensure and Supervision after consultation with the State Board of Pharmacy on the Physician Assistant Drug Formulary.

(2) A physician assistant may write an order for a Schedule II drug for immediate or ongoing administration on site. Prescriptions and orders for Schedule II drugs written by a physician assistant must be included a written protocol determined by the supervising physician and approved by the medical staff committee of the facility or by direct verbal order of the supervising physician. Physician assistants may not dispense drugs, but may request, receive, and sign for professional samples and may distribute professional samples to patients.

E. A physician assistant may perform health care services in patient care settings as authorized by the supervising physician.

F. A physician assistant shall obtain approval from the State Board of Medical Licensure and Supervision prior to practicing in remote patient care settings. Such approval requires documented experience in providing a comprehensive range of primary care services, under the direction of a supervising physician, for at least one (1) year prior to practicing in such settings and such other requirement as the Board may require. The Board is granted the authority to waive this requirement for those applicants possessing equivalent experience and training as recommended by the Committee.

G. Each physician assistant licensed under the Physician Assistant Act shall keep his or her license available for inspection at the primary place of business and shall, when engaged in professional activities, identify himself or herself as a physician assistant.

OKLAHOMA STAT. ANN. TIT. 59 SEC. 519.6

(a) The health care services performed by a physician assistant shall be done under the supervision of a physician who retains responsibility for patient care, although the physician need not be physically present at each activity of the physician assistant nor be specifically consulted before each delegated task is performed.

(b) A physician assistant must function only under the supervision of a licensed physician. Nothing in the Physician Assistant Act shall be construed to permit physician assistants to provide health care services independent of physician supervision. Physician supervision shall be conducted in accordance with the following standards:

(1) The supervising physician is responsible for the formulation or approval of all orders and protocols (whether standing orders, direct orders, or any other orders or protocols) that

directs the delivery of health care services, and the supervising physician shall periodically review such orders and protocols.

(2) The supervising physician regularly reviews the health care services provided by the physician assistant and any problems or complications encountered.

(3) The supervising physician or alternate supervising physician is available physically or through direct telecommunications for consultation, assistance with medical emergencies or patient referral.

(4) The supervising physician or alternate supervising physician routinely is present in the facility to provide medical care to patients.

(5) In remote patient care settings, the supervising physician shall be present in the facility at least one-half day each week the facility is in operation. The Committee may recommend that the physician be present more than one-half day each week the facility is in operation based upon the training and experience of the physician assistant and other factors the Committee shall review. This shall be subject to Board review and approval.

(6) The physician assistant is an agent of the supervising physician and shall not be the employer of the supervising physician.

(c) Any waivers of this section may require personal appearance before the Committee, and the Board if so required by the Committee, by the physician assistant and the primary supervising physician to justify the request.

OKLAHOMA ADMIN. CODE SEC. 435:15-5-1

OREGON

(1) The supervising physician is responsible for the direction and regular review of the medical services provided by the physician assistant.

(2) The type of supervision and maintenance of supervision provided for each physician assistant shall be described in the practice description and approved by the Board. The supervising physician or designated agent shall provide for maintenance of verbal communication with the physician assistant at all times, whether the supervising physician and physician assistant practice in the same practice location or a practice location separate from each other, as described in the following:

(a) The practice is listed in the practice description of the physician assistant and is pre-approved by the Board.

(b) In any instance where the supervising physician or designated agent is not providing direct or personal supervision of the physician assistant as defined in OAR 847-050-0010(8)(a) and (c), the supervising physician or designated agent shall provide for the maintenance of direct, verbal communication by telephone, radio, radio telephone, television or similar means but is not required to be physically present at the practice site.

(c) The supervising physician or designated agent will provide a minimum of four hours of on-site supervision every two weeks.

(d) The supervising physician or designated agent will provide chart review of a number or a percentage of the patients the physician assistant has seen during each month as stated in the practice description as approved by the Board.

(3) The degree of independent judgment that the physician assistant may exercise shall be in accordance with the Board approved practice description and supervision. The supervising physician may limit the degree of independent judgment that the physician assistant uses but may not extend it beyond the limits of the practice description.

OREGON ADMIN. RULES SEC. 847-050-0037

PENNSYLVANIA

A primary physician assistant supervisor shall assume the following responsibilities. The supervisor shall:

(1) Monitor the compliance of all parties to the written agreement with the standards contained in the written agreement, the act and this subchapter.

(2) Advise any party to the written agreement of the failure to conform with the standards contained in the written agreement, the act and this subchapter.

(3) Arrange for a substitute physician assistant supervisor. See § 18.154 (relating to substitute physician assistant supervisor).

(4) See each patient in his office every third visit, but at least once a year.

(5) See each patient while hospitalized at least once.

(6) Provide access to the written agreement upon request and provide clarification of orders and prescriptions by the physician assistant relayed to other health care practitioners.

(7) Accept full professional and legal responsibility for the performance of the physician assistant and the care and treatment of his patients.

PENNSYLVANIA ADMIN. CODE SEC. 18.144

Osteopathic

The supervising physician shall monitor and supervise the activities of the physician assistant and review documentation prepared by the physician assistant which should include organized medical records with symptoms, pertinent physical findings, impressions and treatment plans indicated. Also the supervising physician shall provide written protocols for the use of the physician assistant in the performance of delegated tasks. These established protocols may be modified to require additional steps to be followed by the physician assistant in the performance of delegated tasks. The modifications do not require prior approval by the Board. However, an expansion of the protocol to provide for the delegation of additional services or responsibilities does require prior approval by the Board as set forth in § 25.162(c) (relating to criteria for registration as supervising physician). The established protocol shall be available for public inspection upon request and may be reviewed by the Board or its agents without prior notice.

PENNSYLVANIA OSTEO. ADMIN. CODE SEC. 25.173

RHODE ISLAND

"Supervision," pursuant to section 5-54-2 of the Act, means overseeing the activities of, and accepting the responsibility for, the medical services rendered by the physician assistants.

Supervision shall be continuous and under the direct control of a licensed physician expert in the field of medicine in which the physician assistants practice.

The constant physical presence of the supervising physician or physician designee is not required. It is the responsibility of the supervising physician and physician assistant to assure an appropriate level of supervision depending upon the services being rendered. Each physician or group of physicians, or other health care delivery organization excluding licensed hospitals or licensed health care facilities controlled or operated by a licensed hospital employing physician assistant(s), must have on file at the primary practice site a copy of a policy in the form of an agreement between the supervising physician(s) and physician assistant(s) delineating:

a) the level of supervision provided by the supervising physician(s) or designee(s) with particular reference to differing levels of supervision depending on the type of patient services provided and requirements for communication between the supervising physician(s) or designee(s) and the physician assistant.

b) a job description for the physician assistant listing patient care responsibilities and procedures to be performed by the physician assistant.

c) a program for quality assurance for physician assistant services including requirements for periodic review of the physician assistant services.

Requirements for supervision of physician assistants employed or extended medical staff privileges by licensed hospitals or other licensed health care facilities or employed by other health care delivery agencies shall be delineated by the medical staff bylaws and/or applicable governing authority of the facility. The supervising physician or physician designee must be available for easy communication and referral at all times.

RHODE ISLAND R5-54-PA-1.12

SOUTH CAROLINA

(A) The supervising physician is responsible for all aspects of the physician assistant's practice. Supervision must be continuous but must not be construed as necessarily requiring the physical presence of the supervising physician at the time and place where the services are rendered, except as otherwise required for limited licensees. The supervising physician shall identify the physician assistant's scope of practice and determine the delegation of medical tasks. All tasks must be defined in approved written guidelines which must be appropriate to the physician assistant's ability and knowledge.

(B) The supervising physician or alternate supervising physician must be physically present at least seventy-five percent of the time the physician assistant is providing services. A physician assistant must have six months' clinical experience with the current supervising physician before being permitted to practice in the absence of the supervising physician. The physician assistant may provide services in the absence of his or her supervising physician or alternate supervising physician for a period not to exceed seven consecutive days without prior written permission from the board.

(C) A physician assistant may not practice at any location more than forty-five miles or sixty minutes travel time from the supervising physician without written approval of the board. The supervising physician or alternate must review, initial, and date the charts within seventy-two hours of patients seen by the physician assistant when the supervising physician or alternate was not present at the practice site. A supervising physician may not supervise more than two physician assistants.

(D) Upon written request, and recommendation of the committee, the board may authorize exceptions to the requirements of this section.

SOUTH CAROLINA PA PRAC. ACT SEC. 40-47-955

SOUTH DAKOTA

The physician, by direct and indirect supervision, continuous monitoring, and evaluation accepts initial and continuing responsibility for
the physician assistant or assistants responsible to the physician until
such relationship is terminated. This supervision may be by personal
contact or indirect contact by telecommunication. If the office of a
physician assistant is separate from the main office of the supervising
physician, the supervision shall include at least one-half business day
per week of on-site personal supervision by a supervising physician.
A physician assistant who is issued a temporary permit pursuant to §
36-4A-8.1 shall initially receive thirty days of on-site, direct supervision by a supervising physician. Thereafter, and until expiration of the
temporary permit, the supervision shall include at least two one-half
business days per week of on-site personal supervision by a supervising physician.

SOUTH DAKOTA CODIFIED LAWS 36-4A-29

TENNESSEE

(1) The range of services which may be provided by a physician assis-
    tant shall be set forth in a written protocol, jointly developed and
    signed by the physician assistant and the supervising physician
    and maintained at the physician assistant's practice location.
(2) A physician assistant is authorized to perform the services out-
    lined in his or her protocol under the supervision of a supervising
    physician who complies with all the requirements of 0880-2-.18.
(3) Each physician assistant shall have a designated primary supervis-
    ing physician and shall notify the Committee of the name, address,
    and license number of his/her primary supervising physician and
    shall notify the Committee of any change in such primary super-
    vising physician within fifteen (15) days of the change.

RRT SEC.0880-3-10

TEXAS

(a) Supervision shall be continuous, but shall not be construed as
    necessarily requiring the constant physical presence of the super-
    vising physician at a place where physician assistant services are
    performed while the services are performed. Telecommunication
    shall always be available.
(b) It is the obligation of each team of physician(s) and physician
    assistant(s) to ensure that:

(1) the physician assistant's scope of practice is identified;
(2) delegation of medical tasks is appropriate to the physician assistant's level of competence;
(3) the relationship between the members of the team is defined;
(4) the relationship of, and access to, the supervising physician is defined;
(5) a process for evaluation of the physician assistant's performance is established; and
(6) the physician assistant's annual registration permit is current.

(c) A physician assistant may have more than one supervising physician.

(d) Physician assistants must utilize mechanisms which provide medical authority when such mechanisms are indicated, including, but not limited to, standing delegation orders, standing medical orders, protocols, or practice guidelines.

TEXAS CODE ANN. SEC. 185.14

UTAH

In accordance with Section 58-70a-501, the working relationship and delegation of duties between the supervising physician and the physician assistant are specified as follows:

(1) The supervising physician shall provide supervision to the physician assistant to adequately serve the health care needs of the practice population and ensure that the patient's health, safety and welfare will not be adversely compromised. The degree of on-site supervision shall be outlined in the Delegation of Services Agreement maintained at the site of practice. Physician assistants may authenticate with their signature any form that may be authenticated by a physician's signature.

(2) There shall be a method of immediate consultation by electronic means whenever the physician assistant is not under the direct supervision of the supervising physician.

(3) The supervising physician shall review and co-sign sufficient numbers of patient charts and medical records to ensure that the patient's health, safety, and welfare will not be adversely compromised. The Delegation of Services Agreement, maintained at the site of practice, shall outline specific parameters for review that are appropriate for the working relationship.

(4) A supervising physician shall not supervise more than two full time equivalent (FTE) physician assistants without the prior approval of the division and the board, and if patient health, safety, and welfare will not be adversely compromised.

UTAH ADMIN. CODE R58-70A-501

VERMONT

The Supervising physician shall:

(a) Supervise physician assistants only in the field(s) of medicine in which he or she is qualified and actively practices;

(b) Approve and sign the PA's scope of practice as described in Rule 7.3.

(c) Outline in detail how he or she will be available for consultation and review of work performed by the physician assistant;

(d) Supervise no more physician assistants concurrently than have been approved by the board after review of the system of care delivery;

(e) Furnish copies of the physician assistant's scope of practice to any medical facilities with which the physician assistant is affiliated or employed;

(f) Notify the board immediately in writing of termination of the physician assistants employment contract and the reason(s) for termination. Similar notification is required if the scope of practice changes, the employer(s) change, or there is a change in the primary or secondary supervising physician(s). Prior Board approval must be received. Documents already on file with the Board need not be resubmitted.

(g) Sign a statement certifying that the primary supervising physician has read the statutes and Board rules governing physician assistants.

VERMONT RULES OF THE BD. OF MED. SEC. II.7.1

Supervision shall include;

Regular and effective access to the supervising physician for consultation regarding on-going patient care while they are being treated by the PA

Regular retrospective review by the supervising physician with documentation of such review

Regularly scheduled and documented discussion of cases chosen by either the PA or the supervising physician. These may be cases which the PA handled, or cases which the supervising physician handled and believes may be instructive for the PA

Review of PA referrals outside the normal practice referral pattern as defined in the scope of practice.

Methods for in-practice consultation for patients not improving in a reasonable manner or time frame

Review of the record of services rendered the patient by the physician assistant and sign such records within 72 hours after any such care was rendered by a physician assistant

VERMONT RULES OF THE BD. OF MED. SEC. II.7.5

VIRGINIA

The supervising physician shall:

1. See and evaluate any patient who presents the same complaint twice in a single episode of care and has failed to improve significantly. Such physician involvement shall occur not less frequently than every fourth visit for a continuing illness.
2 Be responsible for all invasive procedures.
   a. Under general supervision, a physician assistant may insert a nasogastric tube, bladder catheter, needle, or peripheral intravenous catheter, but not a flow-directed catheter, and may perform minor suturing, venipuncture, and subcutaneous intramuscular or intravenous injection.
   b. All other invasive procedures not listed above must be performed under direct supervision unless, after directly supervising the performance of a specific invasive procedure three times or more, the supervising physician attests to the competence of the physician assistant to perform the specific procedure without direct supervision by certifying to the board in writing the number of times the specific procedure has been performed and that the physician assistant is competent to perform the specific procedure. After such certification has been accepted and approved by the board, the physician assistant may perform the procedure under general supervision.
3. Be responsible for all prescriptions issued by the assistant and attest to the competence of the assistant to prescribe drugs and devices.

18 VIRGINIA ADMIN. CODE SEC. 85-50-110

WASHINGTON

A physician assistant and supervising physician shall ensure that, with respect to each patient, all activities, functions, services and treatment measures are immediately and properly documented in written form by the physician assistant. Every written entry shall be reviewed and countersigned by the supervising physician within two working days unless a different time period is authorized by the commission.

It shall be the responsibility of the physician assistant and the supervising physician to ensure that adequate supervision and review of the work of the physician assistant are provided.

In the temporary absence of the supervising physician, the supervisory and review mechanisms shall be provided by a designated alternate supervisor(s).

The physician assistant, at all times when meeting or treating patients, must wear a badge identifying him or her as a physician assistant.

No physician assistant may be presented in any manner which would tend to mislead the public as to his or her title.

WASHINGTON ANN. CODE SEC. 246-918-130

WEST VIRGINIA

The physician assistant, whether employed by a health care facility or the supervising physician, shall perform only under the supervision and control of the supervising physician. Supervision and control of a physician assistant certified by the NCCPA requires the availability of a physician for consultation and direction of the actions of the physician assistant. It does not necessarily require the personal presence of the supervising physician at the place or places where services are rendered, if the physician assistant certified by the NCCPA is performing (specified) duties at the direction of the supervising physician. In the case of a physician assistant who has not been certified by the NCCPA, the presence of the supervising physician or alternate supervising physician on the premises where the noncertified assistant performs delegated medical tasks is required. The physician assistant may function in any setting within which the supervising physician routinely practices, but in no instance shall a separate place of work for the physician assistant be established. The supervising physician shall be a physician permanently licensed in this State.

WEST VIRGINIA RULES SEC. 11-1B-6

The supervising physician is responsible for observing, directing and evaluating the work, records and practices performed by the physician assistant.

The supervising physician shall notify the Board in writing of any termination of the employment of his or her physician assistant within ten (10) days of the termination.

The legal responsibility for any physician assistant remains that of his or her supervising physician at all times. Also, in temporary situations not to exceed twenty one (21) days, when a licensed and fully qualified physician is substituting for another licensed physician, the acts and omissions of the physician assistant are the legal responsibility of the absent physician assistant's designated supervising physician.

The temporary change in supervisory responsibility shall be provided to the Board in writing, within ten (10) days of the effective date of the substitution, signed by the affected supervising physicians and physician assistants, and clearly specifying the dates of substitution.

WEST VIRGINIA RULES SEC. 11-1B-9

WISCONSIN

(1) No physician may concurrently supervise more than 2 physician assistants unless the physician submits a written plan for the supervision of more than 2 physician assistants and the board approves the plan. A physician assistant may be supervised by more than one physician.

(2) Another licensed physician may be designated by the supervising physician to supervise a physician assistant for a period not to exceed 8 weeks per year. Except in an emergency, the designation shall be made in writing to the substitute supervising physician and the physician assistant. The supervising physician shall file with the board a copy of the substitution agreement before the beginning date of the period of his or her absence.

(3) The supervising physician or substitute supervising physician shall be available to the physician assistant at all times for consultation either in person or within 15 minutes of contact by telephone or by 2-way radio or television communication.

(4) A supervising physician shall visit and conduct an on-site review of facilities attended by the physician assistants at least once a month. Any patient in a location other than the location of the supervising physician's main office shall be attended personally by the physician consistent with his or her medical needs.

WISCONSIN ADMIN. CODE SEC. 8.10

WYOMING

"Supervision" means the ready availability of the supervising physician for consultation and direction of the activities of the physician assistant. Contact with the supervising physician by telecommunications is sufficient to show ready availability, if the board finds that such contact is sufficient to provide quality medical care;

WYOMING STAT. ANN. SEC. 33-26-501

Sample Written Agreements

SAMPLE WRITTEN AGREEMENT #1

PRIMARY CARE PRACTICE

JOB SUMMARY: The Physician Assistant shall augment the physician's data gathering abilities and assist the supervising physician in reaching decisions and instituting care plans for the physician's patients.

RESPONSIBILITY: The PA shall have the knowledge and competency to perform the following functions:

CLINICALLY:
1. Screen patients to determine need for physician attention.
2. Review patient records to determine health status.
3. Take a patient history.
4. Perform a physical examination.
5. Perform developmental screening exams on children.
6. Record pertinent patient data.
7. Make decisions regarding data gathering and appropriate management and treatment for the initial evaluation of a problem or the follow-up of a previously diagnosed condition.
8. Prepare patient summaries.
9. Initiate requests for commonly performed laboratory and radiographic studies.
10. Collect specimens for and carry out commonly performed analysis and office cultures.
11. Identify normal and abnormal findings on history, physical examination, and commonly performed laboratory and radiographic studies.
12. Initiate appropriate evaluation and emergency management for emergency situations, for example: cardiac arrest.

13. Perform clinical procedures such as:
   (A) Venipuncture
   B. Intradermal Test
   C. Electrocardiogram
   D. Care and Suturing of Minor Lacerations
   E. Casting and Splinting
   F. Pulmonary Function Screening Tests
   G. Allergy Testing
   H. Control of Hemorrhage
   I. Application of Dressing and Bandages
   J. Removal of Superficial Foreign Bodies
   K. Removal of Dermatologic Abnormalities
   L. Cardiopulmonary Resuscitation, Adult and Infant
   M. Audiometric Screening
   N. Visual Screening
   O. Carrying Out Aseptic and Isolation Techniques
   P. Insertion of IUD

14. Provide counseling and instruction regarding common patient problems.

15. Assist in monitoring obstetrical patients prenatally and during labor and delivery. Evaluation, monitoring, and caring for the newborn including resuscitation.

16. The PA may function as an assistant in the operating room.

17. The PA may execute and relay those medical regimens as dictated by the supervising physician and/or described in this work agreement.

ADMINISTRATIVELY:

1. Maintain journal article file.

2. Coordinate school health and preparticipation athletic physicals with all related groups.

3. Participate in decisions concerning daily operations.

4. Evaluate flow sheets including immunization records and pediatric development charts.

5. Participate in professional activities which will advance the PA profession on a local, state, and federal level.

6. Participate in all required continuing medical education activities to maintain national certification.

7. Provide other services as directed by the primary supervising physician.

Primary supervision will be performed in the office, hospital or off-site settings by the employer, Dr. A, with personal contact on a nearly daily basis. For those absences longer than three days, alternate supervision will be performed by the substitute physician assistant supervisors who meet all requirements of chart review and have personal contact with the PA at least weekly. Problem cases and those of educational interest will be discussed daily. Immediate access via telecommunications is always available.

List office and hospital addresses.

Other related practice sites: Local school districts, fire companies, sport facilities, and in patients homes due to health, transportation, or convenience reasons as an extension of office, school, or in the hospital.

List names of all substitute physician supervisors.

AFFIRMATION: This written agreement has been read and understood by those signed below. Utilization of the physician assistant is based upon this document, the Medical Practice Act, institutional privileges, and the clinical judgments of the physician assistant and the supervising physician based on the welfare of the patient.

Sample provided by the Pennsylvania Society of Physician Assistants

SAMPLE WRITTEN AGREEMENT #2

Physician Assistant

WRITTEN AGREEMENT

1. Function/Tasks
   a. The above named Physician Assistant will perform and record history and physical examinations in both the inpatient and outpatient setting. This will include both initial evaluations and follow-up visits. Findings not within normal limits shall be reported to the Supervising or substitute Supervising Physician as soon as possible, but not later than 12 hours.
   b. The Physician Assistant will record history and physicals, consultations and progress notes in the patients' charts. All history and physical findings will be reviewed directly by the Supervising Physician prior to any major diagnostic intervention outside the normal scope of practice of a physician assistant, or within 24 hours, but not later than 24 hours. The Supervising Physician will directly confirm all history and physical findings on new patients at the time they are seen. Any abnormal findings or significant changes in patients on follow-up examinations will be reported directly to the Supervising Physician at the time they are noted.
   c. All hospital inpatients will be seen by the Supervising Physician on the same working day. All notes on inpatient charts will be countersigned by the Supervising Physician, usually on the same working day and always within 24 hours.
   d. Initial diagnostic workup and treatment plans will be formulated jointly and will be reviewed directly by the Supervising Physician prior to implementation. In the absence of the Supervising Physician, patient emergencies deemed to be life threatening may be treated pursuant to State Regulations regarding treatment and prescribing by Physician Assistants and thereby accepted ACLS/BCLS protocols while the Supervising Physician is being contacted. He/she will perform CPR when appropriate in accordance with American Heart Association guidelines. He/she will operate Doppler measuring equipment for measurement of blood pressure according to protocol.
   e. The Physician Assistant will dictate histories and physicals, including treatment plans, consults, discharge summaries, letters to referring physicians, and procedure reports in accordance with Medical Center guidelines. The content of all of these will be reviewed by the Supervising Physician prior to dictation. All dictated notes will be reviewed and countersigned by the

Supervising Physician when they become available from transcription.

f. The Physician Assistant will coordinate care for patients admitted to the hospital or seen in consultation in the hospital, including patients admitted for all procedures. This will include:

1. Assuring that an appropriate history and physical examination is on the chart.

2. Ordering appropriate diagnostic studies and assuring that the results are available on the chart and are within normal limits per procedure. All abnormalities will be reported directly to the Supervising Physician prior to the procedure.

3. The Physician Assistant will assist in scheduling the timing of patients procedures with the appropriate area of the hospital.

4. The Physician Assistant will assure that appropriate patient education occurs both pre- and postprocedure.

5. The Physician Assistant will coordinate obtaining appropriate follow-up, consultations, and postprocedure examinations.

6. He/she will coordinate hospitalization of patients admitted for cardiac catheterization, pacemaker or automatic implantable defibrillator (AICD) insertion, Tilt Table testing or invasive electrophysiologic (EPS) testing, also including postcatheterization orders and review of discharge instructions with patients.

7. He/she will check on patients' postoperative or postcatheterization status and record appropriate vital signs and physical findings. Any abnormalities will be reported to the Supervising Physician or Substitute Supervising Physician as soon as possible.

g. He/she will write orders for medications under the direction of the Supervising Physician or Substitute Supervising Physician within hospital pharmacy dosing guidelines. (See Attachment A.)

Frequent contact throughout the day between the physician(s) and the physician assistant will occur. It is expected that daily review of the notes and orders by the physician assistant will occur.

h. Informed Consent for each procedure will be obtained directly by the Supervising Physician.

i. Medications and diagnostic agents will be prescribed by the Physician Assistant in accordance with applicable State law. All new prescriptions for outpatients and any changes in chronically prescribed medications for outpatients other than substitution of "therapeutically" equivalent drugs will be confirmed with the Supervising Physician prior to implementation.

j. Initiate routine orders such as laboratory, X-ray studies, and consultations which will be written as indicated or requested by the Supervising Physician or Substitute Supervising Physician. These will include but may not be limited to:

1. Ultrasound and Doppler study
2. Chest X-ray
3. Abdominal X-rays
4. X-rays of any suspected fracture site
5. Stress testing
6. Cultures and antibiotic sensitivities
7. Vital signs
8. Laxative of choice
9. Pulmonary function studies
10. Medication blood levels
11. CBC
12. Urinalysis
13. Coagulation studies
14. Chemistry profiles
15. Electrocardiograms and signal-averaged electrocardiograms
16. Activity orders
17. Arterial blood gases
18. Diet orders
19. Blood glucose monitoring
20. Foley catheterization
21. Ordering of medications taken at home

All orders written in inpatient charts will be reviewed and counter-signed by the Supervising Physician within 24 hours.

j. Appropriate postprocedure wound management will be performed by the Physician Assistant including:

1. Appropriate monitoring of the wound itself
2. Appropriate monitoring the patient's vital signs and heart rhythm
3. Removal of vascular sheaths and indwelling catheters under the Supervising Physician's supervision
4. Removal of sutures and staples
5. Obtaining cultures and sensitivity specimens if indicated
6. Any abnormalities or wound-related complications will be reported immediately to the Supervising Physician.

k. Performance of certain diagnostic procedures such as, but not limited to, heart rhythm monitoring, exercise stress testing, pacemaker monitoring and programming, monitoring of therapeutic agents such as anticoagulants. These procedures will only be delegated to the Physician Assistant after appropriate education has been obtained and the Physician Assistant has shown with sufficient proficiency in each individual area. All abnormal or questionable findings will be reviewed by the Supervising Physician prior to release of the patient and all recordings and results will be reviewed by the Supervising Physician prior to generation of any final reports.

2. Time, Place, and Manner of Supervision

It is anticipated that the Physician Assistant and Supervising Physician will jointly admit patients in the morning prior to the scheduled start times in the Laboratory. Admission, H & Ps will be dictated, and admission orders will be generated.

During the course of time that the Physician is in the Laboratory of Medical Center performing procedures and/or while in the adjacent offices seeing out-patients, the Physician Assistant will have various delegated responsibilities including admissions of Inpatients, rounds, and/or providing initial contact on consultations with subsequent evaluation of ongoing patient problems and required therapeutic interventions.

These patients will be discussed by telephone and/or in person while the Physician is in either the Laboratory or the office seeing patients and later that day seen by myself, preferably jointly with the Physician Assistant after completion of Laboratory Procedure(s) and/or scheduled office hours.

It is anticipated that the Physician and the Physician Assistant would round in the early evening after completion of the Laboratory hours or the office. Very close telephone contact and a minimum of several times daily personal contact between the Physician and Physician Assistant are anticipated.

All therapeutic interventions will be discussed with the Physician by the Physician Assistant.

PRESCRIBING/DISPENSING DRUGS BY PA

Appendix A

List of medications from which Physician Assistant is likely to prescribe under supervision.

1. Aspirin
2. Persantine
3. Coumadin
4. Heparin
5. Ticlopidine

Analgesics

1. Tylenol—extra strength or with Codeine
2. Darvocet N 100

Antacids

1. Riopan
2. Mylanta
3. Maalox
4. Mylicon
5. Amphojel

Antiemetics

1. Compazine
2. Tigan
3. Reglan
4. Phenergan
5. Etc.

Nonsteroidal anti-inflammatory agents

1. Anaprox
2. Motrin
3. Naprosyn
4. Relafen
5. Toradol

Hematinics

1. Ferrous Sulfate

Antibiotics

1. First-generation cephalosporins
2. Erythromycin and derivatives
3. Biaxin
4. Zithromax
5. Penicillin, Augmentin
6. Sulfonamides, such as Bactrim
7. Tetracycline's and derivatives

Anticholinergics

1. Levsinex

Antihistamines

1. Benadryl
2. Dimetapp
3. Phenergan
4. Allegra

Antihypertensive Medications*

1. Beta blockers
2. Calcium channel blockers
3. Ace inhibitors
4. Alpha amid beta adrenergic blockers
5. Angiotensin II receptor antagonist
6. Vasodilators

*Under especially close physician supervision with discussion of same.

Antiasthmatic Medications

1. Asthmacort
2. Beconase
3. Alupent
4. Vanceril
5. Beclovent
6. Atrovent

Antilipemic

1. Lopid
2. Mevacor
3. Zocor
4. Pravachol
5. Lescol
6. Nicobid
7. Tricor

Antiarrhythmics

1. Lidocaine
2. Mexitil
3. Norpace
4. Quinidine
5. Procainamide
6. Flecainide*
7. Ethmozine*
8. Propafenone* (Rythmol)
9. Amiodarone*
10. Sotalol*
11. Dilantin
12. Lanoxim

* Only after preliminary close discussion with physician.

Antidiarrheals

1. Imodium

Antidotes

1. Digibind*

*Only after direct preliminary discussion with physician.

Laxatives

1. Milk of Magnesia
2. Cascara
3. Dulcolax
4. Metamucil
5. Fleets Enema

Premedications

1. Versed*
2. Atropine
3. Benadryl
4. Valium*

*Only after direct discussion with physician.

Sedatives

1. Restoril
2. Ambien
3. Ativan
4. Xanax
5. Benadryl

Antianginals

1. Beta blockers
2. Calcium channel blockers
3. Nitrates (oral, topical, and intravenous)

Diuretics

1. Dyazide
2. Maxide
3. Bumex
4. Lasix
5. Aldactone

Antitussives

1. Phenergan DM
2. Robitussin DM

Decongestants

1. Entex
2. Humibid

Topical Agents

1. 1% Hydrocortisone cream
2. Silvadene cream

Supplements

1. Potassium
2. Magnesium
3. Iron
4. Vitamins

Electrolyte Agents

1. Florinef

Antidysautonoimic Agents

1. Florinef
2. Pro-Amatine* (Midodrine)
3. Norpace
4. Beta blockers
5. Ritalin*
6. Effexor
7. Zoloft

*Only after direct preliminary discussion with physician.

Enteral Therapeutic Agents*

1. Ensure
2. Ensure Plus
3. Pulmocare
4. Jevity
5. Osmolite

*Only after direct preliminary discussion with physician.

Topical Anti-Infectives

1. Neosporin

Antipsychotic Medication*

1. Haldol

*Only after direct preliminary discussion with physician.

Limited Hormone Preparations and Synthetic Substitutes

1. Synthroid

SAMPLE WRITTEN AGREEMENT #3

WRITTEN AGREEMENT

PRIMARY PHYSICIAN ASSISTANT SUPERVISOR

PHYSICIAN ASSISTANT

INSTRUCTIONS: Please provide the following information for questions 1 and 2 on 8 1/2 x 11 sheets and attach to this form. Number each section on the attachment. The information on this agreement must be identical for all supervisors listed on page 2.

1. Describe the functions/tasks to be delegated to the physician assistant, including the manner in which the physician assistant will be assisting each named physician, instructions for the use of the physician assistant in the performance of delegated functions/tasks and medical regimens to be administered or relayed by the physician assistant.

2. Describe the time, place, and manner of supervision and direction you will provide the physician assistant, including the frequency of personal contact with the physician assistant.

3. Identify the location and practice setting (i.e., hospital, private practice, group practice, etc.) where the physician assistant will serve.

4. Is/are the name(s) of physician(s) who is/are willing to act as a substitute physician assistant supervisor in your absence listed on page 2 of this application?

Yes _____ No_____

5. Will the physician assistant prescribe and dispense drugs?

Yes _____ No_____

If yes, will Schedule III, IV, and/or V controlled substances be prescribed and dispensed? Yes _____ No_____ (Note: Physician assistants are not permitted to prescribe Schedule I and II controlled substances.)

PHYSICIAN ASSISTANT PRACTICE GUIDELINES AND PHYSICIAN AGREEMENTS

The following paragraphs describe the Practice Guidelines for Physician Assistants employed by XYZ Associates. These guidelines include all requirements for the practice as a Physician Assistant in the State of (   ) as regulated by the (   ) State Board of Medicine. In addition, specific practice protocols developed by Supervising Physicians and employed Physician Assistants of XYZ Associates are also outlined. These practice protocols may be more restrictive than the State Regulations for Physician Assistant practice, but under no circumstances shall they be less restrictive than the (   ) State Board of Medicine allows.

REQUIREMENTS FOR EMPLOYMENT AS A PHYSICIAN ASSISTANT WITH XYZ ASSOCIATES

Physician Assistants employed by XYZ Associates must be certified by the National Commission for the Certification of Physician Assistants (NCCPA) and maintain documentation of valid current certification. In order to maintain current National Certification the PA must earn 100 hours of Continuing Medical Education (CME) every 2 years, with at least 50 hours in American Medical Association Category I or the equivalent. The documentation of CME hours earned is to be maintained as part of the PA practice site record.

Employed Physician Assistants must hold a current Certificate of Approval from the (   ) State Board of Medicine. All related materials are to be maintained at the practice site for easy reference and availability to the (   ) State Board of Medicine and other appropriate authorities overseeing the practice and employment of Physician Assistants.

SCOPE OF PRACTICE

The Physician Assistant employed by XYZ Associates may be asked to perform duties at several practice sites and must apply and be approved for privileges at these particular sites. In no instance shall a PA employed by XYZ Associates practice in or at sites other than those approved by the Supervising Physicians. If a PA is also employed by another practice, this must be made known to XYZ Associates and the name of the Supervising Physician(s) in that practice must be divulged. Physician Assistants employed by XYZ Associates will generally be responsible for attending daily rounds, writing daily progress notes, performing admission histories and physical examinations, and dictating Admission and Discharge Summaries. PAs would also be expected to notify the Supervising Physician of any acute change in a patient's status and carry out instructions for the care and disposition of such patient. Routine duties would also include ordering medications and diagnostic tests, developing treatment plans with review of laboratory data and diagnostic testing, and recording these in the patient's medical record. The PA is also expected to participate in team conferences and interact with other team members, patients, family members, as well as other persons deemed appropriate to the care of the patients

The Supervising Physician may ask the PA to perform other duties as needed in carrying out the responsibilities of his/her practice. In no instance will the Physician Assistant be asked to perform tasks that are beyond the scope of practice that the Physician Assistant has been trained in or is uncomfortable in performing without training.

Medical records, including progress notes and "Physician's Orders," are to be countersigned by the Supervising Physician within a time frame of not greater than 7 days from the time they are written by the PA. A Supervising Physician will always be available by pager within 30 minutes for consultation and recommendations regarding patient care.

PRESCRIBING PRIVILEGES

Physician Assistants employed by XYZ Associates may write orders for medications in patients' charts in all covered practice locations. Medication orders are reviewed and countersigned by the Supervising Physicians on at least a weekly basis. Written prescriptions may be issued by Physician Assistants to patients discharged from the practice settings. These medications are limited to those previously approved by the physician, or their equivalent. Most written prescriptions are limited to a 1 month supply with 1 (one) refill.

Prescriptions for controlled substances are limited to those medications previously approved by the Supervising Physician. Only Physician Assistants who have a current DEA number and abide by the following requirements set by the (   ) State Board of Medicine may prescribe controlled substances. The following documentation will be on file at the practice site:

(1) A statement signed by the PA and Supervising Physician that each has read and understands the DEA Mid-Level Practitioner Manual. A copy of the DEA Mid-Level Practitioner Manual will be maintained on file. A copy of the PA's DEA # and approval form will also be maintained in this file.

(2) Documentation of a least 3 hours of CME every 2 years regarding the Medical and the Social Effects of Misuse and Abuse of Alcohol, Nicotine, Prescription Drugs (to include Controlled Substances) and Illicit Drugs. PAs will maintain a file of all certificates indicating completion of such training.

CHAPTER 3

Maintaining Certification and Licensure

Maintaining NCCPA Certification • Continuing Medical Education • Recertification Examination • Regaining Certification • Unprofessional Conduct • Discipline and Sanctions • **Appendix 3A** State-by-State License Requirements • **Appendix 3B** State-by-State Temporary License Requirements • **Appendix 3C** State-by-State Continuing Medical Education Requirements

A physician assistant (PA) must be licensed, certified, or registered by the state prior to beginning to practice. All states require that a PA pass the national certification exam, administered by the NCCPA. Only graduates from an accredited PA program are eligible to sit for the Physician Assistant National Certification Exam (PANCE). The majority of states have statutory or regulatory provisions that allow graduates of accredited PA programs to obtain temporary licensure. (See Appendix 3-B.) PAs can practice under a temporary license until they receive their exam scores. Upon passing PANCE, a PA is issued NCCPA certification and the PA should immediately apply for state licensure. If a PA does not sit for the exam or does not obtain a passing score, the temporary state licensure is revoked and the PA can no longer practice.

MAINTAINING NCCPA CERTIFICATION[1]

After obtaining initial certification from the NCCPA a PA is eligible to use the initials *PA-C*. A PA enters into a 6-year certification maintenance cycle. Every 2 years, a physician assistant must log 100 hours of continuing medical education with the NCCPA. By the end of the 6-year cycle, a physician assistant must pass a recertification exam.

CONTINUING MEDICAL EDUCATION

Continuing medical education (CME) means clinical or professional educational activities that increase the knowledge and skills that a physician assistant uses in his or her day-to-day professional activities and patient care.

Continuing medical education credits must be earned by June 30 of the calendar year in which the PA's certification expires. Each PA must earn a total of 100 hours of continuing medical education during each 2-year cycle. Of the 100 hours of CME credits, half must be Category I (preapproved by one of several sponsoring organizations) and the others may be Category II (elective). Acceptable CME sponsors for Category I credits include the American Academy of Physician Assistants (AAPA), the American Medical Association (AMA), the American Osteopathic Association on Continuing Medical Education (AOACME), the American Academy of Family Physicians (AAFP), and Category I CME credits for the Physician's Recognition Award (PRA) from the organizations accredited by the Accreditation Council on Continuing Medical Education (ACCME).

The remaining 50 CME credits can be Category II (elective). Acceptable Category II activities include any medical program that has not been approved as Category I CME, any self-learning activity (for example, reading journals or medical texts or precepting students), or any medically related postgraduate course excluding those taken in the PA program. Category II hours are recorded on an hourly basis.

There are no minimum requirements for professional educational activities. Any nonclinical educational activity that can be related to the PA profession is considered professional education. Some examples of professional education include educational programs on reimbursement for services, privacy issues, medical malpractice issues, managed-care topics, PA legislative issues, faculty development, and the use of electronic charting.

The 100 hours of CME must be logged by September 30 of the year in which the PA's certification expires in order to avoid a late processing fee. All CME must be logged by December 31 in order to avoid a lapse in certification. It is important to keep original documentation of all attendance at Category I CME activities. This documentation will be required in the event of an audit of CME activities by the NCCPA.

RECERTIFICATION EXAMINATION

By the end of the 6-year certification maintenance cycle, a PA must also pass a recertification examination. A PA may choose to sit for the traditional Physician Assistants National Recertification Exam (PANRE) or elect to take the Pathway II examination. The PANRE is a multiple-choice exam designed to assess general medical and surgical knowledge and is offered at testing centers throughout the United States. The Pathway II exam is a take-home exam in which PAs are allowed to utilize medical texts in order to answer the multiple-choice questions.

In order to be eligible for the Pathway II exam applicants must have earned an additional 100 hours of CME over the past 6-year period in addition to the 100 hours of CME required every 2 years to maintain certification. An applicant for the Pathway II exam must have earned a total of 400 CME credits in the 6-year cycle. The additional 100 hours of CME can be earned in one of nine categories:

- Clinical Category I (preapproved) CME credits that were not part of the 300 required credits (50-point maximum)
- Clinical skills training (50-point maximum)
- Medical teaching (50-point maximum)
- Publications (40-point maximum)
- Postgraduate courses (40-point maximum)
- Professionally relevant postgraduate degree (50-point maximum)
- NCCPA's surgery exam (25-point maximum)
- Self-assessments and specialty review (40-point maximum)
- Other clinically relevant activities not included in the above list (point value is determined on a case-by-case basis)[1]

The recertification exam can be taken in the fifth or sixth year of the maintenance cycle. If a PA does not pass the exam by the end of the sixth year, he or she will lose certification. In order to regain certification the PA will have to pass the PANCE.

Following the completion of the CME logging requirements and the passage of the recertification exam, the certification maintenance cycle begins again.

REGAINING CERTIFICATION

If a PA fails to earn 100 hours of CME credit during any 2-year period or fails to pass the recertification exam, the only way to regain certification is to pass an exam.

Failure to log CME credits in a timely fashion or failure to pay the appropriate fees to NCCPA will also result in loss of certification. For loss of certification for an administrative reason, a PA can file paperwork and pay an additional fee to NCCPA within 6 months of the due date for the original paperwork and/or fee and regain certification without being required to take an exam. Once all the paperwork and fees have been paid, a new certificate will be issued. However, this will not remedy the lapse of certification.

A PA who loses certification cannot work in most states until it is regained because he or she would no longer meet state licensure requirements.

UNPROFESSIONAL CONDUCT

A state can refuse to grant a license or can revoke a previously issued license if a PA engages in unprofessional conduct. I have included a representative example below.

Colorado's statute states that:

(1) The board may refrain from issuing a license or may grant a license

subject to terms of probation if the board determines that an applicant for a license:

    (a) Does not possess the qualifications required by this article;

    (b) Has engaged in unprofessional conduct, as defined in section 12-36-117;

    (c) Has been disciplined in another state or foreign jurisdiction with respect to his or her license to practice medicine or license to practice as a physician assistant; or

    (d) Has not actively practiced medicine or practiced as a physician assistant for the two-year period immediately preceding the filing of such application or otherwise maintained continued competency during such period, as determined by the board.

(2) For purposes of this section, *discipline* includes any matter that must be reported pursuant to 45 CFR 60.8 and is substantially similar to unprofessional conduct, as defined in section 12-36-117.

(3) An applicant whose application is denied or whose license is granted subject to terms of probation may seek review pursuant to section 24-4-104 (9), C.R.S.; except that, if an applicant accepts a license that is subject to terms of probation, such acceptance shall be in lieu of and not in addition to the remedies set forth in section 24-4-104 (9), C.R.S.

C.R.S. SEC. 12-36-116.

Colorado defines *unprofessional conduct* as:

(1) *Unprofessional conduct* as used in this article means:

    (a) Resorting to fraud, misrepresentation, or deception in applying for, securing, renewing, or seeking reinstatement of a license to practice medicine or a license to practice as a physician assistant in this state or any other state, in applying for professional liability coverage, required pursuant to section 13-64-301, C.R.S., or privileges at a hospital, or in taking the examination provided for in this article;

    (b) Procuring, or aiding or abetting in procuring, criminal abortion;

    (c) to (e) Repealed.

    (f) Any conviction of an offense of moral turpitude, a felony, or a crime that would constitute a violation of this article. For purposes of this paragraph (f), *conviction* includes the entry of a plea of guilty or nolo contendere or the imposition of a deferred sentence.

    (g) Administering, dispensing, or prescribing any habit-forming drug, as defined in section 12-22-102 (13), or any controlled substance, as defined in section 12-22-303 (7), other than in the course of legitimate professional practice;

(h) Any conviction of violation of any federal or state law regulating the possession, distribution, or use of any controlled substance, as defined in section 12-22-303 (7), and, in determining if a license should be denied, revoked, or suspended, or if the licensee should be placed on probation, the board shall be governed by section 24-5-101, C.R.S. For purposes of this paragraph (h), *conviction* includes the entry of a plea of guilty or nolo contendere or the imposition of a deferred sentence.

(i) Habitual intemperance or excessive use of any habit-forming drug, as defined in section 12-22-102 (13), or any controlled substance, as defined in section 12-22-303 (7);

(j) Repealed.

(k) The aiding or abetting, in the practice of medicine, of any person not licensed to practice medicine as defined under this article or of any person whose license to practice medicine is suspended;

(l) Repealed.

(m) (I) Except as otherwise provided in section 25-3-103.7 and section 25-3-314, C.R.S., practicing medicine as the partner, agent, or employee of, or in joint adventure with, any person who does not hold a license to practice medicine within this state, or practicing medicine as an employee of, or in joint adventure with, any partnership or association any of whose partners or associates do not hold a license to practice medicine within this state, or practicing medicine as an employee of or in joint adventure with any corporation other than a professional service corporation for the practice of medicine as described in section 12-36-134. Any licensee holding a license to practice medicine in this state may accept employment from any person, partnership, association, or corporation to examine and treat the employees of such person, partnership, association, or corporation.

(II) (A) Nothing in this paragraph (m) shall be construed to permit a professional services corporation for the practice of medicine, as described in section 12-36-134, to practice medicine.

(B) Nothing in this paragraph (m) shall be construed to otherwise create an exception to the corporate practice of medicine doctrine.

(n) Violating, or attempting to violate, directly or indirectly, or assisting in or abetting the violation of or conspiring to violate any provision or term of this article;

(o) Such physical or mental disability as to render the licensee unable to perform medical services with reasonable skill and with safety to the patient;

(p) Any act or omission which fails to meet generally accepted standards of medical practice;

(q) Repealed.

(r) Engaging in a sexual act with a patient during the course of patient care or within six months immediately following the termination of the licensee's professional relationship with the patient. *Sexual act*, as used in this paragraph (r), means sexual contact, sexual intrusion, or sexual penetration as defined in section 18-3-401, C.R.S.

(s) Refusal of an attending physician to comply with the terms of a declaration executed by a patient pursuant to the provisions of article 18 of title 15, C.R.S., and failure of the attending physician to transfer care of said patient to another physician;

(t) (I) Violation of abuse of health insurance pursuant to section 18-13-119, C.R.S.; or

(II) Advertising through newspapers, magazines, circulars, direct mail, directories, radio, television, or otherwise that the licensee will perform any act prohibited by section 18-13-119 (3), C.R.S.;

(u) Violation of any valid board order or any rule or regulation promulgated by the board in conformance with law;

(v) Dispensing, injecting, or prescribing an anabolic steroid as defined in section 18-18-102 (3), C.R.S., for the purpose of the hormonal manipulation that is intended to increase muscle mass, strength, or weight without a medical necessity to do so or for the intended purpose of improving performance in any form of exercise, sport, or game;

(w) Dispensing or injecting an anabolic steroid as defined in section 18-18-102 (3), C.R.S., unless such anabolic steroid is dispensed from a pharmacy prescription drug outlet pursuant to a prescription order or is dispensed by any practitioner in the course of his professional practice;

(x) Prescribing, distributing, or giving to a family member or to oneself except on an emergency basis any controlled substance as defined in section 18-18-204, C.R.S., or as contained in schedule II of 21 U.S.C. sec. 812, as amended;

(y) Failing to report to the board any adverse action taken against the licensee by another licensing agency in another state or country, any peer review body, any health care institution, any professional or medical society or association, any governmental agency, any law enforcement agency, or any court for acts or conduct that would constitute grounds for action as described in this article;

(z) Failing to report to the board the surrender of a license or other authorization to practice medicine in another state or jurisdiction or the surrender of membership on any medical staff or in any medical or professional association or society while under investigation by any of those authorities or bodies for acts or conduct similar to acts or conduct that would constitute grounds for action as defined in this article;

(aa) Failing to accurately answer the questionnaire accompanying the renewal form as required pursuant to section 12-36-123 (1) (b);

(bb) (I) Engaging in any of the following activities and practices: Willful and repeated ordering or performance, without clinical justification, of demonstrably unnecessary laboratory tests or studies; the administration, without clinical justification, of treatment which is demonstrably unnecessary; the failure to obtain consultations or perform referrals when failing to do so is not consistent with the standard of care for the profession; or ordering or performing, without clinical justification, any service, X-ray, or treatment which is contrary to recognized standards of the practice of medicine as interpreted by the board.

(II) In determining which activities and practices are not consistent with the standard of care or are contrary to recognized standards of the practice of medicine, the board of medical examiners shall utilize, in addition to its own expertise, the standards developed by recognized and established accreditation or review organizations which organizations meet requirements established by the board by rule and regulation. Such determinations shall include but not be limited to appropriate ordering of laboratory tests and studies, appropriate ordering of diagnostic tests and studies, appropriate treatment of the medical condition under review, appropriate use of consultations or referrals in patient care, and appropriate creation and maintenance of patient records.

(cc) Falsifying or repeatedly making incorrect essential entries or repeatedly failing to make essential entries on patient records;

(dd) Committing a fraudulent insurance act, as defined in section 10-1-128, C.R.S.;

(ee) Failing to establish and continuously maintain financial responsibility, as required in section 13-64-301, C.R.S.;

(ff) Any violation of the provisions of section 12-36-202 or any rule or regulation of the board adopted pursuant to that section;

(gg) Failing to respond in an honest, materially responsive, and timely manner to a complaint issued pursuant to section 12-36-118 (4);

(hh) Advertising in a manner that is misleading, deceptive, or false;

(ii) Entering into or continuing a collaborative agreement pursuant to sections 12-38-111.6 (4) (d) (IV) and 12-36-106.3 that fails to meet generally acceptable standards of medical practice.

(jj) Any act or omission in the practice of telemedicine that fails to meet generally accepted standards of medical practice.

(1.5) (a) A licensee shall not be subject to disciplinary action by the board solely for prescribing controlled substances for the relief of intractable pain.

(b) For the purposes of this subsection (1.5), *intractable pain* means a pain state in which the cause of the pain cannot be removed and which in the generally accepted course of medical practice no relief or cure of the cause of the pain is possible or none has been found after reasonable efforts including, but not limited to, evaluation by the attending physician and one or more physicians specializing in the treatment of the area, system, or organ of the body perceived as the source of the pain.

(2) The discipline of a license to practice medicine or of a license to practice as a physician assistant in another state, territory, or country shall be deemed to be unprofessional conduct. For purposes of this subsection (2), discipline includes any sanction required to be reported pursuant to 45 CFR 60.8. This subsection (2) shall apply only to discipline that is based upon an act or omission in such other state, territory, or country that is defined substantially the same as unprofessional conduct pursuant to subsection (1) of this section.

(3) (a) For purposes of this section, *alternative medicine* means those health care methods of diagnosis, treatment, or healing that are not generally used but that provide a reasonable potential for therapeutic gain in a patient's medical condition that is not outweighed by the risk of such methods. A licensee who practices alternative

medicine shall inform each patient in writing, during the initial patient contact, of such licensee's education, experience, and credentials related to the alternative medicine practiced by such licensee. The board shall not take disciplinary action against a licensee solely on the grounds that such licensee practices alternative medicine.

(b) Nothing in paragraph (a) of this subsection (3) shall. be construed to prevent disciplinary action against a licensee for practicing medicine or practicing as a physician assistant in violation of this article.

C.R.S. SEC. 12-36-117.

DISCIPLINE AND SANCTIONS

A PA who does not maintain certification may be disciplined. Sanctions include administrative fines of up to $10,000 in some states for violating board rules, revocation of licensure, injunctions, misdemeanor violations, and possible jail sentences. I have included several representative examples below.

Alabama

Alabama will discipline a PA's license under the following circumstances:

After notice and hearing, the Board, within its discretion, shall suspend, revoke, place on probation or otherwise discipline the license of a physician assistant who is found guilty on the basis of substantial evidence of any of the following acts or offenses:

(1) Conviction of a felony;

(2) Conviction of any crime or other offense, felony or misdemeanor, reflecting on the ability of the individual to render patient care in a safe manner;

(3) Conviction of any violation of state or federal laws relating to controlled substances;

(4) Termination, restriction, suspension, revocation, or curtailment of licensure, registration or certification by another state or other licensing jurisdiction on grounds similar to those stated in these rules;

(5) The denial of a registration, a certification, or a license to practice by another state or other licensing jurisdiction;

(6) Being unable to render patient care with reasonable safety by reason of addiction to alcohol or drugs or by reason of a mental or physical condition or disability;

(7) Revocation, termination, suspension or restriction of hospital privileges;

(8) Knowingly submitting or causing to be submitted any false, fraudulent, deceptive or misleading information to the Board of Medical Examiners in connection with an application for licensure or registration.

(9) That the physician assistant has represented himself or herself or permitted another to represent him or her as a physician.

(10) That the physician assistant has performed otherwise than at the direction and under the supervision of a physician approved by the Board.

(11) That the physician assistant has been delegated and/or has performed or attempted to perform tasks and functions beyond his or her competence.

(12) That the physician assistant has performed or attempted to perform tasks beyond those authorized in the approved job description.

(13) Practicing or permitting another to practice as a physician assistant without the required license and registration from the Board of Medical Examiners.

(14) Prescribing in violation of statutory authority and/or Board rules and/or Board guidelines.

(15) Intentional falsification of a certification of compliance with the continuing medical education requirement for physician assistants established in these rules.

Alabama. Admin. Code r. 540-X-7-.12.

Montana

Montana's statute sets the following requirements:

A person may not be licensed as a physician assistant-certified in this state unless the person:

(1) is of good moral character;

(2) is a graduate of a physician assistant training program approved by the American Medical Association's Committee on Allied Health Education and Accreditation;

(3) has taken and successfully passed an examination recognized by the National Commission on the Certification of Physician Assistants;

(4) holds a current certificate from the National Commission on the Certification of Physician Assistants; and

(5) has submitted to the board detailed information on the person's history, education, and experience.

Montana Code Ann. sec. 37-20-402.

(1) A person who violates a provision of this part is guilty of a misdemeanor and upon conviction shall be fined not more than $500 or imprisoned for not more than 90 days, or both.

(2) The board may enforce any provision of this part by injunction or any other appropriate proceeding.

MONTANA CODE ANN. SEC. 37-19-831.

Missouri

Missouri will discipline physician assistants for any of the following actions:

(1) The board may refuse to issue or renew any physician assistant license required pursuant to this chapter for one (1) or any combination of causes stated in section (2) of this rule. The board shall notify the physician assistant in writing of the reasons for the refusal and shall advise the physician assistant of their right to file a complaint with the Administrative Hearing Commission as provided by Chapter 621, RSMo.

(2) The board may cause a complaint to be filed with the Administrative Hearing Commission as provided by Chapter 621, RSMo, against any holder of any certificate of registration or authority, permit or license required by this chapter or any person who has failed to renew or has surrendered a certificate of registration or authority, permit or license for any one (1) or any combination of the following causes:

   (A) Use of any controlled substance, as defined in Chapter 195, RSMo, or alcoholic beverage to an extent that such use impairs a person's ability to perform the work of any profession licensed or regulated by this chapter;

   (B) The person has been finally adjudicated and found guilty, or entered a plea of guilty or nolo contendere, in a criminal prosecution under the laws of any state or of the United States, for any offense reasonably related to the qualifications, functions or duties of any profession licensed or regulated under this chapter, for any offense an essential element of which is fraud, dishonesty or an act of violence, or for any offense involving moral turpitude, whether or not sentence is imposed;

   (C) Use of fraud, deception, misrepresentation or bribery in securing any certificate of registration or authority, permit or license issued pursuant to this chapter or in obtaining permission to take any examination given or required pursuant to this chapter;

   (D) Misconduct, fraud, misrepresentation, dishonesty, unethical conduct or unprofessional conduct in the performance of the functions or duties of any profession licensed or regulated by this chapter, including, but not limited to the following:

1. Obtaining or attempting to obtain any fee, charge, tuition or other compensation by fraud, deception or misrepresentation; willfully and continually overcharging or overtreating patients; or charging for services which did not occur unless the services were contracted for in advance, or for services which were not rendered or documented in the patient's records;

2. Attempting, directly or indirectly, by way of intimidation, coercion or deception, to obtain or retain a patient or discourage the use of a second opinion or consultation;

3. Willfully and continually performing inappropriate or unnecessary treatment, diagnostic tests or medical or surgical services;

4. Delegating professional responsibilities to a person who is not qualified by training, skill, competency, age, experience, licensure, registration or certification to perform them;

5. Misrepresenting that any disease, ailment or infirmity can be cured by a method, procedure, treatment, medicine or device;

6. Performing or prescribing medical services which have been declared by board rule to be of no medical or osteopathic value;

7. Final disciplinary action by any professional physician assistant association or society or licensed hospital or medical staff of such hospital in this or any other state or territory, whether agreed to voluntarily or not, and including, but not limited to, any removal, suspension, limitation, or restriction of his/her registration, license or staff or hospital privileges, failure to renew such privileges of registration or license for cause, or other final disciplinary action, if the action was in any way related to unprofessional conduct, professional incompetence, malpractice or any other violation of any provision of this chapter;

8. Signing a blank prescription form; or dispensing, prescribing, administering or otherwise distributing any drug, controlled substance or other treatment without sufficient examination, or for other than medically accepted therapeutic or experimental or investigative

purposes duly authorized by a state or federal agency, or not in the course of professional practice, or not in good faith to relieve pain and suffering, or not to cure an ailment, physical infirmity or disease, except as authorized in section 334.104, RSMo;

9. Exercising influence within a physician assistant–patient relationship for purposes of engaging a patient in sexual activity;

10. Terminating the medical care of a patient without adequate notice or without making other arrangements for the continued care of the patient;

11. Failing to furnish details of a patient's medical records to other treating physician assistants, physicians or hospitals upon proper request; or failing to comply with any other law relating to medical records;

12. Failure of any physician assistant or applicant, other than the physician assistant subject of the investigation, to cooperate with the board during any investigation;

13. Failure to comply with any subpoena or subpoena duces tecum from the board or an order of the board;

14. Failure to timely pay license renewal fees specified in this chapter;

15. Violating a probation agreement with this board or any other licensing or regulatory agency;

16. Failing to inform the board of the physician assistant's current residence and business address;

17. Advertising by an applicant or licensed physician assistant which is false or misleading, or which violates any rule of the board, or which claims without substantiation the positive cure of any disease, or professional superiority to or greater skill than that possessed by any other physician assistant. An applicant or licensed physician assistant shall also be in violation of this provision if s/he has a financial interest in any organization, corporation or association which issues or conducts such advertising;

18. Violation of one (1) or any combination of the standards listed in the American Academy of Physician Assistants' Code of Ethics. The board adopts and incorporates by reference the American Academy of Physician Assistants' Code of Ethics. A copy of the American Academy of Physician Assistants' Code of Ethics is retained at the office of the board and is available to any interested

person, upon written request, at a cost not to exceed the actual cost of reproduction; and

19. Loss of national certification, for any reason, shall result in the termination of licensure;

    (A) Any conduct or practice which is or might be harmful or dangerous to the mental or physical health of a patient or the public; or incompetency, gross negligence or repeated negligence in the performance of the functions or duties of any profession licensed or regulated by this chapter. For the purposes of this subsection, *repeated negligence* means the failure, on more than one (1) occasion, to use that degree of skill and learning ordinarily used under the same or similar circumstances by the member of the applicant's, registrant's or licensee's profession;

    (B) Violation of, or attempting to violate, directly or indirectly, or assisting or enabling any person to violate, any provision of this chapter, or of any lawful rule or regulation adopted pursuant to this chapter;

    (C) Impersonation of any person holding a certificate of registration or authority, permit or license or allowing any person to use his/her certificate of registration or authority, permit, license or diploma from any school;

    (D) Revocation, suspension, restriction, modification, limitation, reprimand, warning, censure, probation or other final disciplinary action against the holder of or applicant for licensure or other right to practice any profession regulated by this chapter by another state, territory, federal agency or country, whether or not voluntarily agreed to by the physician assistant or applicant, including, but not limited to, the denial of licensure or registration, surrender of the license or registration, allowing physician assistant license or registration to expire or lapse, or discontinuing or limiting the practice of the physician assistant while subject to an investigation or while actually under investigation by any licensing authority, medical facility, branch of the armed forces of the United States of America, insurance company, court, agency of the state or federal government, or employer;

(E) A person is finally adjudged incapacitated or disabled by a court of competent jurisdiction;

(F) Assisting or enabling any person to practice or offer to practice any profession licensed or regulated by this chapter who is not licensed and currently eligible to practice under this chapter; or knowingly performing any act which in any way aids, assists, procures, advises, or encourages any person to practice who is not licensed and currently eligible to practice under this chapter;

(G) Issuance of a certificate of registration or authority, permit or license based upon a material mistake of fact;

(H) Failure to display a valid license as required by this chapter;

(I) Violation of the drug laws or rules and regulations of this state, any other state or the federal government;

(J) Knowingly making, or causing to be made, or aiding, or abetting in the making of, a false statement in any birth, death or other certificate or document executed in connection with the practice of his/her profession;

(K) Soliciting patronage in person or by agents or representatives, or by any other means or manner, under his/her own name or under the name of another person or concern, actual or pretended, in such a manner as to confuse, deceive, or mislead the public as the need or necessity for or appropriateness of health care services for all patients, or the qualifications of an individual person(s) to diagnose, render or perform health care services;

(L) Using, or permitting the use of, his/her name under the designation of physician assistant, licensed physician assistant, physician assistant-certified, or any similar designation with reference to the commercial exploitation or product endorsement of any goods, wares or merchandise;

(M) Knowingly making, or causing to be made, a false statement or misrepresentation of a material fact, with intent to defraud, for payment under the provisions of Chapter 208, RSMo, or Chapter 630, RSMo, or for payment from Title XVIII or Title XIX of the federal Medicare program;

(N) Failure or refusal to properly guard against contagious, infectious or communicable diseases or the spread thereof; maintaining an unsanitary office or performing professional services under unsanitary conditions; or failure to report the existence of an unsanitary condition in the office of a physician or in any health care facility to the board, in writing, within thirty (30) days after the discovery thereof;

(O) Any person licensed to practice as a physician assistant, requiring, as condition of the physician assistant–patient relationship, that the patient receive prescribed drugs, devices or other professional services directly from facilities of that physician assistant's office or other entities under the supervising physician's or physician assistant's ownership or control. A physician assistant shall provide the patient with a prescription which may be taken to the facility selected by the patient;

(P) A pattern of personal use or consumption of any controlled substance unless it is prescribed, dispensed or administered by a physician who is authorized by law to do so;

(Q) Practicing outside the scope of practice of the physician assistant as referenced in the physician assistants' supervision agreement;

(R) For a physician assistant to operate, conduct, manage, practice or establish an abortion facility, or for a physician assistant to perform an abortion in an abortion facility, if such facility comes under the definition of an ambulatory surgical center pursuant to sections 197.200 to 197.240, RSMo, and such facility has failed to obtain or renew a license as an ambulatory surgical center; and

(S) Being unable to practice as a physician assistant or with a specialty with reasonable skill and safety to patients by reasons of medical or osteopathic incompetency, or because of illness, drunkenness, excessive use of drugs, narcotics, chemicals, or as a result of any mental or physical condition.

MISSOURI CODE OF REGS. TIT. 4 SEC. 150-7.140.

1. In enforcing this paragraph the board shall, after a hearing by the board, upon a finding of probable cause, require a physician assis-

tant to submit to a reexamination for the purpose of establishing his/her competency to practice as a physician assistant or with a specialty conducted in accordance with rules adopted for this purpose by the board, including rules to allow the examination of the pattern and practice of said physician assistant's professional conduct, or to submit to a mental or physical examination or combination thereof by at least three (3) physician assistants, one (1) selected by the physician assistant compelled to take the examination, one (1) selected by the board, and one (1) selected by the two (2) physician assistants so selected who are graduates of a professional school approved and accredited by the Commission for the Accreditation of Allied Health Education Programs and has active certification by the National Commission on Certification of Physician Assistants.

2. For the purpose of this paragraph, every physician assistant licensed under this chapter is deemed to have consented to submit to a mental or physical examination when directed in writing by the board and further to have waived all objections to the admissibility of the examining physician's testimony or examination reports on the ground that same is privileged.

3. In addition to ordering a physical or mental examination to determine competency, the board may, notwithstanding any other law limiting access to medical or other health data, obtain medical data and health records relating to a physician assistant or applicant without the physician assistant's or applicant's consent.

4. Written notice of the reexamination or the physical or mental examination shall be sent to the physician assistant, by registered mail, addressed to the physician assistant at his/her last known address. Failure of a physician assistant to designate an examining physician to the board or failure to submit to the examination when directed shall constitute an admission of the allegations against him/her, in which case the board may enter a final order without the presentation of evidence, unless the failure was due to circumstances beyond his/her control. A physician assistant whose right to practice has been affected under this paragraph shall, at reasonable intervals, be afforded an opportunity to demonstrate that s/he can resume competent practice as a physician assistant.

5. In any proceeding under this paragraph neither the record of proceedings nor the orders entered by the board shall be used against a physician assistant in any other proceeding. Proceedings under this paragraph shall be conducted by the board without the filing of a complaint with the Administrative Hearing Commission.

6. When the board finds any person unqualified because of any of the grounds set forth in this paragraph, it may enter an order imposing one (1) or more of the disciplinary measures set forth in section (4) of this rule.

(A) After the filing of such complaint before the Administrative Hearing Commission, the proceedings shall be conducted in accordance with the provisions of Chapter 621, RSMo. Upon a finding by the Administrative Hearing Commission that the grounds, provided in section (2) of this rule, for disciplinary action are met, the board may, singly or in combination, warn, censure or place the person named in the complaint on probation on such terms and conditions as the board deems appropriate for a period not to exceed ten (10) years, or may suspend license, certificate or permit for a period not to exceed ten (10) years, or restrict or limit his/her license, certificate or permit for an indefinite period of time, or revoke his/her license, certificate, or permit for an indefinite period of time, or revoke his/her license, certificate or permit, or administer a public or private reprimand, or deny his/her application for licensure, or permanently withhold issuance of licensure or require the physician assistant to submit to the care, counseling or treatment of physicians designated by the board at the expense of the individual to be examined, or require the physician assistant to attend such continuing educational courses and pass such examinations as the board may direct.

(B) In any order of revocation, the board may provide that the person may not apply for reinstatement of licensure for a period of time ranging from two to seven (2–7) years following the date of the order of revocation. All stay orders shall toll this time period.

(C) Before restoring to good standing a license, certificate or permit issued under this chapter which has been in a revoked, suspended or inactive state for any cause for more than two (2) years, the board may require the applicant to attend such continuing education courses and pass such examinations as the board may direct.

(D) In any investigation, hearing or other proceeding to determine a licensed physician assistant's or applicant's fitness to practice, any record relating to any patient of the licensed physician assistant or applicant shall be discoverable by the board and admissible into evidence, regardless of any statutory or common law privilege which such licensee, applicant, record custodian or patient might otherwise invoke. In addition, no such licensed physician assistant, applicant, or record custodian may withhold records or testimony bearing upon a license's or applicant's fitness to practice on the ground of privilege between such physician assistant licensee, applicant or record custodian and a patient.

MISSOURI CODE OF REGS. TIT. 4 SEC. 150-7.150.

REFERENCES

1. National Commission on Certification of Physician Assistants Web site. CME requirements. Available at http://nccpa.net. Accessed March 2005.

State-by-State License Requirements

ALABAMA

(1) To qualify for a license to practice as a physician assistant an individual must meet the following requirements:

    (a) Provide evidence, satisfactory to the Board, of successful completion of a training program accredited by the Committee on Allied Health Education and Accreditation (CAHEA), or the Commission on Accreditation of Allied Health Education Programs (CAAHEP), or their successor agencies;

    (b) Provide evidence, satisfactory to the Board, of successful completion of the Physician Assistant National Certification Examination (PANCE) as administered by the National Commission on Certification of Physician Assistants (NCCPA);

    (c) Submit an application on forms approved by the Board; and Pay the required license application fee as determined by the Board.

(2) Documentation submitted through the Federation Credentials Verification Service (FCVS) may be accepted to demonstrate compliance with the credentialing requirements of this rule.

ALABAMA ADMIN. CODE R. 540-X-7-.04.

ALASKA

(a) An individual who desires to undertake medical diagnosis and treatment or the practice of medicine in AS 08.64.380(6) or AS 08.64.380(7) as a physician assistant

    (1) shall apply for a permanent renewable license on a form provided by the department;

    (2) shall pay the appropriate fees established in 12 AAC 02.250; and

    (3) must be approved by the board.

   (b) The application must contain documented evidence of
      (1) graduation from a physician assistant program accredited by the American Medical Association Committee on Allied Health Education and Accreditation or its successor, the Commission on Accreditation of Allied Health Education Programs;
      (2) a passing score on the certifying examination administered by the National Commission on Certification of Physician Assistants;
      (3) a current certification issued by the National Commission on Certification of Physician Assistants (NCCPA);
      (4) compliance with continuing medical education standards established by the National Commission on Certification of Physician Assistants; and
      (5) verification of registration or licensure in all other states where the applicant is or has been registered or licensed as a physician assistant or any other health care professional;
      (6) verification of successful completion of a physician assistant program that meets the requirements of this subsection; that verification must be sent directly from the program to the board;
      (7) clearance from the Board Action Data Bank maintained by the Federation of State Medical Boards; and
      (8) clearance from the federal Drug Enforcement Administration (DEA).
   (c) A physician assistant must be licensed under this section at the time the board issues an authorization to practice in this state.

12 ALASKA ADMIN. CODE 40.400.

ARIZONA

   A. An applicant for licensure shall:
      1. Have attended and completed a course of training for physician assistants approved by the board.
      2. Pass a certifying examination approved by the board.
      3. Be physically and mentally able to safely perform health care tasks as a physician assistant.
      4. Have a professional record that indicates that the applicant has not committed any act or engaged in any conduct that constitutes grounds for disciplinary action against a licensee pursuant to this chapter.

5. Not have had a license to practice revoked by a regulatory board in another jurisdiction in the United States for an act that occurred in that jurisdiction that constitutes unprofessional conduct pursuant to this chapter.

6. Not be currently under investigation, suspension or restriction by a regulatory board in another jurisdiction in the United States for an act that occurred in that jurisdiction that constitutes unprofessional conduct pursuant to this chapter. If the applicant is under investigation by a regulatory board in another jurisdiction, the board shall suspend the application process and may not issue or deny a license to the applicant until the investigation is resolved.

7. Not have surrendered, relinquished or given up a license in lieu of disciplinary action by a regulatory board in another jurisdiction in the United Sates for an act that occurred in that jurisdiction that constitutes unprofessional conduct pursuant to this chapter.

B. The board may:

1. Require an applicant to submit written or oral proof of credentials.

2. Make such investigations as it deems necessary to advise itself with respect to the qualifications of the applicant including physical examinations, mental evaluations, written competency examinations or any combination of such examinations and evaluations.

ARIZONA REV. STAT. ANN. SEC. 32-2521.

ARKANSAS

Has successfully completed an educational program for physician assistants or surgeon assistants accredited by the Committee on Allied Health Education and Accreditation or by its successor agency and has passed the Physician Assistant National Certifying Examination administered by the National Commission on Certification of Physician Assistants;

ARKANSAS CODE 17-105-102(3).

CALIFORNIA

The committee shall issue under the name of the Medical Board of California a license to all physician assistant applicants who meet all of the following requirements:

Provide evidence of the following:

(1) Successful completion of an approved program.
(2) Pass required examination
    (a) Not be subject to denial of licensure under Division 1.5 (commencing with Section 475) or Section 3527.
    (b) Pay all fees required under Section 3521.1.

California Bus. & Prof. Code sec. 3519

COLORADO

To become licensed, a physician assistant shall have:
  (I) Successfully completed an education program for physician assistants which conforms to standards approved by the board, which standards may be established by utilizing the assistance of any responsible accrediting organization; and
 (II) Successfully completed the national certifying examination for assistants to the primary care physician which is administered by the National Commission on Certification of Physician Assistants or successfully completed any other examination approved by the board; and
(III) Applied to the board on the forms and in the manner designated by the board and paid the appropriate fee established by the board pursuant to section 24-34-105, C.R.S.; and
(IV) Attained the age of twenty-one years.
    (a) The board may determine whether any applicant for licensure as a physician assistant possesses education, experience, or training in health care that is sufficient to be accepted in lieu of the qualifications required for licensure under subparagraph (I) of paragraph (c) of this subsection (5). Every person who desires to qualify for practice as a physician assistant within this state shall file with the secretary of the board his or her written application for licensure, on which application he or she shall list any act the commission of which would be grounds for disciplinary action against a licensed physician assistant under section 12-36-117, along with an explanation of the circumstances of such act. The board may deny licensure to any applicant who has performed any act that constitutes unprofessional conduct, as defined in section 12-36-117.
    (b) No person licensed as a physician assistant may perform any act that constitutes the practice of medicine within a hospital or nursing care facility that is licensed pursuant to part 1 of article 3 of title 25, C.R.S., or that is required to obtain a certificate of compliance pursuant to section 25-1-107 (1) (l)

(II), C.R.S., without authorization from the governing board of the hospital or nursing care facility. Such governing board shall have the authority to grant, deny, or limit such authority to its own established procedures.

COLORADO REV. STAT. ANN. 12-36-106(5)C

Applicants shall be licensed as physician assistants by the State Board of Medical Examiners upon submission of the following:
 I. A completed Board-approved application form and required fee; and
 II. Proof of satisfactory passage of the national certifying examination for assistants to the primary care physician administered by the National Commission on Certification of Physician Assistants, Inc.

COLORADO CODE REGS. SEC. 400-1

CONNECTICUT

The department may, upon receipt of a fee of one hundred fifty dollars, issue a physician assistant license to an applicant who:
(1) holds a baccalaureate or higher degree in any field from a regionally accredited institution of higher education;
(2) has graduated from an accredited physician assistant program;
(3) has passed the certification examination of the national commission;
(4) has satisfied the mandatory continuing medical education requirements of the national commission for current certification by such commission and has passed any examination or continued competency assessment the passage of which may be required by the national commission for maintenance of current certification by such commission; and
(5) has completed not less than sixty hours of didactic instruction in pharmacology for physician assistant practice approved by the department.

CONNECTICUT GEN. STATUTE SEC. 20-12(B)

DELAWARE

A "physician's assistant" is defined as an individual who has graduated from a physician's or surgeon's assistant program which has been accredited by the Committee on Allied Health Education and Accreditation (CAHEA) of the American Medical Association (AMA), or a successor agency acceptable to and approved by the Board, has passed a national certifying examination acceptable to the Physician's Assistant Advisory Council of the Board and approved by the full

Board, and who is licensed under this chapter to practice as a physician's assistant. Physician's assistants who are currently registered in the State but who are not graduates of an approved program of the type outlined above may be licensed to practice as, and use the title "physician's assistant," provided the individual has successfully passed 1 of the national certifying examinations developed and administered by the National Board of Medical Examiners (NBME) or the National Commission on Certification of Physician's Assistants (NCCPA) on or prior to October 1987, and has maintained Continuing Medical Education (CME) credits as required by rules and regulations developed under this chapter.

TIT. 24 DELAWARE CODE SEC. 1770A-1

DISTRICT OF COLUMBIA

An applicant for a license to practice as a physician assistant shall submit with a completed application three (3) letters of reference from licensed physician assistants or licensed physicians who have personal knowledge of the applicant's abilities and qualifications to practice as a physician assistant.

Educational Requirements

An applicant shall furnish proof satisfactory to the Board that the applicant has successfully completed an educational program to practice as a physician assistant accredited by the Committee on Allied Health Education and Accreditation (CAHEA) of the American Medical Association by submitting to the Board, with a completed application, a certified transcript and an official statement verifying graduation from an educational program.

Examination

An applicant shall receive a passing score on an examination administered by the National Commission on Certification of Physician Assistants (the NCCPA examination).

An applicant who fails the certifying examination three (3) times shall successfully complete for the second time an educational program to practice as a physician assistant accredited by CAHEA in order to be eligible to take the examination a fourth time. An applicant who fails the NCCPA examination (administered in any jurisdiction) six (6) times shall not be eligible for licensure in the District by any means.

TIT. 17 D.C. MUN. REG. SEC. 4900.4, 4902.1, 4903

FLORIDA

Any person desiring to be licensed as a physician assistant must apply to the department. The department shall issue a license to any person certified by the council as having met the following requirements:

1. Is at least 18 years of age.
2. Has satisfactorily passed a proficiency examination by an acceptable score established by the National Commission on Certification of Physician Assistants. If an applicant does not hold a current certificate issued by the National Commission on Certification of Physician Assistants and has not actively practiced as a physician assistant within the immediately preceding 4 years, the applicant must retake and successfully complete the entry-level examination of the National Commission on Certification of Physician Assistants to be eligible for licensure.
3. Has completed the application form and remitted an application fee not to exceed $300 as set by the boards. An application for licensure made by a physician assistant must include:
   a. A certificate of completion of a physician assistant training program specified in subsection (6).
   b. A sworn statement of any prior felony convictions.
   c. A sworn statement of any previous revocation or denial of licensure or certification in any state.
   d. Two letters of recommendation.

FLORIDA STAT. CH. 458.347(7)

GEORGIA

No person shall practice as a Physician's Assistant without Board approval. The requirements for Board approval of a Physician's Assistant are the following:

(a) Good moral character as demonstrated by two (2) acceptable references from licensed physicians, other than from the applying supervising physician(s), who are personally acquainted with the proposed Physician's Assistant. At the option of the Board, the Physician's Assistant and the applying supervising physician(s) will be required to appear before the Board for a personal interview;
(b) Requirements for Board Approval of Physician's Assistant:
   1. A training program approved by the Board.
      (a) The Board has approved or will approve those Physician's Assistants program of training offered by accredited colleges or universities consisting of 2 or more academic years of didactic and clinical experience in a health care

field appropriate to the task of a Physician's Assistant, or a Board-approved equivalent program.

(b) The curriculum of an approved program of training must provide adequate instruction in the basic sciences underlying the medical practice to provide the trainee with an understanding of the nature of disease processes and symptoms, abnormal tests, drug actions, etc. This must be combined with history taking, physical examinations, therapeutic procedures, etc. This should be in sufficient depth to enable the graduate to integrate and organize historical and physical findings. The didactic instruction shall follow a planned and progressive outline and shall include an appropriate mixture of classroom lectures, text assignments, discussions, demonstrations, and similar activities. Instruction shall include clinical experience with qualified supervision sufficient to provide understanding of and skill in performing those clinical functions which the assistant may be asked to perform. There must be sufficient evaluative procedures to assure adequate evidence of competence. "The student may concentrate his efforts and his interest in a particular specialty of medicine and a Type A (Primary Care) student must ensure that he possesses a broad general understanding of medical practice and therapeutic techniques and must be competent in this area. A Physician's Assistant Type B cannot be certified to any physician other than one whose primary specialty is in the specialty in which the Physician's Assistant is trained and the Physician's Assistant's services will not be utilized in any specialty other than in which the Physician's Assistant is trained."

(c) A current list of Board approved Physician's Assistants Programs of study will be made available to the applicant upon request.

2. Effective on or after September 1, 1985, new applicants for certification must submit evidence that the applicant has achieved a passing score on an examination approved or administered by the Board for which the applicant is eligible. The Board approves either:

(a) The certification examination administered by the National Commission for Certification of Anesthesiologist Assistants (NCCAA) or its successor, or

(b) The certification examination administered by the National Commission on Certification of Physician Assistants (NCCPA) or its successor.

(c) The application and/or job description for the proposed Physician's Assistant signed by the applying physician(s) and Physician's Assistant, shall include the following information:

1. Application made by the Physician's Assistant for certification shall include the medical qualifications including related experience possessed by the Physician's Assistant applicant.

2. Application made by the applying supervising physician(s) shall include a detailed description of the medical tasks to be performed by the Physician's Assistant, and the location where such tasks will be usually performed. Attachment of the Basic Job Description shall be deemed adequate compliance with the requirement for a detailed description of medical tasks, unless further tasks are requested.

3. Each physician must indicate the name and location of the medical school from which he was graduated and the date the degree was received. The physician should also indicate the type of practice and a current Georgia medical license number.

Fee to be submitted in the form of a check or money order payable to the Composite State Board of Medical Examiners. A schedule of fees may be obtained from the Board office by request.

The supervising and alternate supervising physician shall at all times maintain on file, readily available for inspection, documentation from the Board evidencing current approval for utilization of the Physician's Assistant and a copy of the applicable approved job description.

GEORGIA COMP. R. AND REGS. R. 360-5.03

HAWAII

(a) The board of medical examiners shall require each person practicing medicine under the supervision of a physician, other than a person licensed under section 453-3, to be licensed as a physician assistant. A person who is trained to do only a very limited number of diagnostic or therapeutic procedures under the direction of a physician shall not be deemed a practitioner of medicine and therefore does not require licensure under this section.

(b) The board shall establish medical educational and training standards with which a person applying for licensure as a physician assistant shall comply. The standards shall be at least equal to recognized national education and training standards for physician assistants.

(c) Upon satisfactory proof of compliance with the required medical educational and training standards, the board may grant state licensure to a person who has been granted certification based upon passage of a national certifying examination and who holds a current certificate from the national certifying entity approved by the board.

HAWAII REV. STAT. SEC. 453-5.3

An application for certification shall be made under oath on a form to be provided by the board. The form may require the applicant to provide:

(1) The appropriate fees including the application fee which shall not be refunded;

(2) The applicant's full name;

(3) Evidence of graduation from a board approved school or training program;

(4) Evidence of passage of the national certification examination developed by the National Commission on Certification of Physician's Assistants (NCCPA);

(5) Evidence of current NCCPA certification;

(6) Information regarding any conviction of any crime which has not been annulled or expunged;

(7) A completed Federation Discipline Report from the Federation of State Medical Boards;

(8) If applicable, evidence of any certifications held or once held in other jurisdictions indicating the status of the certification and documenting any disciplinary action;

(9) Any other information the board may require to investigate the applicant's qualifications for certification;

(10) A statement signed by the licensed physician or group of physicians, as the case may be, stating that the physician or group of physicians will direct and supervise the physician assistant and that the physician assistant will be considered the agent of the physician or group of physicians; and

(11) The name of the employer.

HAWAII ADMIN. R SEC. 16-85-46

IDAHO

License Applications. All applications for licensure as physician assistants shall be made to the Board on forms supplied by the Board.

Reapplication. If more than two (2) years have elapsed since a physician assistant has actively engaged in practice, reapplication to the Board as a new applicant is required. The Board may require evidence of an educational update and close supervision to assure safe and qualified performance.

Requirements for Licensure.

Baccalaureate Degree. Applicants for licensure shall provide evidence of having received a college baccalaureate degree and completed an approved program.

National Certifying Examination. Satisfactory completion and passage of the certifying examination for physician assistants, administered by the National Commission of Certification of Physician Assistants or such other examinations, which may be written, oral or practical, as the Board may require.

Personal Interview. The Board may at its discretion, require the applicant or the supervising physician or both to appear for a personal interview.

Completion Of Form. If the applicant is to practice in Idaho, complete a form provided by the Board indicating:
- The applicant has completed a delegation of services agreement signed by the physician assistant, supervising physician and alternate supervising physicians; and
- The agreement is on file at the Idaho practice sites; or
- Complete a form provided by the Board indicating the applicant is not practicing in Idaho and prior to practicing in Idaho, the applicant will meet the requirements of Subsections 021.04. a. and 021.04.b.

IDAHO ADMIN. CODE SEC. 22.01.03.020-021

ILLINOIS

a) An applicant for licensure as a physician assistant shall file an application on forms provided by the Department. The application shall include:
   1) Certification of graduation from an approved program that meets the requirements set forth in Section 1350.30 of this Part or certification from the National Commission on Certification of Physician Assistants, or its successor agency, that the applicant has substantially equivalent training and experience;

2) Certification of successful completion of the Physician Assistant National Certifying Examination. The certification shall be forwarded to the Department from the National Commission on Certification of Physician Assistants, or its successor agency;

3) A complete work history since graduation from a physician assistant program;

4) Certification, on forms provided by the Department, from all states in which an applicant was licensed and is currently licensed, if applicable, stating:

A) The time during which the applicant was licensed in that state, including the date of the original issuance of the license;

B) Whether the file on the applicant contains any record of disciplinary actions taken or pending;

5) The fee required in Section 1350.25 of this Part.

b) A physician assistant license will be issued when the applicant meets the requirements set forth above. However, a physician assistant may not practice until a notice of employment has been filed in accordance with Section 1350.100 of this Part.

c) The supervising physician shall submit a notice of prescriptive authority indicating the physician assistant has been delegated prescriptive authority. If the physician assistant is supervised by more than one physician, a separate notice of prescriptive authority shall be submitted by each supervising physician. In addition, if prescriptive authority includes Schedule III, IV and/or V controlled substances, the physician assistant will be required to apply for a mid-level practitioner license in accordance with the Illinois Controlled Substances Act.

ILLINOIS ADMIN. CODE TIT. 68 SEC. 1350.40

INDIANA

Certification required; conditions

An individual must be certified by the committee before the individual may practice as a physician assistant. The committee may grant a certificate as a physician assistant to an applicant who does the following:

(1) Submits an application on forms approved by the committee.

(2) Pays the fee established by the board.

(3) Has:

(A) successfully completed an educational program for physician assistants or surgeon assistants accredited by an accrediting agency; and

(B) passed the Physician Assistant National Certifying Examination administered by the NCCPA and maintains current NCCPA certification.

(4) Submits to the committee any other information the committee considers necessary to evaluate the applicant's qualifications.

(5) Presents satisfactory evidence to the committee that the individual has not been:

(A) engaged in an act that would constitute grounds for a disciplinary sanction under IC 25-1-9; or

(B) the subject of a disciplinary action by a licensing or certification agency of another state or jurisdiction on the grounds that the individual was not able to practice as a physician assistant without endangering the public.

INDIANA CODE REV. SEC. 25-27.5-4-1

(a) The application for certification of a physician assistant must be made upon forms supplied by the committee.

(b) Each application for certification as a physician assistant or for a temporary permit while waiting for the next committee meeting shall include all of the following information:

(1) Complete names, address, and telephone number of the physician assistant.

(2) Satisfactory evidence of the following:

(A) Completion of an approved educational program.

(B) Passage of the Physician Assistant National Certifying Examination administered by the NCCPA.

(C) A current NCCPA certificate.

(3) All names used by the physician assistant, explaining the reason for such name change or use.

(4) Date and place of birth of the physician assistant, and age at the time of application.

(5) Citizenship and visa status if applicable.

(6) Whether the physician assistant has been licensed, certified, or registered in any other jurisdiction and, if so, the dates thereof.

(7) Whether the physician assistant has had any disciplinary action taken against the license, certificate, or registration by the licensing or regulatory agency of any other state or jurisdiction, and the details and dates thereof.

(8) A complete listing of all places of employment, including:

(A) the name and address of employers;

(B) the dates of each employment; and

(C) employment responsibilities held or performed; that the

applicant has had since becoming a physician assistant in any state or jurisdiction.

(9) Whether the physician assistant is, or has been, addicted to, or is chemically dependent upon, any narcotic drugs, alcohol, or other drugs, and if so, the details thereof.

(10) Whether the applicant has been denied a license, certificate, approval, or registration as physician assistant by any other state or jurisdiction, and, if so, the details thereof, including the following:

(A) The name and location of the state or jurisdiction denying licensure.

(B) Certification, approval, or registration.

(C) The date of denial of the certification, approval, or registration.

(D) The reasons relating to the denial of certification, approval, or registration.

(11) Whether the physician assistant has been convicted of, or pleaded guilty to, any violation of federal, state, or local law relating to the use, manufacturing, distributing, sale, dispensing, or possession of controlled substances or of drug addiction, and, if so, all of the details relating thereto.

(12) Whether the physician assistant has been convicted of, or pleaded guilty to, any federal or state criminal offense, felony, or misdemeanor, except for traffic violations that resulted only in fines, and, if so, all of the details thereto.

(13) Whether the physician assistant was denied privileges in any hospital or health care facility, or had such privileges revoked, suspended, or subjected to any restriction, probation, or other type of discipline or limitation, and, if so, all of the details relating thereto, including the name and address of the hospital or health care facility, the date of such action, and the reasons therefore.

(14) Whether the physician assistant has ever been admonished, censured, reprimanded, or requested to withdraw, resign, or retire from any hospital or health care facility in which the physician assistant was employed, worked, or held privileges.

(15) Whether the physician assistant has had any malpractice judgments entered against him or her or settled any malpractice action or cause of action, and, if so, a complete, detailed description of the facts and circumstances relating thereto.

(16) A statement from the supervising physician that the physician assistant is, or will be, supervised by that physician.

(17) A description of the setting in which the physician assistant shall be working under the physician supervision.

(18) The name, business address, and telephone number of the physician under whose supervision the physician assistant will be supervised.

(19) One (1) passport-type photo taken of the applicant within the last eight (8) weeks.

(c) All information in the application shall be submitted under oath or affirmation, subject to the penalties of perjury.

(d) Each applicant for certification as a physician assistant shall submit an executed authorization and release form supplied by the committee that:

(1) authorizes the committee or any of its authorized representatives to inspect, receive, and review;

(2) authorizes and directs any:

(A) person;

(B) corporation;

(C) partnership;

(D) association;

(E) organization;

(F) institute;

(G) forum; or

(H) officer thereof;

to furnish, provide, and supply to the committee all relevant documents, records, or other information pertaining to the applicant; and

(3) releases the committee, or any of its authorized representatives, and any:

(A) person;

(B) corporation;

(C) partnership;

(D) association;

(E) organization;

(F) institute;

(G) forum; or

(H) officer thereof;

from any and all liability regarding such inspection, review, receipt, furnishing, or supply of any such information.

(e) Application forms submitted to the committee must be complete in every detail. All supporting documents required by the application must be submitted with the application.

(f) Applicants for a temporary permit to practice as a physician assistant while waiting to take the examination or waiting for results of the examination must submit all requirements of subsection (b), except for subsection (b)(2)(B) and (b)(2)(C), in order to apply for a temporary permit.

(g) A temporary permit becomes invalid if the temporary permit holder fails to sit or fails to register for the next available examination.

Indiana Admin. Code Tit. 844 r. 2.2-1-5

IOWA

a. An applicant shall complete a board-approved application packet. Application forms may be obtained from the board's Web site (http://www.idph.state.ia.us/licensure) or directly from the board office. All applications shall be sent to the Board of Physician Assistant Examiners, Professional Licensure Division, Fifth Floor, Lucas State Office Building, Des Moines, Iowa 50319-0075.

b. An applicant shall complete the application form according to the instructions contained in the application.

c. Each application shall be accompanied by the appropriate fees payable by check or money order to the Iowa Board of Physician Assistant Examiners. The fees are nonrefundable.

d. Each applicant shall provide official copies of academic transcripts that have been sent to the board directly from an approved program for the education of physician assistants. EXCEPTION: An applicant who is not a graduate of an approved program but who passed the NCCPA initial certification examination prior to 1986 is exempt from the graduation requirement.

e. An applicant shall provide a copy of the initial certification from NCCPA, or its successor agency, sent directly to the board from the NCCPA, or its successor agency.

f. Prior to beginning practice, the physician assistant shall notify the board of the identity of the supervising physician(s) on the board-approved form.

Iowa Admin. Code r. 645-326.2

KANSAS

No person shall be licensed as a physician assistant by the state board of healing arts unless such person has:

(1) Presented to the state board of healing arts proof that the applicant has successfully completed a course of education and training approved by the state board of healing arts for the education and training of a physician assistant or presented to the state

board of healing arts proof that the applicant has acquired experience while serving in the armed forces of the United States which experience is equivalent to the minimum experience requirements established by the state board of healing arts;

(2) passed an examination approved by the state board of healing arts covering subjects incident to the education and training of a physician assistant; and

(3) submitted to the state board of healing arts any other information the state board of healing arts deems necessary to evaluate the applicant's qualifications.

(b) The board may refuse to license a person as a physician assistant upon any of the grounds for which the board may revoke such license.

(c) The state board of healing arts shall require every physician assistant to submit with the renewal application evidence of satisfactory completion of a program of continuing education required by the state board of healing arts. The state board of healing arts by duly adopted rules and regulations shall establish the requirements for such program of continuing education as soon as possible after the effective date of this act. In establishing such requirements the state board of healing arts shall consider any existing programs of continuing education currently being offered to physician assistants.

KANS. STAT. ANN. SEC. 65-28A04

KENTUCKY

Certification of physician assistants—Requirements—Endorsement from other state—Renewal of certification.

(1) To be certified by the board as a physician assistant, an applicant shall:
   (a) Submit a completed application form with the required fee;
   (b) Be of good character and reputation;
   (c) Be a graduate of an approved program; and
   (d) Have passed an examination approved by the board within three (3) attempts.

(2) A physician assistant who is authorized to practice in another state and who is in good standing may apply for certification by endorsement from the state of his or her credentialing if that state has standards substantially equivalent to those of this Commonwealth.

(3) A physician assistant's certification shall be renewed upon fulfillment of the following requirements:

(a) The holder shall be of good character and reputation;

(b) The holder shall provide evidence of completion during the previous two (2) years of a minimum of one hundred (100) hours of continuing education approved by the American Medical Association, the American Osteopathic Association, the American Academy of Family Physicians, the American Academy of Physician Assistants, or by another entity approved by the board;

(c) The holder shall provide evidence of completion of a continuing education course on the human immunodeficiency virus and acquired immunodeficiency syndrome in the previous ten (10) years that meets the requirements of KRS 214.610; and

(d) The holder shall provide proof of current certification with the National Commission on Certification of Physician Assistants.

KY. REV. STAT. SEC. 311.844

LOUISIANA

A. Except as otherwise provided for in this Part, an individual shall be licensed by the board before the individual may practice as a physician assistant. The board may grant a license to a physician assistant applicant who:

(1) Submits an application on the forms approved by the board.

(2) Pays the appropriate fee as determined by the board.

(3) Has successfully completed an education program for physician assistants accredited by the Committee on Allied Health Education and Accreditation or its successors and who has passed the physician assistant national certifying examination administered by the National Commission on Certification of Physician Assistants.

(4) Certifies that he is mentally and physically able to engage in practice as a physician assistant.

(5) Has no licensure, certification, or registration as a physician assistant in any jurisdiction under current discipline, revocation, suspension, or probation for cause resulting from the applicant's practice as a physician assistant, unless the board considers such condition and agrees to licensure.

(6) Is of good moral character.

(7) Submits to the board any other information the board deems necessary to evaluate the applicant's qualifications.

(8) Has been approved by the board.

B. A personal interview of a physician assistant applicant shall be required only in those cases where the assistant is making his first application before the board and where discrepancies exist in the application or the applicant has been subject to prior adverse licensure, certification, or registration action.

LOUISIANA REV. STAT. SEC. 1360.24

Qualifications for Licensure

A. To be eligible for licensure under this Chapter, an applicant shall:
    1. be at least 20 years of age;
    2. be of good moral character;
    3. demonstrate his competence to provide patient services under the supervision and direction of a supervising physician by:
        a. presenting to the board a valid diploma certifying that the applicant is a graduate of a physician assistant training program accredited by the Committee on Allied Health Education and Accreditation (CAHEA), or its successors, and by presenting or causing to be presented to the board satisfactory evidence that the applicant has successfully passed the national certification examination administered by the National Commission on Certification of Physician Assistants (NCCPA) or its successors, together with satisfactory documentation of current certification; or
        b. presenting to the board a valid, current physician assistant license, certificate or permit issued by any other state of the United States; provided, however, that the board is satisfied that the certificate, license or permit presented was issued upon qualifications and other requirements substantially equivalent to the qualifications and other requirements set forth in this Chapter;
    4. certify that he is mentally and physically able to engage in practice as a physician assistant;
    5. not, as of the date of application or the date on which it is considered by the board, be subject to discipline, revocation, suspension, or probation of certification or licensure in any jurisdiction for cause resulting from the applicant's practice as a physician assistant; provided, however, that this qualification may be waived by the board in its sole discretion.
B. The burden of satisfying the board as to the eligibility of the applicant for licensure shall be upon the applicant.

LOUISIANA ADMIN. CODE SEC. 1507

MAINE

Except as otherwise provided in this chapter, an individual must be granted a license and a certificate of registration by the Board before the individual may practice as a physician assistant.

A. LICENSE

The Board may grant a license as a physician assistant to an applicant who:

1. submits an application on forms approved by the Board;
2. pays the appropriate fee as determined by the Board; if appropriate, the Board may prorate the fee for licensure. The manner of proration will be explained in the Board's published schedule of fees;
3. has successfully completed an educational program for physician assistants or surgeons assistants accredited by the American Medical Association Committee on Allied Health Education and Accreditation, or the Commission for Accreditation of Allied Health Education Programs, or their successors;
4. has passed the Physician Assistant National Certifying Examination administered by the National Commission on Certification of Physician Assistants or its successor; and
5. has no license, certification or registration as a physician assistant under current discipline, revocation, suspension or probation for cause resulting from the applicant's practice as a physician assistant, and there are no allegations which could form the basis of disciplinary action pending, unless the Board considers such condition and agrees to licensure.

B. CERTIFICATE OF REGISTRATION

Except as otherwise provided in these rules, in order to practice as a physician assistant the individual must have both a license and a certificate of registration. To obtain a certificate of registration, an individual must complete the following:

1. obtain a license as provided in subsection A;
2. submit at least one of the following:
    a. if a physician assistant is employed by or a principle in an individual practice, a signed statement from the primary supervising physician agreeing to provide supervision; or
    b. if a physician assistant is to be employed by or a principle in an organized health care delivery system, a statement from the organized health care delivery system certifying employment and signed by a physician in the organized health care delivery system facility who has been approved as a primary supervising physician; or

      c. if a physician assistant is to be employed by or practice in a group practice, a statement from a primary supervising physician in the group practice agreeing to provide supervision; and

   3. comply with the requirements of Section 6. An individual may not practice until granted a license and certificate of registration by the Board.

CODE MAINE R. SEC. 02 373 2

MARYLAND

Qualifications for Certification as a Physician Assistant.

A. Application. Applicants shall:
  (1) Complete an application on a form approved by the Board;
  (2) Pay an application fee of $150;
  (3) Be at least 18 years old;
  (4) Be of good moral character, and identify two individuals who have known the applicant for 5 years and can attest to the applicant's reputation for honesty and credibility;
  (5) Demonstrate oral and written competency in English by:
    (a) Graduating from an English-speaking professional school, or
    (b) Receiving a grade of 220 on the Test of Spoken English and a grade of 550 on the Test of English as a Foreign Language, Test P.

B. Education.
  (1) Before October 1, 2003, an applicant shall be a graduate from a physician assistant training program that is:
    (a) Accredited by the American Medical Association Committee on Allied Health Education and Accreditation; or
    (b) Equivalent to a program accredited by the American Medical Association Committee on Allied Health Education and Accreditation, and approved by the Board.
  (2) After October 1, 2003, an applicant who graduates from a physician assistant training program shall have:
    (a) A baccalaureate degree; or
    (b) The education equivalent to a baccalaureate degree as determined by the Board.

C. Examination. An applicant shall:
  (1) Pass the national certifying examination for physician assistants given by the NCCPA or an equivalent national certifying examination approved by the Board;
  (2) Receive 100 percent of the minimal composite NCCPA score,

after adjustment for error, in order to pass the examination, or the equivalent score on an equivalent examination; and

(3) Waive the applicant's right to confidentiality of the grade in order that the testing service may submit the grade to the Board.

MARYLAND REGS. CODE TIT. 10. SEC. 32.03.04

MASSACHUSETTS

Requirements for Registration

(1) Any person who commenced practice as a physician assistant in the Commonwealth of Massachusetts prior to January 1, 1990, shall be granted a certificate of registration as a physician assistant by the Board upon submission of proof satisfactory to the Board that:

(a) he or she is of good moral character;

(b) he or she has graduated from a physician assistant training program which holds a valid certificate of program approval issued by the Board;

(c) he or she has passed the certifying examination of the National Commission on Certification of Physician Assistants; and

(d) he or she has been practicing as a physician assistant under the supervision of a registered physician.

(2) Any person who commenced practice as a physician assistant in the Commonwealth of Massachusetts on or after January 1, 1990, shall be granted a certificate of registration as a physician assistant by the Board upon submission of proof satisfactory to the Board that:

(a) he or she is of good moral character;

(b) he or she possesses a baccalaureate degree from an educational institution on the list of accredited colleges of the United States Office of Education, or any like institution approved by the Board;

(c) he or she has graduated from a physician assistant training program which holds a valid certificate of program approval issued by the Board; and

(d) he or she has passed the certifying examination of the National Commission on Certification of Physician Assistants.

(3) The Board may, in its discretion, grant an applicant credit towards satisfaction of the baccalaureate degree requirement set forth in 263 CMR 3.02(2)(b) for education received at an institution outside of the United States if the applicant submits proof satisfactory to the Board that such foreign education is substantially

equivalent to that provided in a baccalaureate degree program in an institution accredited by the United States Office of Education or otherwise approved by the Board.

CODE MASSACHUSETTS REGS. TIT. 263 SEC. 3.02

MICHIGAN

An applicant for a physician's assistant license by examination shall submit a completed application on a form provided by the department, together with the requisite fee. In addition to meeting the requirements of the code and the administrative rules promulgated pursuant thereto, an applicant shall satisfy both of the following requirements:

(a) The applicant shall have satisfactorily completed a program for the training of physicians' assistants approved by the task force.

(b) The applicant shall have passed the certifying examination conducted and scored by the national commission on certification of physicians' assistants.

MICHIGAN ADMIN. CODE R. 338.6301

An applicant for a physician's assistant license by endorsement shall submit a completed application on a form provided by the department, together with the requisite fee. In addition to meeting the requirements of the code and the administrative rules promulgated pursuant thereto, an applicant shall have passed the certifying examination conducted and scored by the National Commission on Certification of Physicians' Assistants and satisfy the following requirements, as applicable:

(a) If the applicant was first licensed, certified, registered, or otherwise approved to practice as a physician's assistant in another state before July 7, 1986, it will be presumed that the applicant meets the requirements of section 16186(1)(a) and (d) of the code.

(b) If the applicant was first licensed, certified, registered, or otherwise approved to practice as a physician's assistant in another state on or after July 7, 1986, the applicant shall have satisfactorily completed a program for the training of physicians' assistants approved by the task force.

MICHIGAN ADMIN. CODE R. 338.6305

MINNESOTA

Qualifications for registration.

Except as otherwise provided in this chapter, an individual shall be registered by the board before the individual may practice as a physician assistant.

The board may grant registration as a physician assistant to an applicant who:

(1) submits an application on forms approved by the board;

(2) pays the appropriate fee as determined by the board;

(3) has current certification from the National Commission on Certification of Physician Assistants, or its successor agency as approved by the board;

(4) certifies that the applicant is mentally and physically able to engage safely in practice as a physician assistant;

(5) has no licensure, certification, or registration as a physician assistant under current discipline, revocation, suspension, or probation for cause resulting from the applicant's practice as a physician assistant, unless the board considers the condition and agrees to licensure;

(6) has a physician-physician assistant agreement, and internal protocol and prescribing delegation form, if the physician assistant has been delegated prescribing authority, as described in section 147A.18 in place at the address of record;

(7) submits to the board a practice setting description and any other information the board deems necessary to evaluate the applicant's qualifications; and

(8) has been approved by the board.

All persons registered as physician assistants as of June 30, 1995, are eligible for continuing registration renewal. All persons applying for registration after that date shall be registered according to this chapter.

MINNESOTA STAT. ANN. SEC. 147A.02

MISSISSIPPI

(1) The State Board of Medical Licensure shall license and regulate the practice of physician assistants in accordance with the provisions of this act.

(2) All physician assistants who are employed as physician assistants by a Department of Veterans Affairs health care facility, a branch of the United States military, or the Federal Bureau of Prisons, and who are practicing as physician assistants in a federal facility in Mississippi on July 1, 2000, and those physician assistants who trained in a Mississippi physician assistant program and have been continuously practicing as a physician assistant in Mississippi since 1976, shall be eligible for licensure if they submit an application for licensure to the Board by December 31, 2000. Physician assistants licensed under this subsection will be eligible

for license renewal so long as they meet standard renewal requirements.

(3) Before December 31, 2004, applicants for physician assistant licensure, except those licensed under subsection (2) of this section, must be graduates of physician assistant educational programs accredited by the Commission on Accreditation of Allied Health Educational Programs or its predecessor or successor agency, have passed the certification examination administered by the National Commission on Certification of Physician Assistants (NCCPA), have current NCCPA certification, and possess a minimum of a baccalaureate degree. Physician assistants meeting these licensure requirements will be eligible for license renewal so long as they meet standard renewal requirements.

(4) On or after December 31, 2004, applicants for physician assistant licensure must meet all of the requirements in subsection (3) of this section and, in addition, must have obtained a minimum of a master's degree in a health-related or science field.

(5) For new graduate physician assistants and all physician assistants receiving initial licenses in the state, except those licensed under subsection (2) of this section, supervision Mississippi State Board of Medical Licensure Page 26 Rules and Regulations, Laws and Policies shall require the on-site presence of a supervising physician for one hundred twenty (120) days.

MISSISSIPPI CODE ANN. SEC. 573-26-3

1. Pursuant to Section 73-43-11, Mississippi Code (1972) Annotated, all Physician Assistants who are employed as Physician Assistants by a Department of Veterans Affairs health care facility, a branch of the United States military, or the Federal Bureau of Prisons and who are practicing as Physician Assistants in a federal facility in Mississippi on July 1, 2000, and those Physician Assistants who trained in a Mississippi Physician Assistant program and have been continuously practicing as a Physician Assistant in Mississippi since 1976, shall be eligible for licensure if they submit an application for licensure to the Board by December 31, 2000, and meet the following additional requirements:

   a. Satisfies the Board that he is at least twenty-one (21) years of age and of good moral character.

   b. Submits an application for license on a form supplied by the Board, completed in every detail with a recent photograph (wallet-size/passport type) attached. A Polaroid or informal snapshot will not be accepted.

   c. Pays the appropriate fee as determined by the Board.

    d. Presents a certified copy of birth certificate.

    e. Proof of legal change of name if applicable (notarized or certified copy of marriage or other legal proceeding).

    f. Provides information on registration or licensure in all other states where the applicant is or has been registered or licensed as a Physician Assistant.

    g. Must have favorable references from two (2) physicians licensed in the United States with whom the applicant has worked or trained.

    h. No basis or grounds exist for the denial of licensure as provided at Article N below.

Physician Assistants licensed under this subsection will be eligible for license renewal so long as they meet standard renewal requirements.

2. Before December 31, 2004, applicants for Physician Assistant licensure, except those licensed pursuant to the paragraph above, must be graduates of Physician Assistant educational programs accredited by the Commission on Accreditation of Allied Health Educational Programs or its predecessor or successor agency, have passed the certification examination administered by the National Commission on Certification of Physician Assistants (NCCPA), have current NCCPA certification, and possess a minimum of a baccalaureate degree, and meet the following additional requirements:

    a. Satisfies the Board that he is at least twenty-one (21) years of age and of good moral character.

    b. Submits an application for license on a form supplied by the Board, completed in every detail with a recent photograph (wallet-size/passport type) attached. A Polaroid or informal snapshot will not be accepted.

    c. Pays the appropriate fee as determined by the Board.

    d. Presents a certified copy of birth certificate.

    e. Proof of legal change of name if applicable (notarized or certified copy of marriage or other legal proceeding).

    f. Provides information on registration or licensure in all other states where the applicant is or has been registered or licensed as a Physician Assistant.

    g. Must have favorable references from two (2) physicians licensed in the United States with whom the applicant has worked or trained.

    h. No basis or grounds exist for the denial of licensure as provided at Article N below.

Mississippi State Board of Medical Licensure

Physician Assistants meeting these licensure requirements will be eligible for license renewal so long as they meet standard renewal requirements.

3. On or after December 31, 2004, applicants for Physician Assistant licensure must meet the following requirements:
   a. Satisfies the Board that he is at least twenty-one (21) years of age and of good moral character.
   b. Submits an application for license on a form supplied by the Board, completed in every detail with a recent photograph (wallet-size/passport type) attached. A Polaroid or informal snapshot will not be accepted.
   c. Pays the appropriate fee as determined by the Board.
   d. Presents a certified copy of birth certificate.
   e. Proof of legal change of name if applicable (notarized or certified copy of marriage or other legal proceeding).
   f. Possesses a master's degree in a health-related or science field.
   g. Has successfully completed an educational program for Physician Assistants accredited by CAAHEP or its predecessor or successor agency.
   h. Passed the certification examination administered by the NCCPA and have current NCCPA certification.
   i. Provides information on registration or licensure in all other states where the applicant is or has been registered or licensed as a Physician Assistant.
   j. Must have favorable references from two (2) physicians licensed in the United States with whom the applicant has worked or trained.
   k. No basis or grounds exist for the denial of licensure as provided at Article N below.

MISSISSIPPI RULES, CH. XXII SEC. 1 (C)

MISSOURI

(1) Applicants shall furnish satisfactory evidence as to their good moral character including a letter of reference from the director of their physician assistant program.

(2) Applicants must present satisfactory evidence of completion of a physician assistant program accredited by the Committee on Allied Health Education and Accreditation of the American Medical Association or by its successor agency the Commission for the Accreditation of Allied Health Education Programs or its

successor agency. A photostatic copy of the applicant's diploma shall be submitted as evidence of satisfactory completion.

(3) Applicants who did not complete a physician assistant program and were employed as physician assistants for three (3) years prior to August 28, 1989, shall have written verification of employment, made under oath, submitted to the board from the physician who supervised the applicant. The supervising physician shall also submit a letter of reference documenting the performance of the physician assistant during the employment period. This verification of employment and letter of reference shall be accepted in lieu of the requirements in section (1) and (2) of this rule.

(4) Applicants shall, upon a form provided by the board, designate any and all physicians who will serve as their supervising physician. A change of physician supervision, for any reason, must be submitted to the board within fifteen (15) days of such occurrence.

(5) Applicants shall have verification of passage of the certifying examination and active certification submitted to the board from the National Commission on Certification of Physician Assistants.

(6) Applicants are required to make application upon forms prepared by the board.

(7) No application will be considered unless fully and completely made out on the specified form and properly attested.

(8) Applicants shall attach to the application a recent unmounted photograph not larger than three and one-half inches by five inches (3 1/2" × 5").

(9) Applications shall be sent to the State Board of Registration for the Healing Arts, P.O. Box 4, Jefferson City, MO 65102.

(10) Applicants shall submit the licensure application fee in the form of a cashier's check or money order drawn on or through a United States bank made payable to the State Board of Registration for the Healing Arts. Personal checks will not be accepted.

(11) Applicants shall have verification of licensure, registration and/or certification submitted from every state and/or country in which the applicants have ever held privileges to practice. This verification must be submitted directly from the licensing agency and include the type of license, registration or certification, the issue and expiration date, and information concerning any disciplinary or investigative actions.

(12) Applicants must submit a complete curriculum vitae from high school graduation to the date of application submission. This

document shall include the name(s) and address(es) of all employers and supervisors, dates of employment, job title, and all professional and nonprofessional activities.

(13) When an applicant has filed an application and an appropriate fee, to be established by the board in conjunction with the director of the Division of Professional Registration for licensure and the application is denied by the board or subsequently withdrawn by the applicant, that fee will be retained by the board as a service charge.

(14) The board may require the applicant to make a personal appearance before the board and/or commission prior to rendering a final decision regarding licensure.

(15) An applicant may withdraw an application for licensure anytime prior to the board's vote on the applicant's candidacy for licensure.

MISSOURI CODE OF REGS. TIT. 4 SEC. 150-7.100

MONTANA

A person may not be licensed as a physician assistant-certified in this state unless the person:

(1) is of good moral character;

(2) is a graduate of a physician assistant training program approved by the American Medical Association's committee on allied health education and accreditation;

(3) has taken and successfully passed an examination recognized by the National Commission on Certification of Physician Assistants;

(4) holds a current certificate from the National Commission on the Certification of Physician Assistants; and

(5) has submitted to the board detailed information on the person's history, education, and experience.

MONTANA CODE ANN. SEC. 37-20-402

NEBRASKA

(1) The board shall issue licenses to persons who are graduates of physician assistant programs approved by the board and have satisfactorily completed a proficiency examination.

(2) The board shall issue temporary licenses to persons who have successfully completed an approved program for the education and training of physician assistants but have not yet passed a proficiency examination. Any temporary license issued pursuant to this

subsection shall be issued for a period not to exceed one year and under such conditions as the board determines, with the approval of the department. The temporary license may be extended by the board, with the approval of the department, upon a showing of good cause.

(3) The board may recognize groups of specialty classifications of training for physician assistants. These classifications shall reflect the training and experience of the physician assistant. The physician assistant may receive training in one or more such classifications which shall be shown on the license issued.

NEBRASKA REV. STAT. SEC. 71-1.107.19

An applicant for licensure as a physician assistant must submit the following:

1. An application for a license to practice as a physician assistant may be submitted on a form provided by the Department or on an alternate format.

   The application must include the following information:
   a. Legal name, first, last, middle/maiden
   b. Mailing address
   c. Permanent address
   d. Telephone number (optional)
   e. E-mail address/fax number (optional)
   f. Place and date of birth
   g. Social Security Number
   h. Official documentation showing successful completion of an approved program for the education of physician assistants sent directly to the Department from the institution.
   i. Certifications of licensure submitted directly to the Department from all states where licensed, certified, or registered as a physician assistant.

   A licensure certification must include the following information:
   (1) Applicant's name;
   (2) License number;
   (3) Date of license issuance and date of expiration;
   (4) Answer the following questions either yes or no; if you answer yes; explain the circumstances and outcome:
       (a) Has the applicant's license ever been suspended?
       (b) Has the applicant's license ever been revoked?
       (c) Has the applicant's license ever had any other disciplinary action(s) taken against it?
       (d) As far as the licensing agency's records are concerned, is the applicant entitled to your endorsement?

    (5) The nature of disciplinary actions, if any, taken against the applicant's license, certificate, or registration;

    (6) Date certification was prepared;

    (7) Signature of official from licensing agency;

    (8) Printed name and title of official from licensing agency;

    (9) Name and address of licensing agency;

    (10) Seal of the licensing agency.

  j. Official documentation showing successful completion of the proficiency examination submitted directly to the Department from the examination entity.

  k. Answer the following questions either yes or no; if you answer yes; explain the circumstances and outcome:

    (1) Has any state or territory of the U.S. ever taken any of the following actions against your license, certificate, or registration? Denied Suspended Revoked Limited

    (2) Has any licensing or disciplinary authority ever taken any of the following actions against your license, certificate, or registration? Denied Suspended Revoked Limited

    (3) Has any licensing or disciplinary authority placed your license, certificate or registration on probation?

    (4) Have you ever voluntarily surrendered a license, certificate, or registration issued to you by a licensing or disciplinary authority?

    (5) Have you ever been voluntarily limited in any way by a license, certificate or registration issued to you by a licensing or disciplinary authority?

    (6) Have you ever been requested to appear before any licensing agency?

    (7) Have you ever been notified of any charges or complaints filed against you by any licensing or disciplinary authority or criminal prosecution authority?

    (8) Have you ever been addicted to, dependent upon or chronically impaired by alcohol, narcotics, barbiturates, or other drugs which may cause physical and/or psychological dependence?

    (9) During the past ten years, have you voluntarily entered or been involuntarily admitted to an institution or health care facility for treatment of a mental or emotional disorder/condition?

    (10) During the last ten years, have you been diagnosed with or treated for bipolar disorder, schizophrenia, or any psychotic disorder?

    (11) Have you ever been convicted of a felony?

(12) Have you ever been convicted of a misdemeanor?

(13) Have you ever been denied a Federal Drug Enforcement Administration (DEA) registration or State controlled substances registration?

(14) Have you ever been called before any licensing agency or lawful authority concerned with DEA controlled substances?

(15) Have you ever surrendered your State or Federal controlled substances registration for reasons other than a move to a state where controlled substances registration was not required?

(16) Have you ever had your State or Federal controlled substances registration restricted in any way?

(17) Have you ever been notified of any malpractice claim against you?

l. List in chronological order all medical activities since graduation, including absences from work except incidental sick leave and usual vacation;

m. Notarized statement from the applicant that states, the statements on the application are true and complete; and

n. The required licensure fee and Licensee Assistance Program (LAP) fee as prescribed in 172 NAC 90-013. 90-003.01B The Department must act within 150 days upon all completed applications for licensure.

172 NEBRASKA CODE ANN. SEC. 90-003

NEVADA

An applicant for licensure as a physician assistant must have the following qualifications:

1. If he has not practiced as a physician assistant for 12 months or more before applying for licensure in this state, he must, at the order of the board, have taken and passed the same examination to test medical competency as that given to applicants for initial licensure.

2. Be able to communicate adequately orally and in writing in the English language.

3. Be of good moral character and reputation.

4. Have attended and completed a course of training in residence as a physician assistant approved by the Committee on Allied Health Education and Accreditation, the Commission on Accreditation of Allied Health Education Programs or the Accreditation Review Committee on Education for the Physician Assistant, which are affiliated with the American Medical Association.

5. Be certified by the National Commission on Certification of Physician Assistants.
6. Possess a high school diploma, general equivalency diploma or post-secondary degree.

NEVADA ADMIN. CODE SEC. 630.280

1. An application for licensure as a physician assistant must be made on a form supplied by the board. The application must state:
   (a) The date and place of the applicant's birth, his sex, the various places of his residence from the date of graduation from high school and at least two references from persons who have knowledge of the applicant's training or experience;
   (b) The applicant's education, including, without limitation, high schools and postsecondary institutions attended, the length of time in attendance at each and whether he is a graduate of those schools and institutions;
   (c) Whether the applicant has ever applied for a license or certificate as a physician assistant in another state and, if so, when and where and the results of his application;
   (d) The applicant's practical training and experience;
   (e) Whether the applicant has ever been investigated for misconduct as a physician assistant or had a license or certificate as a physician assistant revoked, modified, limited or suspended or whether any disciplinary action or proceedings have ever been instituted against him by a licensing body in any jurisdiction;
   (f) Whether the applicant has ever been convicted of a felony or an offense involving moral turpitude; and
   (g) Whether the applicant has ever been investigated for, charged with or convicted of the use or illegal sale or dispensing of controlled substances.
2. The application must also include:
   (a) The name and address of the practice of each supervising physician and the type of practice of the applicant;
   (b) The address of each location where the applicant will practice;
   (c) A description of the medical services to be performed by the physician assistant, including, but not limited to, those medical services to be performed in the supervising physician's office, in a hospital and in other settings; and
   (d) A list of any poisons, controlled substances, dangerous drugs or devices which the supervising physician prohibits the physician assistant to prescribe, possess, administer or dispense in or out of the presence of the supervising physician.

3. An applicant must submit to the board:
   (a) Proof of completion of a training program as a physician assistant which is approved by the Committee on Allied Health Education and Accreditation or the Commission on Accreditation of Allied Health Education Programs, both of which are affiliated with the American Medical Association;
   (b) Proof of passage of the examination given by the National Commission on Certification of Physician Assistants; and
   (c) Such further evidence and other documents or proof of qualifications as required by the board.
4. Each application must be signed by the applicant and sworn to before a notary public or other officer authorized to administer oaths.
5. The application must be accompanied by the applicable fee.
6. An applicant shall pay the reasonable costs of any examination required for licensure.

NEVADA ADMIN. CODE SEC. 630.290

NEW HAMPSHIRE

(a) Applicants for licensure as a physician assistant shall file an application supplied by the board which includes the following:
   (1) Name, home address and telephone number of the applicant;
   (2) Date of birth and sex of the applicant;
   (3) Name, address and telephone number of the applicant's proposed place of employment and registered supervising physician;
   (4) Certification from the RSP or ARSP that he or she has accepted supervisory responsibility for the physician assistant, including the proposed date on which the relationship will commence;
   (5) Documentation of completion of an approved program of education as defined in Med 601.03;
   (6) Verification from the licensing authority of any other state license ever held by the applicant which shows such license to be in good standing;
   (7) Documentation that the applicant has passed an initial examination administered by the NCCPA and continues to hold a valid national certificate issued by that organization or its successor agency; and
   (8) A statement indicating whether the applicant has ever been refused a license or certification by any other licensing or certifying body and if so, the circumstances of the incident;

(9) A statement indicating whether the applicant has ever been or has reason to believe that he or she is, or will soon be, the subject of any kind of disciplinary investigation or action by any hospital, healthcare organization or licensing or certifying body and if so, the nature of the allegations and the subsequent disposition of the action;

(10) A statement indicating whether the applicant has ever been convicted of a felony or misdemeanor, and, if so, the name of the court, the details of the offense, the date of conviction and the sentence imposed;

(11) A statement indicating whether the applicant has been treated for drug or alcohol abuse, or has been hospitalized for any mental illness within the year preceding the filing of the application, or whether the applicant has ever had such treatment or hospitalization for a condition which affected his or her ability to perform the functions of a physician assistant.

(12) A statement that the applicant has arranged for the direct submission of letters of reference from 2 physicians, who have served in an advisory capacity to the applicant. Such letters of reference shall be original, signed documents submitted directly to the board on professional letterhead.

(13) A statement as to whether the applicant is also seeking a temporary license under Part Med 606.

(14) Signature and 3 × 5 inch full face photograph of the applicant.

NEW HAMPSHIRE CODE ADMIN. R. ANN. (MED) SEC. 604.01

NEW JERSEY

a. The board shall issue a license as a physician assistant to an applicant who has fulfilled the following requirements:

(1) Is at least 18 years of age;

(2) Is of good moral character;

(3) Has successfully completed an approved program; and

(4) Has passed the national certifying examination administered by the National Commission on Certification of Physician Assistants, or its successor.

b. In addition to the requirements of subsection a. of this section, an applicant for renewal of a license as a physician assistant shall:

(1) Execute and submit a sworn statement made on a form provided by the board that neither the license for which renewal is sought nor any similar license or other authority issued by another jurisdiction has been revoked, suspended or not renewed; and

(2) Present satisfactory evidence that any continuing education requirements have been completed as required by this act.

c. The board, in consultation with the committee, may accept, in lieu of the examination required by paragraph (4) of subsection a. of this section, proof that an applicant for licensure holds a current license in a state which has standards substantially equivalent to those of this State.

d. The board shall issue a temporary license to an applicant who meets the requirements of paragraphs (1), (2) and (3) of subsection a. of this section and who is either waiting to take the first scheduled examination following completion of an approved program or is awaiting the results of the examination. The temporary license shall expire upon the applicants receipt of notification of failure to pass the examination.

New Jersey Stat. Ann. sec. 45: 9-27.13

NEW MEXICO

The board may license as a physician assistant a qualified person who has graduated from a physician assistant or surgeon assistant program accredited by the national accrediting body as established by rule and has passed a physician assistant national certifying examination as established by rule. The board may also license as a physician assistant a person who passed the physician assistant national certifying examination administered by the National Commission on Certification of Physician Assistants prior to 1986.

New Mexico Stat. Ann. sec. 61-6-7

NEW YORK

1. To qualify for registration as a physician assistant or specialist assistant, each person shall pay a fee of one hundred fifteen dollars to the department for admission to a department conducted examination, a fee of forty-five dollars for each reexamination and a fee of seventy dollars for persons not requiring admission to a department-conducted examination and shall also submit satisfactory evidence, verified by oath or affirmation, that he or she:

   a. at the time of application is at least twenty-one years of age;
   b. is of good moral character;
   c. has successfully completed a four-year course of study in a secondary school approved by the board of regents or has passed an equivalency test;

    d. has satisfactorily completed an approved program for the training of physician assistants or specialist assistants. The approved program for the training of physician assistants shall include not less than forty weeks of supervised clinical training and thirty-two credit hours of classroom work. The commissioner is empowered to determine whether an applicant possesses equivalent education and training, such as experience as a nurse or military corpsman, which may be accepted in lieu of all or part of an approved program; and

    e. in the case of an applicant for registration as a physician assistant, has obtained a passing score on an examination acceptable to the department.

2. The department shall furnish to each person applying for registration hereunder an application form calling for such information as the department deems necessary and shall issue to each applicant who satisfies the requirements of subdivision one of this section a certificate of registration as a physician assistant or specialist assistant in a particular medical specialty for the period expiring December thirty-first of the first odd-numbered year terminating subsequent to such registration.

3. Every registrant shall apply to the department for a certificate of registration. The department shall mail to every registered physician assistant and specialist assistant an application form for registration, addressed to the registrant's post office address on file with the department. Upon receipt of such application properly executed, together with evidence of satisfactory completion of such continuing education requirements as may be established by the commissioner of health pursuant to section thirty-seven hundred one of the public health law, the department shall issue a certificate of registration. Registration periods shall be triennial and the registration fee shall be forty-five dollars.

NEW YORK STAT. C. L. SEC. 6541

NORTH CAROLINA

Except as otherwise provided in this Subchapter, an individual shall obtain a license from the Board before the individual may practice as a physician assistant. The Board may grant a license as a physician assistant to an applicant who has met all the following criteria:

(1) submits a completed application on forms provided by the Board;

(2) pays the fee established by Rule .0121(1) in this Section;

(3) has successfully completed an educational program for physician

assistants or surgeon assistants accredited by the Commission on Accreditation of Allied Health Education Programs or its predecessor or successor agencies and; if licensed in North Carolina after June 1, 1994, has successfully completed a licensing examination approved by the Board;

(4) certifies that he or she is mentally and physically able to engage safely in practice as a physician assistant;

(5) has no license, certificate, or registration as a physician assistant currently under discipline, revocation, suspension or probation for cause resulting from the applicant's practice as a physician assistant;

(6) has good moral character;

(7) submits to the Board any other information the Board deems necessary to evaluate the applicants qualifications; and

(8) if two years or more have passed since graduation from an approved program, the applicant must submit documentation of the completion of at least 100 hours of continuing medication education (CME) during the preceding two years.

21 North Carolina Ann. Code 32 sec. .0102

NORTH DAKOTA

No physician assistant may be employed in the state until the assistant has passed the certifying examination of the National Commission on Certification of Physician Assistants or other certifying examinations approved by the North Dakota state board of medical examiners.

North Dakota Admin. Code sec. 50-03-01-02

Every applicant for licensure shall file a written application, on forms provided by the board, showing to the board's satisfaction that the applicant is of good moral character and satisfies all of the requirements of this chapter including:

a. Successful completion of a medical licensure examination satisfactory to the board;

b. Physical, mental, and professional capability for the practice of medicine in a manner acceptable to the board; and

c. A history free of any finding by the board, any other state medical licensure board, or any court of competent jurisdiction of the commission of any act that would constitute grounds for disciplinary action under North Dakota law; the board may modify this restriction for cause.

http://www.ndbomex.com/MD-Req.htm

OHIO

An individual seeking a certificate of registration as a physician assistant shall file with the state medical board a written application on a form prescribed and supplied by the board. The application shall include all of the following:

(1) Satisfactory proof that the applicant is at least eighteen years of age and of good moral character;

(2) The status of the applicant with respect to eligibility for and application to take, or satisfactory completion of, the examination of the National Commission on Certification of Physician Assistants or a successor organization that is recognized by the board;

(3) Any other information the board requires.

(B) The board shall review all applications received under this section. The board shall determine whether an applicant meets the requirements to receive a certificate of registration not later than sixty days after receiving a complete application. The affirmative vote of not fewer than six members of the board is required to determine that an applicant meets the requirements for a certificate.

A certificate of registration shall not be issued to an applicant unless the applicant is certified by the National Commission on Certification of Physician Assistants or a successor organization that is recognized by the board, except that the board may issue a temporary certificate of registration to an applicant who has not yet taken the examination of the commission or its successor organization but is eligible for and has made application to take the examination. A temporary certificate shall be valid only until the results of the next examinations are available to the board.

(C) At the time of making application for a certificate of registration, the applicant shall pay the board a fee of one hundred dollars, no part of which shall be returned. Such fees shall be deposited in accordance with section 4731.24 of the Revised Code

OHIO REV. CODE SEC. 4730.10

OKLAHOMA

To be eligible for licensure as a physician assistant pursuant to the provisions of Section 519.1 et seq. of this title an applicant shall:

1. Be of good moral character;

2. Have graduated from an accredited physician assistant program recognized by the State Board of Medical Licensure and Supervision; and

3. Successfully pass an examination for physician assistants recognized by the Board.

OkLouisiana Stat. Ann. Tit. 59 sec. 519.4

(a) A Physician Assistant license shall only be issued by the Board upon application filed by the physician assistant.
(b) All applicants for Physician Assistant licenses shall meet the following qualifications:
   (1) Graduation from an accredited Physician Assistant Program recognized by the Board.
   (2) A passing score on the Physician Assistant National Certifying Examination administered by the National Commission on the Certification of Physician Assistants, or its successor. The Board may recognize another national examination to determine the qualifications of the applicant to practice as a physician assistant when such examination has documented its ability to measure such skills and abilities. The applicant must bear the cost of the examination.
   (3) Applicants must be of good moral character.
   (4) Applicants must meet other requirements as determined by the Board.

OKLAHOMA ADMIN. CODE SEC. 435:15-3-1

OREGON

To be licensed by the Board, a physician assistant must have a supervising physician. The supervising physician must be actively licensed in Oregon and in good standing with the Board:
(1) Each application for the licensure of a physician assistant must be signed by the physician assistant and include the following information:
   (a) Specific detailed information relating to the type of supervision to be provided by the supervising physician is to be set forth in the practice description submitted for the applicant by the physician who shall supervise. The practice description must be signed by the supervising physician. All such practice descriptions are subject to Board approval;
   (b) The specialty, type of degree, professional address, and type of practice of the supervising physician;
   (c) All information required by ORS 677.510(1);
   (d) The applicant must provide the Board with sufficient evidence of good moral character.
(2) No applicant shall be entitled to licensure who:

(a) Has failed an examination for licensure in the State of Oregon;

(b) Has had his license or certificate revoked or suspended in this or any other state unless the said license or certificate has been restored or reinstated and the applicant's license or certificate is in good standing in the state which had revoked the same;

(c) Has been refused a license or certificate in any other state on any grounds other than failure in a medical licensure examination; or

(d) Has been guilty of conduct similar to that which would be prohibited by or to which ORS 677.190 would apply.

(3) A person applying for licensure under these rules who has not completed the licensure process within a 12-month consecutive period from date of receipt of the application shall file a new application, documents, letters and pay a full filing fee as if filing for the first time.

OREGON ADMIN. RULES SEC. 847-050-0015

On or after July 12, 1984, an applicant for original licensure as a physician assistant in this state must possess the following qualifications:

(1) Have successfully completed a course in physician assistant training which is approved by the American Medical Association Committee on Allied Health Education and Accreditation (C.A.H.E.A.), the Commission on Accreditation for Allied Health Education Programs (C.A.A.H.E.P.), or the Accreditation Review Commission on Education for the Physician Assistant (A.R.C.P.A.).

(2) Have passed the Physician Assistant National Certifying Examination (PANCE) given by the National Commission on Certification of Physician Assistants (N.C.C.P.A.). Those who have met the requirements of section (1) of this rule may make application for a Limited License, Postgraduate before passing the aforementioned examination with the stipulation that if the examination is not passed within one year from the date of application, the Board shall withdraw its approval.

(3) Applicants that apply for prescription privileges must meet the requirements specified in OAR 847-050-0041.

OREGON ADMIN. RULES SEC. 847-050-0020

PENNSYLVANIA

The Board will approve for certification as a physician assistant an applicant who:

(1) Satisfies the certification requirements in § 16.12 (relating to general qualifications for licenses and certificates).
(2) Has graduated from a physician assistant program approved by the Board.
(3) Has submitted a completed application together with the required fee, under § 16.13 (relating to licensure, certification, examination and registration fees).
(4) Has passed the physician assistant examination.

The Board will approve for certification as a physician assistant an applicant who:
(1) Satisfies the certification requirements in § 16.12 (relating to general qualifications for licenses and certificates).
(2) Has graduated from a physician assistant program approved by the Board.
(3) Has submitted a completed application together with the required fee, under § 16.13 (relating to licensure, certification, examination and registration fees).
(4) Has passed the physician assistant examination.

PENNSYLVANIA ADMIN. CODE SEC. 18.141

Osteopathic

(a) The Board has approved as a proficiency examination the national certification examination on primary care developed by the NCCPA. The Board will maintain a current register of approved proficiency examinations. This register will list the full name of the examination, the organization giving the examination, the mailing address of the examination organization and the date the proficiency examination received Board approval. This register shall be available for public inspection.

(b) The clinical experience required by the Board is at present identical to the clinical experience required by the NCCPA for taking the NCCPA examination on primary care. To qualify for an NCCPA proficiency examination, the applicant's employment history must be verified by the NCCPA in cooperation with the Board and must be evaluated by the NCCPA in relation to specific work criteria.

(c) The Board will approve for certification as a physician assistant an applicant who:
(1) Is of good moral character and reputation.
(2) Has graduated from a physician assistant training program certified by the Board.
(3) Has submitted a completed application detailing his education and work experience, together with the required fee.

(4) Has passed a proficiency examination approved by the Board.

(d) The physician assistant may amend information regarding his education and work experience submitted under the requirements of subsection (c)(3), by submitting to the Board in writing additional detailed information. No additional fee will be required. The file for each physician assistant will be reviewed by the Board to determine whether the physician assistant possesses the necessary skills to perform the tasks that a physician, applying for registration to supervise and utilize the physician assistant, intends to delegate to him as set forth in the protocol contained in the physician's application for registration.

(e) A person who has been certified as a physician assistant by the State Board of Medicine shall make a separate application to the Board if he intends to provide physician assistant services for a physician licensed to practice osteopathic medicine and surgery without restriction.

(f) An application for certification as a physician assistant by the Board may be obtained by writing to the Harrisburg office of the Board.

PENNSYLVANIA STATE BOARD OF OSTEOPATHIC REGS. SEC. 25.161

Note: PAs in Pennsylvania are currently licensed under the state boards of medicine. New regulatory/statutory language is not yet available.

RHODE ISLAND

An applicant seeking licensure to practice in this state as a physician assistant must:

a) be of good character and reputation;

b) have been graduated from a physician assistant training program certified by the AMA's Committee on Allied Health, Education and Accreditation its successor, the Commission on Accreditation of Allied Health Education Programs (CAAHEP) or its successor;

c) have passed a certifying examination approved by the National Commission on Certification of Physician Assistants, or any other national certifying exam approved by the Board, and

d) have submitted a completed application together with the required fee of sixty-two dollars and fifty cents ($62.50).

RHODE ISLAND R5-54-PA-3.1

SOUTH CAROLINA

An application must be submitted to the board on forms supplied by the board. The application must be complete in every detail before it may be approved and must be accompanied by a nonrefundable fee. As part of the application process, the supervising physician and physician assistant must clearly specify in detail those tasks for which approval is being sought. The specific tasks must be included in the scope of practice guidelines and the scope of practice guidelines must accompany the application. When the administrative staff of the board has reviewed the entire application for completeness and correctness, has found the applicant eligible, and the supervising physician and physician assistant have appeared before the committee or a designated board member, a temporary license may be issued. At the next committee meeting the entire application, including scope of practice guidelines, must be considered and, if qualified, the committee may recommend to the board that a permanent license be issued to the physician assistant. If the committee declines to recommend issuance of a permanent license, the committee may extend or withdraw the temporary license.

SOUTH CAROLINA PA PRAC. ACT SEC. 40-47-940

Except as otherwise provided in this article, an individual must obtain a license from the board before the individual may practice as a physician assistant. The board shall grant a license as a physician assistant to an applicant who has:

(1) submitted a completed application on forms provided by the board;

(2) paid the nonrefundable application fees established in this article;

(3) successfully completed an educational program for physician assistants approved by the Commission on Accredited Allied Health Education Programs or its successor organization;

(4) successfully completed the NCCPA certifying examination and provide documentation that he or she possesses a current, active, NCCPA certificate;

(5) certified that he or she is mentally and physically able to engage safely in practice as a physician assistant;

(6) no licensure, certificate, or registration as a physician assistant under current discipline, revocation, suspension, probation, or investigation for cause resulting from the applicant's practice as a physician assistant;

(7) good moral character;

(8) submitted to the board any other information the board considers necessary to evaluate the applicant's qualifications;

(9) appeared before a board member with his or her supervising physician and all original diplomas and certificates and demonstrated knowledge of the contents of this article;

(10) successfully completed an examination administered by the committee on the statutes and regulations regarding physician assistant practice and supervision.

SOUTH CAROLINA PA PRAC. ACT SEC. 40-47-945

SOUTH DAKOTA

The board shall license as a physician assistant and issue an appropriate license to any person who files a verified application with the board signed by both the proposed supervising physician and the physician assistant to be licensed, upon a form prescribed by the board, renders payment of the required fee, and furnishes evidence to the board that the physician assistant applying for licensure:

(1) Is at least eighteen years of age;

(2) Is of good moral character;

(3) Is a resident of South Dakota;

(4) Has completed a course of study approved by the board at an accredited university, college, or school which includes the subjects of anatomy, physiology, biochemistry, pathology, pharmacology, microbiology, medicine, surgery, pediatrics, psychiatry, and obstetrics, and possesses a license of completion of the physician assistant courses of study from the institution;

(5) Has had at least two years' experience with patients in a clinical setting in an associated field such as military medicine, nursing, dentistry, pharmacy, etc. The board shall decide in each individual case as to what experience would be recognized as fulfillment of the requirement;

(6) Has passed an impartially administered examination given and graded by the board or one of equivalency authorized by the board. Such examination may be in writing or oral, or both, and shall fairly test the applicant's knowledge in theoretical and applied primary medical care as it applies to the practice of the physician assistant in at least the subjects of physical diagnosis, laboratory procedures, common childhood diseases and common medical diseases, emergency care and treatment, minor surgery, emergency obstetrics, and common psychiatric disorders. The applicant's professional skill and judgment in the utilization of medical and surgical techniques may also be examined; and

(7) Deleted by SL 1999, ch 192, § 2.

(8) Has submitted verification that neither the physician assistant applicant nor the supervising physician named in the practice agreement are subject to any disciplinary proceeding or pending

complaint before any medical or other licensing board unless such pending complaint is waived by the licensing board.

SOUTH DAKOTA CODIFIED LAWS 36-4A-8

TENNESSEE

(1) Pursuant to T.C.A. §63-19-105, the Committee and Board shall license no person as a physician assistant unless:
   (a) The person is a graduate of a physician assistant training program accredited by C.A.H.E.A., C.A.A.H.E.P. or A.R.C.-P.A.; and
   (b) The person has successfully completed the examination of the National Commission on Certification of Physician Assistants.
(2) Alternatively to 0880-3-.04(1), any person licensed/certified/registered as a physician assistant in another state may be licensed as a physician assistant in Tennessee if both of the following requirements are met:
   (a) The person is a graduate of a physician assistant program accredited by C.A.H.E.A., C.A.A.H.E.P. or A.R.C.-P.A. at the time of graduation; and
   (b) Has practiced as a physician assistant in another state for a period of ten (10) consecutive years immediately prior to seeking licensure in the State of Tennessee.
   (c) All persons licensed pursuant to 0880-3-.04(2) must provide letters of verification of employment. All expenses of verification will be the applicant's responsibility.

RRT SEC. 0880-3-04

To become licensed as a physician assistant in Tennessee, a person must comply with the following procedures and requirements:
(1) Physician Assistant—Licensure by examination:
   (a) An application packet shall be requested from the Committee's administrative office.
   (b) An applicant shall respond truthfully and completely to every question or request for information contained in the application form and submit it along with all documentation and fees required by the form and rules to the Committee's Administrative Office. It is the intent of this rule that activities necessary to accomplish the filing of the required documentation be completed prior to filing an application and that all documentation be filed simultaneously.
   (c) An applicant shall submit with his application a signed and notarized passport type photograph taken within the preceding

12 months and the photo must be affixed to the proper page of the application.

(d) It is the applicant's responsibility to request that a graduate transcript, from an education program approved by the C.A.H.E.A., C.A.A.H.E.P. or A.R.C.-P.A., be submitted directly from the program to the Committee's Administrative Office. The transcript must show that graduation has been completed and carry the official seal of the institution.

(e) An applicant shall submit evidence of good moral character. Such evidence shall be two recent (within the preceding 12 months) original letters from medical professionals, attesting to the applicant's personal character and professional ethics on the signatory's letterhead.

(f) If the applicant intends to immediately commence practice upon licensure he or she must designate a primary supervising physician. Any change in the primary supervising physician must be reported in writing submitted directly to the Committee's Administrative Office by the physician assistant.

(g) An applicant shall disclose the circumstances surrounding any of the following:
    1. Conviction of any criminal law violation of any country, state or municipality, except minor traffic violations.
    2. The denial of professional licensure/certification application by any other state or the discipline of licensure/certification in any state.
    3. Loss or restriction of licensure/certification.
    4. Any civil suit judgment or civil suit settlement in which the applicant was a party defendant including, without limitation, actions involving malpractice, breach of contract, antitrust activity or any other civil action remedy recognized under the country's or state's statutory common or case law.
    5. Failure of any licensure or certification examination.

(h) If an applicant holds or has ever held a license/certificate to practice any profession in any other state, the applicant shall cause to be submitted the equivalent of a Tennessee Certificate of Endorsement (verification of licensure/certification) from each such licensing board which indicates the applicant holds or held an active license/certificate and whether it is in good standing presently or was at the time it became inactive.

(i) An applicant shall submit the Application Fee and State Regulatory Fee as provided in Rule 0880-3-.06.

(j) All applicants shall cause to be submitted documentation of successful completion of the examination for licensure as governed by Rule 0880-3-.08 once the exam has been successfully completed. This verification must be submitted by the examining agency directly to the Committee's Administrative Office.

(k) When necessary, all required documents shall be translated into English and such translation and original document certified as to authenticity by the issuing source. Both versions must be submitted.

(l) Personal resumes are not acceptable and will not be reviewed.

(m) Application review and licensure decisions shall be governed by Rule 0880-3-.07.

(n) All documents submitted for qualification of licensure become the property of the State of Tennessee and will not be returned.

(o) The application form is not acceptable if any portion has been executed and dated prior to one year before filing with the Committee. As used in this part, application means the application form approved by the Committee and shall include, as appropriate:

1. Attached current, notarized passport photograph;
2. Official transcript from physician assistant training program;
3. Verification of N.C.C.P.A. exam;
4. Two (2) original letters of professional recommendation;
5. Certificate of completion or diploma from an approved physician assistant program; and
6. Certification/licensure from other state boards.

(p) All applications shall be sworn to and signed by the applicant and notarized.

RRT SEC. 0880-3-05

TEXAS

(a) Except as otherwise provided in this section, an individual shall be licensed by the board before the individual may function as a physician assistant. A license shall be granted to an applicant who:

(1) submits an application on forms approved by the board;

(2) pays the appropriate application fee as prescribed by the board;

(3) has successfully completed an educational program for physician assistants or surgeon assistants accredited by the

Commission on Accreditation of Allied Health Education Programs, or by that committee's predecessor or successor entities, and holds a valid and current certificate issued by the National Commission on Certification of Physician Assistants ("NCCPA");

(4) certifies that the applicant is mentally and physically able to function safely as a physician assistant;

(5) does not have a license, certification, or registration as a physician assistant in this state or from any other licensing authority that is currently revoked or on suspension or the applicant is not subject to probation or other disciplinary action for cause resulting from the applicant's acts as a physician assistant, unless the board takes that fact into consideration in determining whether to issue the license;

(6) is of good moral character;

(7) submits to the board any other information the board considers necessary to evaluate the applicant's qualifications; and

(8) meets any other requirement established by rules adopted by the board.

(b) The following documentation shall be submitted as a part of the licensure process:

(1) Name Change. Any applicant who submits documentation showing a name other than the name under which the applicant has applied must present certified copies of marriage licenses, divorce decrees, or court orders stating the name change. In cases where the applicant's name has been changed by naturalization the applicant should send the original naturalization certificate by certified mail to the board for inspection.

(2) Certification. Each applicant for licensure must submit:

(A) a letter of verification of current NCCPA certification sent directly from NCCPA, and

(B) a certificate of successful completion of an educational program submitted directly from the program on a form provided by the board.

(3) Verification from other states. Each applicant for licensure who is licensed, registered, or certified in another state must have that state submit directly to the board, on a form provided by the board, that the physician assistant's license, registration, or certification is current and in full force and that the license, registration, or certification has not been restricted, canceled, suspended, or revoked. The other state shall also include a description of any sanctions imposed by or disciplinary matters pending in the state.

(4) State License Registration. Each applicant, if licensed, registered, or certified in another state as a physician assistant, must submit a copy of the license registration certificate to the board. The license, registration, or certificate number and the date of expiration must be visible on the copy.

(5) Arrest Records. If an applicant has ever been arrested, a copy of the arrest and arrest disposition needs to be requested from the arresting authority and that authority must submit copies directly to the board.

(6) Malpractice. If an applicant has ever been named in a malpractice claim filed with any liability carrier or if an applicant has ever been named in a malpractice suit, the applicant must:

(A) have each liability carrier complete a form furnished by this board regarding each claim filed against the applicant's insurance;

(B) for each claim that becomes a malpractice suit, have the attorney representing the applicant in each suit submit a letter directly to the board explaining the allegation, dates of the allegation, and current status of the suit. If the suit has been closed, the attorney must state the disposition of the suit, and if any money was paid, the amount of the settlement. The letter shall be accompanied by supporting documentation including court records if applicable. If such letter is not available, the applicant will be required to furnish a notarized affidavit explaining why this letter cannot be provided; and

(C) provide a statement, composed by the applicant, explaining the circumstances pertaining to patient care in defense of the allegations.

(7) Additional Documentation. Additional documentation as is deemed necessary to facilitate the investigation of any application for licensure must be submitted.

(c) The executive director shall review each application for licensure and shall recommend to the board all applicants eligible for licensure. The executive director also shall report to the board the names of all applicants determined to be ineligible for licensure, together with the reasons for each recommendation. An applicant deemed ineligible for licensure by the executive director may request review of such recommendation by a committee of the board within 20 days of receipt of such notice, and the executive director may refer any application to said committee for a recommendation concerning eligibility. If the committee finds the applicant ineligible for licensure, such recommendation, together with the reasons therefor, shall be submitted to the board unless the applicant requests a hearing within 20 days of receipt of notice of the committee's determination. The hearing shall be before an administrative law judge of the State Office of Administrative Hearings and shall comply with the Administrative Procedure Act and its subsequent amendments and the rules of the State Office of Administrative Hearings and the board. The committee may refer any application for determination of eligibility to the full board. The board shall, after receiving the administrative law judge's proposed findings of fact and conclusions of law, determine the eligibility of the applicant for licensure. A physician assistant whose application for licensure is denied by the board shall receive a written statement containing the reasons for the board's action. All reports received or gathered by the board on each applicant are confidential and are not subject to disclosure under the Public Information Act. The board may disclose such reports to appropriate licensing authorities in other states.

(d) All physician assistant applicants shall provide sufficient documentation to the board that the applicant has, on a full-time basis, actively practiced as a physician assistant, has been a student at an acceptable approved physician assistant program, or has been on the active teaching faculty of an acceptable approved physician assistant program, within either of the last two years preceding receipt of an application for licensure. The term "full-time basis," for purposes of this section, shall mean at least 20 hours per week for 40 weeks duration during a given year. Applicants who do not meet the requirements of subsections (a) and (b) of this section may, in the discretion of the board, be eligible for an unrestricted license or a restricted license subject to one or more of the following conditions or restrictions as set forth in paragraphs (1)–(4) of this subsection:

(1) completion of specified continuing medical education hours approved for Category 1 credits by a CME sponsor approved by the American Academy of Physician Assistants;

(2) limitation and/or exclusion of the practice of the applicant to specified activities of the practice as a physician assistant;

(3) remedial education; and

(4) such other remedial or restrictive conditions or requirements which, in the discretion of the board are necessary to ensure protection of the public and minimal competency of the applicant to safely practice as a physician assistant.

(e) Applicants for licensure:

(1) whose application for licensure which has been filed with the

board office and which is in excess of two years old from the date of receipt, shall be considered inactive. Any fee previously submitted with the application shall be forfeited. Any further application procedure for licensure will require submission of a new application and inclusion of the current licensure fee;

(2) who in any way falsify the application may be required to appear before the board;

(3) on whom adverse information is received by the board may be required to appear before the board;

(4) shall be required to comply with the board's rules and regulations which are in effect at the time the completed application form and fee are filed with the board;

(5) may be required to sit for additional oral or written examinations that, in the opinion of the board, are necessary to determine competency of the applicant;

(6) must have the application of licensure complete in every detail 20 days prior to the board meeting in which they are considered for licensure. Applicants may qualify for a Temporary License prior to being considered by the board for licensure, as required by §185.7 of this title (relating to Temporary License);

(7) who previously held a Texas health care provider license may be required to complete additional forms as required.

TEXAS CODE ANN. SEC. 185.4

UTAH

Each applicant for licensure as a physician assistant shall:
(1) submit an application in a form prescribed by the division;
(2) pay a fee determined by the department under Section 63-38-3.2;
(3) be of good moral character;
(4) have successfully completed a physician assistant program accredited by the Commission on Accreditation of Allied Health Education Programs;
(5) have passed the licensing examinations required by division rule made in collaboration with the board;
(6) meet with the board and representatives of the division, if requested, for the purpose of evaluating the applicant's qualifications for licensure; and
(7) (a) if the applicant desires to practice in Utah, complete a form provided by the division indicating:
(i) the applicant has completed a delegation of services agreement signed by the physician assistant, supervising physician, and substitute supervising physicians; and

(ii) the agreement is on file at the Utah practice sites; or

(b) complete a form provided by the division indicating the applicant is not practicing in Utah and, prior to practicing in Utah, the applicant will meet the requirements of Subsection (7)(a).

UTAH CODE ANN. SEC. 58-70A-302

VERMONT

Applicants for initial certification as a physician assistant shall be interviewed by a board member and may be interviewed by the licensing committee and/or the Board; and shall submit:

(a) The Board's application form, completed in full;

(b) Certified copy of birth certificate;

(c) Verification of certification or licensure in all other states where currently or ever certified or licensed;

(d) Two reference forms from allopathic or osteopathic physicians with whom the applicant has recently worked, including one from the most recent supervising physician. If the applicant has recently graduated from a Board-approved physician assistant program, one form must be from the Director of the program. If the applicant has recently completed a Board-approved apprenticeship program, one form must be from the primary training physician;

(e) Either (1) documentation of completion of a Board-approved physician assistant program sponsored by an institution of higher education and proof of satisfactory completion of the certification examination given by the NCCPA; or (2) documentation of completion of a Board-approved apprenticeship program, including the evaluation conducted by the Board;

(f) Application by the proposed supervising physician(s), including a statement that the physician will be personally responsible for all the medical acts of the physician assistant;

(g) Application by the proposed secondary supervising physician(s), including a statement that the secondary physician will be personally responsible for all the medical acts of the physician assistant only when the supervising physician is unavailable and only when consulted by the physician assistant;

(h) A scope of practice as defined by Rule 5.2(k) and described in Rule 7.3.

(i) A completed applicant's employment contract (form provided by the Board);

(j) The required fee.

Regarding the above items, except the required fee, the Board shall have discretion to require additional information.

VERMONT RULES OF THE BD. OF MED. SEC. II.5.4

VIRGINIA

The applicant seeking licensure as a physician assistant shall submit:
1. A completed application and fee as prescribed by the board.
2. Documentation of successful completion of an educational program as prescribed in §54.1-2951.1 of the Code of Virginia.
3. Documentation of passage of the certifying examination administered by the National Commission on Certification of Physician Assistants.
4. Documentation that the applicant has not had a license or certification as a physician assistant suspended or revoked and is not the subject of any disciplinary proceedings in another jurisdiction.

18 VIRGINIA ADMIN. CODE SEC. 85-50-50

WASHINGTON

Physician assistant qualifications effective July 1, 1999. Individuals applying to the commission under chapter 18.71A RCW after July 1, 1999, must have graduated from an accredited physician assistant program approved by the commission and be certified by successful completion of the NCCPA examination: EXCEPT those applying for an interim permit under RC\V 18.7 1A.020(1) who will have one year from issuance of the interim permit to successfully complete the examination.

WASHINGTON ANN. CODE SEC. 246-918-050

Credentialing of physician assistants. All completed applications for licensure shall be reviewed by a member of the commission or a designee authorized in writing by the commission, prior to licensure.

WASHINGTON ANN. CODE SEC. 246-918-070

Physician assistant—Licensure.
(1) Application procedure. Applications may be made jointly by the physician and the physician assistant on forms supplied by the commission. Applications and supporting documents must be on file in the commission office prior to consideration for a license or interim permit.
(2) No physician assistant or physician assistant-surgical assistant shall begin practice without commission approval of the practice plan of that working relationship. Practice plans must be submitted on forms provided by the commission.
(3) Changes or additions in supervision. In the event that a physician assistant or physician assistant-surgical assistant who is currently

credentialed desires to become associated with another physician, he or she must submit a new practice plan. See WAC 246-918-110 regarding termination of working relationship.

WASHINGTON ANN. CODE SEC. 246-918-080

WEST VIRGINIA

4.1. An application completed by the applicant and a job description signed by the supervising physician listing in numerical order the duties which will be performed by the physician assistant must be in the office of the Board of Medicine, 101 Dee Drive, Charleston, West Virginia 25311, thirty (30) days prior to a Board meeting. Meetings are held bimonthly or as needed, beginning in January. The filing of an application and job description does not entitle a physician assistant to licensure. The Board is the only legal authority for approval and licensure.

4.2. Applications for licensure and the proposed job description shall be accompanied by proof of qualifications as follows:

   a. documentation that the applicant graduated from an approved program,

   b. documentation that the applicant attained a baccalaureate or masters degree,

   c. the required fee,

   d. documentation that the applicant has unencumbered licensure or certification status in all states where he or she was previously licensed or certified, and

   e. documentation that the applicant passed the NCCPA examination. Noncertified physician assistants who are issued a temporary license under W. Va. Code §30-3-16(f) shall sit for and obtain a passing score on the examination next offered following graduation from an approved program. No applicant shall receive a temporary license who, following graduation from an approved program, has sat for and not obtained a passing score on the NCCPA examination.

4.3. The Board may provide interim approval to a physician to supervise a currently licensed physician assistant provided that:

   a. A completed application and proposed job description has been received at the office of the Board of Medicine;

   b. The skills and training of the prospective supervising physician are appropriate to supervise the range of medical services provided for in both the proposed and previously approved job descriptions;

   c. The physician assistant is limited to performing those medical services provided for in the previously approved job description, until the Board has approved the proposed job description; and

d. The licenses of the prospective supervising physician and the physician assistant are in good standing.

4.4. Application for changes to the standard approved job description as provided for in subdivision 13.1. of this rule or a previously approved job description shall be made by the physician assistant or supervising physician thirty (30) days prior to a Board meeting. The proposed job description shall be signed by the supervising physician and physician assistant.

WEST VIRGINIA RULES SEC. 11-1B-4

WISCONSIN

An applicant for examination for licensure as a physician assistant shall submit to the board:

(a) An application on a form prescribed by the board.
Note: An application form may be obtained upon request to the Medical Examining Board office located at 1400 East Washington Avenue, P.O. Box 8935, Madison, Wisconsin 53708.

(b) After July 1, 1993, proof of successful completion of an educational program, as defined in ss. Med 8.02 (4) and 8.04.

(c) Proof of successful completion of the national certifying examination.
(1) Proof that the applicant is currently certified by the National Commission on Certification of Physician Assistants or its successor agency.

(d) The fee specified in s. 440.05 (1), Stats.

(e) An unmounted photograph, approximately 8 by 12 cm., of the applicant taken no more than 60 days prior to the date of application which has on the reverse side a statement of a notary public that the photograph is a true likeness of the applicant.

(2) EXAMINATIONS, PANEL REVIEW OF APPLICATIONS.
(a) All applicants shall complete the written examination under this section, and an open book examination on statutes and rules governing the practice of physician assistants in Wisconsin.

(b) An applicant may be required to complete an oral examination if the applicant:
1. Has a medical condition which in any way impairs or limits the applicant's ability to practice as a physician assistant with reasonable skill and safety.

2. Uses chemical substances so as to impair in any way the applicant's ability to practice as a physician assistant with reasonable skill and safety.

3. Has been disciplined or had certification denied by a licensing or regulatory authority in Wisconsin or another jurisdiction.

4. Has been convicted of a crime, the circumstances of which substantially relate to the practice of physician assistants.

5. Has not practiced as a physician assistant for a period of 3 years prior to application, unless the applicant has been graduated from an approved educational program for physician assistants within that period.

6. Has been found to have been negligent in the practice as a physician assistant or has been a party in a lawsuit in which it was alleged that the applicant has been negligent in the practice of medicine.

7. Has been diagnosed as suffering from pedophilia, exhibitionism or voyeurism.

8. Has within the past 2 years engaged in the illegal use of controlled substances.

9. Has been subject to adverse formal action during the course of physician assistant education, postgraduate training, hospital practice, or other physician assistant employment.

(c) An application filed under this chapter shall be reviewed by an application review panel of at least 2 council members designated by the chairperson of the board to determine whether an applicant is required to complete an oral examination under par.

(d) If the application review panel is not able to reach unanimous agreement on whether an applicant is eligible for licensure without completing an oral examination, the application shall be referred to the board for a final determination.

(e) Where both written and oral examinations are required they shall be scored separately and the applicant shall achieve a passing grade on both examinations to qualify for a license.

1. EXAMINATION FAILURE. An applicant who fails to receive a passing score on an examination may reapply by payment of the fee specified in sub. (1) (d). An applicant may reapply twice at not less than 4-month intervals. If an applicant fails the examination 3 times, he or she may not be admitted to an examination unless the applicant submits proof of having

completed further professional training or education as the board may prescribe.

WISCONSIN ADMIN. CODE SEC. 8.05

WYOMING

Has graduated from a physician assistant program accredited by CAAHEP or its predecessor or successor organization;

Has satisfactorily completed a certification examination administered by NCCPA or other national certifying agency established for such purposes which has been reviewed and approved by the board and is currently certified;

WYOMING STAT. ANN. SEC. 33-26-504

State-by-State Temporary License Requirements

ALABAMA

(a) The board may, in its discretion, grant a temporary license to an applicant who meets the qualifications for licensure as an assistant to physician except that the applicant has not taken the Physician Assistant National Certification Examination (PANCE) or the National Certifying Examination for Anesthesiologist Assistants (NCEAA) for the first time or the applicant has taken the PANCE or the NCEAA for the first time and is awaiting the results. A temporary license is valid:

    (1) For one year from the date issued, or

    (2) Until the results of an applicant's examination are available, or

    (3) Until the board makes a final decision on the applicant's request for licensure as an assistant to physician, whichever comes first.

(b) Assistants to physicians granted a temporary license will not be granted prescriptive privileges, allowed to practice without direct, on-site physician supervision, or allowed to practice in a remote practice site.

(c) The board, in its discretion, may waive the requirements in subsection (b).

(d) An assistant to physician who is granted a temporary license shall not practice or offer to practice in this state unless he or she is registered by the board in accordance with this article and the rules of the board.

(e) There shall be no independent unsupervised practice by an assistant to physician who is granted a temporary license.

ALABAMA CODE SEC. 34-24-301

ALASKA

(a) A member or designee of the board may approve a temporary physician assistant license of an applicant who meets the requirements of 12 AAC 40.400 and 12 AAC 40.408 and pays the fee set out in 12 AAC 02.250.

(b) Temporary license is valid for eight months or until the board meets and considers the application for permanent renewable license, whichever occurs first.

(c) The board will, in its discretion, renew a temporary license once only, based on good cause.

(d) An applicant who has been denied authorization to practice by the board under 12 AAC 40.408 is not entitled to temporary license or to renew a temporary license.

12 ALASKA ADMIN. CODE 40.405

GRADUATE PHYSICIAN ASSISTANT LICENSE.

(a) An applicant for a license to practice as a graduate physician assistant
  (1) shall apply on a form provided by the department;
  (2) shall pay the fees established in 12 AAC 02.250; and
  (3) must be approved by the board.

(b) The application must include
  (1) evidence of having graduated from a physician assistant program accredited by the American Medical Association's Committee on Allied Health Education and Accreditation or the Commission on Accreditation of Allied Health Education Programs; and
  (2) evidence of having been accepted to take the next entry level examination of the National Commission on Certification of Physician Assistants, Inc. (NCCPA) for initial certification.

(c) A graduate physician assistant license is automatically suspended on the date the board receives notice that the applicant failed to take or failed to pass the NCCPA certifying examination required under (b)(2) of this section.

(d) Upon request, the board will reissue a graduate physician assistant license only if the licensee was prevented from taking a scheduled examination.

(e) A licensed graduate physician assistant must be authorized to practice under 12 AAC 40.447 and be under the continuous on-site supervision of a licensed physician assistant authorized to practice under 12 AAC 40.408 or a physician licensed in this state.

AUTHORIZATION TO PRACTICE AS A GRADUATE PHYSICIAN ASSISTANT.

(a) Before an individual can practice as a graduate physician assistant the individual shall

    (1) apply on the form provided by the department;

    (2) pay the collaborative relationship fee established in 12 AAC 02.250;

    (3) hold a graduate physician assistant license issued under 12 AAC 40.445;

    (4) submit documented evidence of an established collaborative relationship under 12 AAC 40.410 and 12 AAC 40.980; and

    (5) be approved by a member or designee of the board.

(b) When licensed and authorized to practice, the licensee shall display a nameplate designating that person as a "graduate physician assistant."

12 ALASKA ADMIN. CODE 40.445

ARIZONA

A. The board may issue a temporary license to an applicant who meets all the qualifications prescribed in section 322521, subsection A, paragraphs 1, 3, 4 and 5, submits evidence to the board that the applicant is eligible to take the certifying examination and pays the prescribed application fee. The applicant shall have the national commission on the certification of physician assistants submit to the board a letter that verifies the applicant's registration to sit for the physician assistant national certifying examination.

B. A temporary license is not effective for a term of more than sixteen months and expires on the occurrence of any one of the following:

    1. Issuance of a regular license.

    2. Failure to pass the certifying examination.

    3. Expiration of the term for which the temporary license was issued.

C. The board shall not issue a temporary license to an applicant who has failed the National Commission on Certification of Physician Assistants examination.

D. A physician assistant who holds a temporary license shall have the National Commission on The Certification of Physician Assistants submit verification directly to the board of that person's successful passage or failure of the physician assistant national certifying examination.

E. A physician assistant who holds a temporary license shall not prescribe any controlled substance as defined in the federal controlled substances act of 1970 (P.L. 91-513; 84 Stat. 1242; 21 United States code section 801).

F.   Before being granted a temporary license, an applicant for a temporary license shall enter into a written agreement with the board to perform health care tasks only at the same geographic work site where the physician assistant's supervising physician sees patients.

ARIZONA REV. STAT. ANN. SEC. 32-2524

ARKANSAS

The Arkansas State Medical Board may grant a graduate license to an applicant who meets the qualifications for licensure, except that the applicant has not yet taken the national certifying examination or the applicant has taken the national certifying examination and is awaiting the results.

A graduate license is valid:

(1) For one (1) year from the date of issuance;

(2) Until the results of an applicant's examination are available; or until the board makes a final decision on the applicant's request for licensure, whichever comes first.

ARKANSAS CODE 17-105-102

CALIFORNIA

An application with the committee may, between the date of receipt of notice that the application is on file and the date of receipt of his or her license, practice as a physician assistant on interim approval under the supervision of an approved physician. Applicants shall notify the committee in writing of any and all supervising physicians under whom they will be performing services prior to practicing under interim approval. If the applicant shall fail to take the next succeeding licensure examination or fails to pass the examination or fails to receive a license, all privileges under this section shall automatically cease upon written notification sent to the applicant by the committee. In the event the licensure examination required by the committee is under a uniform examination system, the applicant shall provide evidence satisfactory to the committee (a) that an application has been filed and accepted for the examination and (b) that the organization administering the examination has been requested to transmit the applicant's scores to the committee in order for the applicant to maintain interim approval. The applicant shall be deemed to have failed the examination unless the applicant provides evidence to the committee within 30 days after scores have been released that he or she has passed the examination.

CALIFORNIA BUS. & PROF. CODE SEC. 3517

COLORADO

No provision in statutes or regulations.

Program graduates who have not taken PANCE can function as a "Physician Extender" under the delegatory authority of the physician. On-site supervision is required and prescribing and dispensing medication is prohibited.

COLORADO BOARD POLICY 20-13

CONNECTICUT

The department may, upon receipt of a fee of seventy-five dollars, issue a temporary permit to an applicant who
(1) is a graduate of an accredited physician assistant program;
(2) has completed not less than sixty hours of didactic instruction in pharmacology for physician assistant practice approved by the department; and
(3) if applying for such permit on and after September 30, 1991, holds a baccalaureate or higher degree in any field from a regionally accredited institution of higher education. Such temporary permit shall authorize the holder to practice as a physician assistant only in those settings where the supervising physician is physically present on the premises and is immediately available to the physician assistant when needed, but shall not authorize the holder to prescribe or dispense drugs. Such temporary permit shall be valid from the date of issuance of same until the date of issuance of the results of the first certification examination scheduled by the national commission following the applicant's graduation from an accredited physician assistant program. Such permit shall become void and shall not be reissued in the event that the applicant fails to pass such examination. Violation of the restrictions on practice set forth in this subsection may constitute a basis for denial of licensure as a physician assistant.

No license or temporary permit shall be issued under this section to any applicant against whom professional disciplinary action is pending or who is the subject of an unresolved complaint.

No person shall practice as a physician assistant or represent himself as a physician assistant unless he holds a license or temporary permit pursuant to this section or training permit issued pursuant to section 20-12h.

CONNECTICUT GEN. STATUTE SEC. 20-12B (B)

DELAWARE

Notwithstanding any provision of this section to the contrary, the Board may grant a temporary license to an individual who has graduated from a physician's or surgeon's assistant program which has been accredited by the Committee on Allied Health Education and Accreditation (CAHEA) of the American Medical Association (AMA) and who otherwise meets the qualifications for licensure but who has not sat for a national certifying examination; provided, that the individual shall sit for the next scheduled national certifying examination. Any temporary license granted by the Board pursuant to this subsection shall be valid until the results of said examination are available from the certifying agency. In the event that the applicant fails to pass the national certifying examination, any temporary license granted by the Board pursuant to this subsection shall be immediately rescinded until such time as the applicant can successfully qualify for licensure as otherwise provided by this chapter. (68 Del. Laws, c. 147, § 2; 68 Del. Laws, c. 345, § 1; 69 Del. Laws, c. 355, §§ 3-5; 71 Del. Laws, c. 102, § 26.)

TIT. 24 DELAWARE CODE SEC. 1770-3A-3(F)

DISTRICT OF COLUMBIA

No provision

FLORIDA

The department may grant to a recent graduate of an approved program, as specified, who expects to take the first examination administered by the National Commission on Certification of Physician Assistants available for registration after the applicant's graduation, a temporary license. The temporary license shall expire 30 days after receipt of scores of the proficiency examination administered by the National Commission on Certification of Physician Assistants. Between meetings of the council, the department may grant a temporary license to practice based on the completion of all temporary licensure requirements. All such administratively issued licenses shall be reviewed and acted on at the next regular meeting of the council. The recent graduate may be licensed prior to employment, but must comply with paragraph (e). An applicant who has passed the proficiency examination may be granted permanent licensure. An applicant failing the proficiency examination is no longer temporarily licensed, but may reapply for a 1-year extension of temporary licensure. An applicant may not be granted more than two temporary licenses and may not be licensed as a physician assistant until he or she passes the examination administered by the National Commission on Certification of Physician Assistants. As prescribed by board rule, the council may require an applicant who does not pass the licensing examination after five or more attempts to complete additional remedial education or training. The council shall prescribe the additional requirements in a manner that permits the applicant to complete the requirements and be reexamined within 2 years after the date the applicant petitions the council to retake the examination a sixth or subsequent time.

FLORIDA STAT. CH. 458.347

GEORGIA

The Board may issue a permit of temporary certification to any applicant who has otherwise met the requirements for Board certification and who has either applied to take the next available examination or has already taken the examination and is awaiting the results thereof, with the following conditions:

1. The applicant must request this permit in writing.
2. The applicant must be issued a permit of temporary certification before performing the duties of a physician's assistant.
3. The applicant's duties must be limited to those contained in the basic job description which is approved by the Board.
4. The permit shall expire upon notification of the applicant's failure to achieve a satisfactory score.
5. The applicant must demonstrate to the satisfaction of the Board that he/she has made or intends to make application for the next examination approved by the Board for which the applicant is eligible.
6. The permit of temporary certification may be issued only one time.

GEORGIA COMP. R. AND REGS. R. 360-5.03(E)

HAWAII

The board shall approve temporary licensure of an applicant under this section. The applicant shall have graduated from a board-approved training program within twelve months of the date of application and never taken a national certifying examination approved by the board but otherwise meets the requirements of this section. The applicant shall file a complete application with the board and pay all required fees. If the applicant fails to apply for, or to take, the first examination scheduled by the board following the issuance of the temporary license, fails to pass the examination, or fails to receive licensure, all privileges under this section shall automatically cease upon written notification sent to the applicant by the board. A temporary license shall be issued only once to each person.

Prior to practicing under temporary licensure, holders of temporary licenses shall notify the board in writing of any and all supervising physicians under whom they will be performing services.

HAWAII REV. STAT. SEC. 453-5.3 (D-E)

An application for a temporary certificate shall be made under oath on a form to be provided by the board. The form shall require the applicant to provide verification from the NCCPA that the applicant is scheduled to take the next scheduled examination. Graduation from a board-approved school or training program shall have occurred within twelve months of the date of application.

HAWAII ADMIN. R. SEC. 16-85-46 (B)

IDAHO

GRADUATE PHYSICIAN ASSISTANT

Certification Examination. Any person who has graduated from an approved program and meets all requirements, but has not yet taken and passed the certification examination, may be licensed with the Board as a graduate physician assistant. Such license shall automatically be canceled upon receipt of the certification examination score if the graduate physician assistant fails to pass the certifying examination.

Board Consideration. Registration as a graduate physician assistant may also be considered by the Board when:

All application requirements have been met as set forth in Subsection 021.01, except receipt of a baccalaureate degree; and

A personal interview with the applicant or the supervising physician or both may be required and will be conducted by a designated member of the Board.

A plan shall be submitted and approved by the Board for the completion of the baccalaureate degree.

No Prescribing Authority. Physician assistants operating under a graduate physician assistant license shall not be entitled to write any prescriptions and shall be required to have a weekly record review by their supervising physician.

IDAHO ADMIN. CODE SEC. 22-01.03.036.01

ILLINOIS

a) A person may obtain a temporary certificate pursuant to Section 14 of the Act by filing an application for physician assistant licensure in accordance with Section 1350.40. In lieu of the certification of successful completion of the examination required in Section 1350.40(a)(2), the applicant shall submit:

   1) Proof of admission to the Physician Assistant National Certifying Examination given by the National Commission on Certification of Physician Assistants or its successor agency; and

   2) An authorization to release examination scores from the National Commission on Certification of Physician Assistants, or its successor agency, to the Department.

b) Qualified applicants shall receive a temporary certificate which shall be valid until:

   1) Notification of failure of the examination;

   2) Certification from the National Commission on Certification of Physician Assistants of passage of the examination, at which time the physician assistant license will be issued; or

   3) 15 months has elapsed.

c) A physician assistant may not practice on a temporary certificate until a notice of employment has been filed in accordance with Section 1350.100 of this Part.

d) Prescriptive authority may not be delegated to a holder of a temporary certificate.

ILLINOIS ADMIN. CODE TIT. 68 SEC. 1350.50

INDIANA

(a) The application for certification of a physician assistant must be made upon forms supplied by the committee.

(b) Each application for certification as a physician assistant or for a temporary permit while waiting for the next committee meeting shall include all of the following information:

   (1) Complete names, address, and telephone number of the physician assistant.

   (2) Satisfactory evidence of the following:

       (A) Completion of an approved educational program.

    (B) Passage of the Physician Assistant National Certifying Examination administered by the NCCPA.

    (C) A current NCCPA certificate.

(3) All names used by the physician assistant, explaining the reason for such name change or use.

(4) Date and place of birth of the physician assistant, and age at the time of application.

(5) Citizenship and visa status if applicable.

(6) Whether the physician assistant has been licensed, certified, or registered in any other jurisdiction and, if so, the dates thereof.

(7) Whether the physician assistant has had any disciplinary action taken against the license, certificate, or registration by the licensing or regulatory agency of any other state or jurisdiction, and the details and dates thereof.

(8) A complete listing of all places of employment, including:

    (A) the name and address of employers;

    (B) the dates of each employment; and

    (C) employment responsibilities held or performed;

that the applicant has had since becoming a physician assistant in any state or jurisdiction.

(9) Whether the physician assistant is, or has been, addicted to, or is chemically dependent upon, any narcotic drugs, alcohol, or other drugs, and if so, the details thereof.

(10) Whether the applicant has been denied a license, certificate, approval, or registration as physician assistant by any other state or jurisdiction, and, if so, the details thereof, including the following:

    (A) The name and location of the state or jurisdiction denying licensure.

    (B) Certification, approval, or registration.

    (C) The date of denial of the certification, approval, or registration.

    (D) The reasons relating to the denial of certification, approval, or registration.

(11) Whether the physician assistant has been convicted of, or pleaded guilty to, any violation of federal, state, or local law relating the use, manufacturing, distributing, sale, dispensing, or possession of controlled substances or of drug addiction, and, if so, all of the details relating thereto.

(12) Whether the physician assistant has been convicted of, or pleaded guilty to, any federal or state criminal offense, felony, or misdemeanor, except for traffic violations that resulted only in fines, and, if so, all of the details thereto.

(13) Whether the physician assistant was denied privileges in any hospital or health care facility, or had such privileges revoked, suspended, or subjected to any restriction, probation, or other type of discipline or limitation, and, if so, all of the details relating thereto, including the name and address of the hospital or health care facility, the date of such action, and the reasons therefore.

(14) Whether the physician assistant has ever been admonished, censured, reprimanded, or requested to withdraw, resign, or retire from any hospital or health care facility in which the physician assistant was employed, worked, or held privileges.

(15) Whether the physician assistant has had any malpractice judgments entered against him or her or settled any malpractice action or cause of action, and, if so, a complete, detailed description of the facts and circumstances relating thereto.

(16) A statement from the supervising physician that the physician assistant is, or will be, supervised by that physician.

(17) A description of the setting in which the physician assistant shall be working under the physician supervision.

(18) The name, business address, and telephone number of the physician under whose supervision the physician assistant will be supervised.

(19) One (1) passport-type photo taken of the applicant within the last eight (8) weeks.

(c) All information in the application shall be submitted under oath or affirmation, subject to the penalties of perjury.

(d) Each applicant for certification as a physician assistant shall submit an executed authorization and release form supplied by the committee that:

(1) authorizes the committee or any of its authorized representatives to inspect, receive, and review;

(2) authorizes and directs any:

(A) person;

(B) corporation;

(C) partnership;

(D) association;

(E) organization;

(F) institute;

(G) forum; or

(H) officer thereof; to furnish, provide, and supply to the committee all relevant documents, records, or other information pertaining to the applicant; and

(3) releases the committee, or any of its authorized representatives, and any:

(A) person;

(B) corporation;

(C) partnership;

(D) association;

(E) organization;

(F) institute;

(G) forum; or

(H) officer thereof;

from any and all liability regarding such inspection, review, receipt, furnishing, or supply of any such information.

(e) Application forms submitted to the committee must be complete in every detail. All supporting documents required by the application must be submitted with the application.

(f) Applicants for a temporary permit to practice as a physician assistant while waiting to take the examination or waiting for results of the examination must submit all requirements of subsection (b), except for subsection (b) (2) (B) and (b) (2) (C), in order to apply for a temporary permit.

(g) A temporary permit becomes invalid if the temporary permit holder fails to sit or fails to register for the next available examination.

INDIANA ADMIN. CODE TIT. 844 R. 2.2-1-5

IOWA

A temporary license may be issued for an applicant who has not taken the NCCPA initial certification examination or successor agency examination or is waiting for the results of the examination.

A temporary license shall be valid for one year from the date of issuance.

The temporary license shall be renewed only once upon the applicant's showing proof that, through no fault of the applicant, the applicant was unable to take the certification examination recognized by the board. Proof of inability to take the certification examination shall be submitted to the board office with written request for renewal of a temporary license, accompanied by the temporary license renewal fee.

If the temporary licensee fails the certification examination, the temporary licensee must cease practice immediately and surrender the temporary license by the next business day.

IOWA ADMIN. CODE R. 645-326.3

KANSAS

(a) The state board of healing arts shall provide for the temporary licensure of any physician assistant who has made proper application for licensure, has the required qualifications for licensure, except for examination, and has paid the prescribed license fee. Such temporary license shall authorize the person so licensed to provide patient services within the limits of the temporary license.

(b) A temporary license is valid (1) for one year from the date of issuance or (2) until the state board of healing arts makes a final determination on the applicant's request for licensure. The state board of healing arts may extend a temporary license, upon a majority vote of the members of the board, for a period not to exceed one year.

KANS. ADMIN. REGS. 65-28A07

KENTUCKY

If grounds for denial of certification do not exist, a temporary certificate may be issued by the board's executive director to a physician assistant after graduation from an approved program and prior to taking the first available approved examination after graduation. This temporary certificate shall enable the holder to practice as a certified physician assistant pursuant to 201 KAR 9:175 only under the direct supervision of a supervising physician at the same practice location. The holder of this temporary certificate shall take the first available approved examination after graduation. If the holder receives a passing score on this examination, the temporary certificate shall be effective until the board approves the holder for permanent certification. If the holder receives a failing score, or fails to take the first available approved examination after graduation, the temporary certificate shall automatically expire. This temporary certificate shall not be renewed or reissued subsequent to expiration or cancellation. The executive director may also issue a temporary certificate to an applicant who otherwise meets all requirements of 201 KAR 9:175, Section 2 (1). The temporary certificate shall remain in effect until the board approves the holder for permanent certification. This temporary certificate shall allow the applicant to practice as a physician assistant pursuant to 201 KAR 9:175, Section 6. However, under no circumstances shall this temporary certificate remain in effect for longer than six (6) months and the temporary certificate shall not be renewable. Any temporary certificate may be cancelled at any time, without a hearing, for reasons deemed sufficient to the executive director, and who shall cancel it immediately upon direction by the board or the board's physician assistant advisory committee or upon the board's denial of the holder's application for permanent certification. When canceling a temporary certificate, the executive director shall promptly notify, by certified United States mail, the holder of the temporary certificate, at the last known address as reflected by the files of the board, and the temporary certificate shall become terminated and of no further force and effect upon receipt of the notice.

201 KAR 9:175 (2)

LOUISIANA

The board may grant a working permit, which is valid for one year but may be renewed by one additional year, to a physician assistant applicant who meets the qualifications for licensure except that the applicant has not yet taken the national certifying examination or the applicant has taken the national certifying examination and is awaiting the results.

A working permit is valid only until the following occur:

(1) The results of an applicant's examination are available.

(2) The board makes a final decision on the applicant's request for licensure.

LOUISIANA REV. STAT. SEC. 1360.24 c

MAINE

TEMPORARY LICENSE

The Board may grant a temporary license to an applicant who meets the qualifications for licensure except that the applicant has not yet taken the national certifying examination or the applicant has taken the national certifying examination and is awaiting the results. A temporary license is valid:

1. for a period not to exceed 18 months from the date of issuance; or

2. until the results of an applicant's examination are available; and

3. until the Board makes a final decision on the applicant's request for licensure whichever comes first.

TEMPORARY LICENSE EXTENSION

A licensee may apply for an extension of a temporary license by submitting an updated application and a written request, which explains the reason for the extension to the Board. If the temporary licensee has not passed a portion of the certifying exam, the request must include:

1. a plan of registration for the next available certifying exam;
2. a statement from the primary supervising physician regarding the capability of the candidate; and any revisions to the plan of supervision during the extension period.

The Board may extend a temporary license, upon a majority vote of the Board members, for a period not to exceed one year. Under no circumstances will the board grant more than one extension of a temporary license.

CODE MAINE R. SEC. 02 373 3

MARYLAND

A. Qualification. The Board may grant a temporary certificate to an applicant who has met all requirements for certification but has not yet taken a national certifying examination if the individual applies for a temporary certificate within 6 months of meeting all other requirements for certification.

B. Duration.
   (1) A temporary certificate is effective until the results of the first examination are available to the Board.
   (2) If an applicant takes and fails the required examination or fails to take the required examination, the temporary certificate shall be withdrawn and the individual shall cease practicing.
   (3) A physician assistant with a temporary certificate may not be permitted to write medication orders.

C. Extension.
   (1) The applicant may apply to the Board for an extension of a certificate.
   (2) An extension will be granted only in extraordinary circumstances when the individual has been prevented, through no fault of the individual, from taking the required examination.
   (3) An application for an extension shall be made as soon as the individual is aware that the individual cannot take the required examination.

MARYLAND REGS. CODE TIT. 10 SEC. 32.03.05

MASSACHUSETTS

Temporary Practice Certificates

(1) Any individual who holds a baccalaureate degree from an accredited educational institution, as defined in 263 CMR 3.02 (2),

and who has completed a physician assistant training program approved by the Board, but who has not yet passed the certifying examination of the National Commission on Certification of Physician Assistants, may obtain a temporary certificate of registration if:

(a) He or she graduated from said physician assistant training program not more than two years prior to the date of his or her application for said temporary certificate;

(b) He or she submits proof satisfactory to the Board that he or she meets all of the requirements for registration as a physician assistant set forth in 263 CMR 3.02 (2) except for passage of the certifying examination; and

(c) He or she certifies in writing, under the pains and penalties of perjury, that he or she will register for and take the next available administration of the certifying examination of the National Commission on Certification of Physician Assistants.

(2) In the event that an individual who obtains a temporary certificate of registration pursuant to 263 CMR 3.04 (1) passes the certifying examination of the National Commission on Certification of Physician Assistants, said temporary certificate of registration shall remain valid and in effect until such time as the Board has issued a permanent certificate of registration to said individual.

(3) In the event that an individual who obtains a temporary certificate of registration pursuant to 263 CMR 3.04 (1) fails the certifying examination of the National Commission on Certification of Physician Assistants, said temporary certificate of registration shall remain valid and in effect, provided that said individual submits a new written certification, under the pains and penalties of perjury, that he or she has registered to retake said certifying examination on a date not more than two years from the date of his or her graduation from an approved physician assistant training program. Upon submission of such proof of registration to retake the certifying examination, the temporary certificate of registration issued to said individual shall remain valid and in effect until the results of said re-examination are published. In the event that said individual fails the second administration of the certifying examination, he or she shall cease practice as a physician assistant immediately upon receipt of the examination results.

(4) An application for a temporary certificate of registration pursuant to this section shall be accompanied by a check or money order made payable to the Commonwealth of Massachusetts in the amount of any application and temporary certificate fees

established by the Commissioner of Administration and Finance pursuant to M.G.L. c. 7, § 3B.

CODE MASSACHUSETTS REGS. TIT. 263 SEC. 3.04

MICHIGAN

The Task force may grant a non-renewable temporary license to an applicant who meets all the requirements for licensure except examination. Valid for a period of time determined by the task force, not to exceed one year or until the exam results are available, which ever is sooner.

MICHIGAN COMPILED LAWS SEC. 17072

Osteopathic

No Provision

MINNESOTA

"Temporary registration" means the status of a person who has satisfied the education requirement specified in this chapter; is enrolled in the next examination required in this chapter; or is awaiting examination results; has a physician-physician assistant agreement in force as required by this chapter, and has submitted a practice setting description to the board. Such provisional registration shall expire 90 days after completion of the next examination sequence, or after one year, whichever is sooner, for those enrolled in the next examination; and upon receipt of the examination results for those awaiting examination results. The registration shall be granted by the board or its designee.

MINNESOTA STAT. ANN. SEC. 147A.01 (25)

MISSISSIPPI

a. The Board may grant a temporary license to an applicant who meets the qualifications for licensure except that the applicant has not yet taken the national certifying examination administered by the NCCPA or the applicant has taken the national certifying examination and is awaiting the results.

b. A temporary license is valid:
    (1) for one hundred eighty (180) days from the date of issuance;
    (2) until the results of an applicant's examination are available; or

(3) until the Board makes a final decision on the applicant's request for licensure, whichever comes first. The Board may extend a temporary license, upon a majority vote of the Board members, for a period not to exceed one hundred eighty (180) days. Under no circumstances may the Board grant more than one extension of a temporary license.

MISSISSIPPI RULES CH. XXII SEC. 4

MISSOURI

The board may issue without examination a temporary license to practice as a physician assistant. Upon the applicant paying a temporary license fee and the submission of all necessary documents as determined by the board, the board may grant a temporary license to any person who meets the qualifications provided in section 334.735 which shall be valid until the results of the next examination are announced. The temporary license may be renewed at the discretion of the board and upon payment of the temporary license fee.

MISSOURI REV. STAT. SEC. 334.736

(1) Applicants for temporary licensure are required to make application on forms prepared by the board.
(2) No application will be considered unless fully and completely made out on the specified forms and properly attested.
(3) Applications shall be sent to the State Board of Registration for the Healing Arts, 3605 Missouri Boulevard, P.O. Box 4, Jefferson City, MO 65102.
(4) The fee for temporary licensure shall be an appropriate fee, to be established by the board. The fee shall be sent in the form of a cashier's check or money order drawn on a United States bank or firm; payable to the State Board of Registration for the Healing Arts. Personal and/or corporate checks will not be accepted. No application will be processed until the licensure fee is received.
(5) All applicants shall attach to the application a recent photograph not larger than three and one-half inches by five inches (3 1/2" × 5").
(6) All applicants are required to submit satisfactory evidence of completion of a physician assistant program accredited by the Committee on Allied Health, Education and Accreditation of the American Medical Association, or its successor. Applicants shall submit official transcripts from their school of graduation confirming the degree awarded and date of degree award or a copy of their diploma.

(7) All applicants are required to submit a letter of reference from the director of the physician assistant program from which the applicant graduated as proof of the applicant's moral character.

(8) All applicants are required to submit verification of licensure, registration or certification from every state or territory in which the applicant is or has ever been licensed, registered or certified to practice as a physician assistant; and all other professional licenses, registrations, or certifications issued to the applicant regardless of whether or not such license, registration or certification is current.

(9) All applicants shall submit a complete curriculum vitae. This document must include the names and addresses of all previous employers, supervisors and job titles, from the date of high school graduation to the date of licensure application.

(10) All applicants shall furnish, on forms provided by the board, verification of physician supervision.

(11) Each applicant shall instruct the National Commission on Certification of Physician Assistants to submit the applicant's admission letter for the certification examination; such letter shall specify the date the applicant is scheduled to take the certification examination.

(12) Each applicant shall instruct the National Commission on Certification of Physician Assistants to submit the applicant's certification examination results directly to the board.

(13) The temporary license shall be valid until the examination results are received by the board, not to exceed three weeks following the mailing of the results by the National Commission on Certification of Physician Assistants.

(14) The temporary license shall automatically terminate if the temporary licensee fails the examination or does not sit for the examination as scheduled. The temporary licensee may apply for temporary licensure renewal pursuant to rule 4 CSR 150-7.310.

(15) Temporary licensees may be issued permanent licensure upon successful passage of the National Commission on Certification of Physician Assistants Examination as determined by the National Commission on Certification of Physician Assistants; submission/completion of all the requirements specified in rule 4 CSR 150-7.100, an updated activities statement, the application form and application fee.

(16) When an applicant has filed his/her application and the appropriate fee for temporary licensure, and the applicant is denied by the board pursuant to the provisions of section 334.100, RSMo and/or rule 4 CSR 150-7.140, or is subsequently withdrawn by

the applicant, the fee will be retained by the board pursuant to the provisions of rule 4 CSR 150-7.200.

(17) The board may require the applicant for temporary licensure to make a personal appearance before the advisory commission and/or board before a final decision regarding licensure is rendered.

(18) An applicant may withdraw his/her application for temporary licensure any time prior to the boards vote on his/her candidacy for licensure.

MISSOURI CODE OF REGS. TIT. 4 SEC. 150-7.300

MONTANA

No temporary license granted to person's who have not passed the national certifying exam.

NEBRASKA

(1) The board shall issue licenses to persons who are graduates of physician assistant programs approved by the board and have satisfactorily completed a proficiency examination.

(2) The board shall issue temporary licenses to persons who have successfully completed an approved program for the education and training of physician assistants but have not yet passed a proficiency examination. Any temporary license issued pursuant to this subsection shall be issued for a period not to exceed one year and under such conditions as the board determines, with the approval of the department. The temporary license may be extended by the board, with the approval of the department, upon a showing of good cause.

(3) The board may recognize groups of specialty classifications of training for physician assistants. These classifications shall reflect the training and experience of the physician assistant. The physician assistant may receive training in one or more such classifications which shall be shown on the license issued.

NEBRASKA REV. STAT. SEC. 71-1.107.19

NEVADA

1. The board will issue a temporary license to any qualified applicant who:

   (a) Meets the educational and training requirements for certification as a physician assistant of the National Commission on Certification of Physician Assistants and is scheduled to and does sit for the first proficiency examination offered by the National Commission on Certification of Physician Assistants following the completion of his training;

(b) Has taken the proficiency examination offered by the National Commission on Certification of Physician Assistants but has not yet been notified of the results; or

(c) Is licensed or certified in another state, meets the requirements for licensure pursuant to NAC 630.280 and is scheduled to sit for the next examination offered by the board.

2. A physician assistant with a temporary license may perform services only under the immediate supervision of a supervising physician.

NEVADA ADMIN. CODE SEC. 630.320

NEW HAMPSHIRE

(a) Otherwise qualified graduates of approved physician assistant programs shall be entitled to receive one temporary license permitting them to practice as a physician assistant during the time period between the board's acceptance of an application for licensure, complete except for proof of the NCCPA certification required by Med 604.01(g), and the date the board receives proof of the results of the first examination given by the NCCPA.

(b) In addition to filling the application for licensure required by Med 604.01, complete except for proof of the NCCPA certification required by Med 604.01(g), applicants seeking temporary license shall:

(1) Provide documentation to the board that the applicant has either taken the national certifying examination and is awaiting those results or that the applicant is eligible for and has registered to take the next available national certifying examination; and

(2) Participate in a personal interview with a representative of the board as required in Med 604.02.

(c) Temporary licenses shall be valid for no more than 12 months, or the date the board receives the applicant's NCCPA examination results, whichever period is shorter, and shall not be extended under any circumstances.

(d) The applicant shall arrange for the board to be directly notified of the NCCPA examination results, and shall also personally notify the board of the examination results within 72 hours from the time the applicant receives such results.

(e) The board shall issue an order terminating the applicant's temporary license immediately upon receipt of written notice from the NCCPA that the applicant has failed the national certification examination. The board's termination order shall specify a date certain no more than 5 days following the mailing date of the order upon which the applicant shall cease performing any of the activities of a physician assistant.

(f) Holders of temporary licenses shall adhere to the same rules of professional conduct, and shall be subject to the same disciplinary sanctions, as holders of permanent license.

New Hampshire Code Admin. R. Ann. (Med) sec. 606.01

NEW JERSEY

a. The board shall issue a license as a physician assistant to an applicant who has fulfilled the following requirements:
(1) Is at least 18 years of age;
(2) Is of good moral character;
(3) Has successfully completed an approved program; and
(4) Has passed the national certifying examination administered by the National Commission on Certification of Physician Assistants, or its successor.

b. In addition to the requirements of subsection a. of this section, an applicant for renewal of a license as a physician assistant shall:
(1) Execute and submit a sworn statement made on a form provided by the board that neither the license for which renewal is sought nor any similar license or other authority issued by another jurisdiction has been revoked, suspended or not renewed; and
(2) Present satisfactory evidence that any continuing education requirements have been completed as required by this act.

c. The board, in consultation with the committee, may accept, in lieu of the examination required by paragraph (4) of subsection a. of this section, proof that an applicant for licensure holds a current license in a state which has standards substantially equivalent to those of this State.

d. The board shall issue a temporary license to an applicant who meets the requirements of paragraphs (1), (2) and (3) of subsection a. of this section and who is either waiting to take the first scheduled examination following completion of an approved program or is awaiting the results of the examination. The temporary license shall expire upon the applicants receipt of notification of failure to pass the examination.

New Jersey Stat. Ann. sec. 45: 9-27.13

NEW MEXICO

If an applicant has met all requirements except NCCPA certification because of the administration date of the exam, the board's secretary/treasurer may issue a temporary license, valid until the next NCCPA exam and receipt of certification. If the applicant fails, the temporary license immediately expires and shall not be renewed.

NEW MEXICO ADMIN. CODE 15:7

NEW YORK

Permits limited as to eligibility, practice and duration, shall be issued by the department to eligible applicants, as follows:

1. Eligibility. A person who fulfills all requirements for registration as a physician assistant except that relating to the examination shall be eligible for a limited permit.
2. Limit of practice. A permittee shall be authorized to practice as a physician assistant only under the direct supervision of a physician.
3. Duration. A limited permit shall expire one year from the date of issuance or upon notice to the permittee by the department that the application for registration has been denied. A limited permit shall be extended upon application for one additional year, provided that the permittee's request for such extension is endorsed by a physician who either has supervised or will supervise the permittee, except that such extension may be denied by the department for cause which shall be stated in writing. If the permittee is awaiting the results of a licensing examination at the time such limited permit expires, such permit shall continue to be valid until ten days after notification to the permittee of the result of such examination.
4. Fees. The fee for each limited permit shall be one hundred five dollars.[5]

NEW YORK STAT. C. L. SEC. 6548

NORTH CAROLINA

(a) During the years prior to 2002, the Board may grant a temporary license, valid for a period not to exceed one year, to an applicant who meets the qualifications for a license except that the applicant has not yet passed a licensing examination approved by the Board. The Board shall not grant a temporary license to an applicant who has twice failed a licensing examination approved by the Board.

(b) A temporary license becomes void at the time the Board grants the physician assistant a full license or at the expiration date shown on the temporary license.

(c) A temporary license shall expire 30 days after the physician assistant receives notice of non-passing scores on the second attempt of taking a licensing examination approved by the Board or at the expiration date of the temporary license, whichever is sooner. The licensee must notify the Board within 15 days upon the receipt of scores.

21 NORTH CAROLINA ANN. CODE 32 SEC. .0103

NORTH DAKOTA

No Provision

OHIO

An individual seeking a certificate of registration as a physician assistant shall file with the state medical board a written application on a form prescribed and supplied by the board. The application shall include all of the following:

(1) Satisfactory proof that the applicant is at least eighteen years of age and of good moral character;

(2) The status of the applicant with respect to eligibility for and application to take, or satisfactory completion of, the examination of the National Commission for Certification of Physician Assistants or a successor organization that is recognized by the board;

(3) Any other information the board requires.

(A) The board shall review all applications received under this section. The board shall determine whether an applicant meets the requirements to receive a certificate of registration not later than sixty days after receiving a complete application. The affirmative vote of not fewer than six members of the board is required to determine that an applicant meets the requirements for a certificate.

A certificate of registration shall not be issued to an applicant unless the applicant is certified by the National Commission on Certification of Physician Assistants or a successor organization that is recognized by the board, except that the board may issue a temporary certificate of registration to an applicant who has not yet taken the examination of the commission or its successor organization but is eligible for and has made application to take the examination. A temporary certificate shall be valid only until the results of the next examinations are available to the board.

(B) At the time of making application for a certificate of registra-
     tion, the applicant shall pay the board a fee of one hundred
     dollars, no part of which shall be returned. Such fees shall be
     deposited in accordance with section 4731.24 of the Revised
     Code.

OHIO REV. CODE SEC. 4730.10

OKLAHOMA

No Provision

OREGON

On or after July 12, 1984, an applicant for original licensure as a physician assistant in this state must possess the following qualifications:

(1) Have successfully completed a course in physician assistant
     training which is approved by the American Medical Association
     Committee on Allied Health Education and Accreditation
     (C.A.H.E.A.), the Commission on Accreditation for Allied Health
     Education Programs (C.A.A.H.E.P.), or the Accreditation Review
     Commission on Education for the Physician Assistant
     (A.R.C.P.A.).

(2) Have passed the Physician Assistant National Certifying Exami-
     nation (PANCE) given by the National Commission on Certification
     of Physician Assistants (N.C.C.P.A.). Those who have met the
     requirements of section (1) of this rule may make application for a
     Limited License, Postgraduate before passing the aforementioned
     examination with the stipulation that if the examination is not
     passed within one year from the date of application, the Board
     shall withdraw its approval.

(3) Applicants that apply for prescription privileges must meet the
     requirements specified in OAR 847-050-0041.

OREGON ADMIN. RULES SEC. 847-050-0020

(1) An applicant for a Physician Assistant license who has suc-
     cessfully completed a course in physician assistant training
     approved by the American Medical Association Council on
     Allied Health Education and Accreditation (C.A.H.E.A.), or
     the Commission on Accreditation for Allied Health Education
     Programs (C.A.A.H.E.P.), or the Accreditation Review Commission
     on Education for the Physician Assistant (A.R.C.E.P.A.) but
     has not yet passed the Physician Assistant National Certifying
     Examination (PANCE) given by the National Commission for the
     Certification of Physician Assistants (N.C.C.P.A.) may be issued a

Limited License, Postgraduate, if the following are met:
(a) The application file is complete;
(b) Certification by the N.C.C.P.A. is pending;
(c) The physician assistant's practice description has been submitted;
(d) The supervising physician is in good standing with the Board; and
(e) The applicant has submitted the appropriate form and fee prior to being issued a Limited License, Postgraduate.
(2) Prescription privileges may be granted with a Limited License, Postgraduate if the supervising physician requests prescription privileges for the physician assistant in the practice description;
(3) A Limited License, Postgraduate may be granted for one year, and may not be renewed.
(4) Upon receipt of verification that the applicant has passed the N.C.C.P.A. examination, and if his or her application file is otherwise satisfactorily complete, the applicant will be reviewed at the next regularly scheduled Board meeting for permanent licensure.
(5) The Limited License, Postgraduate will automatically be canceled if the applicant fails the N.C.C.P.A. examination.

OREGON ADMIN. RULES SEC. 847-050-0023

PENNSYLVANIA

Graduates of PA Programs recognized by the board may register with the board and practice under the direct supervision of a physician until certified by a process recognized by the board. Practice is limited to the period between graduation and receipt of results of the first examination offered after graduation. If the exam is failed authority to practice expires. Must use the title "graduate physician assistant." No prescriptive privileges.

PL SEC. 13.2

Osteopathic

No Provision

RHODE ISLAND

Any graduate of an approved physician assistant training program who has filed a completed application (which includes all documents except for examination scores) for licensure may, upon receiving a receipt from the Division of Professional Regulation, perform as a graduate physician assistant. During this period, such an applicant shall identify himself or herself only as a "graduate physician assistant." If such an applicant shall fail to take the next succeeding examination without due cause or fail to pass the examination without due cause and be licensed, all aforementioned privileges shall automatically cease.

The level of supervision for the graduate physician assistant shall be determined by the supervising physician.

RHODE ISLAND R5-54-PA-6.7

SOUTH CAROLINA

(A) The board may issue a limited physician assistant license to an applicant who has:
  (1) submitted a completed application on forms provided by the board;
  (2) paid the nonrefundable application fees established by this regulation;
  (3) successfully completed an educational program for physician assistants approved by the American Medical Association Counsel on Medical Education;
  (4) never previously failed two consecutive NCCPA certifying examinations and has registered for, or intends to register to take the next offering of, the NCCPA examination;
  (5) certified that he or she is mentally and physically able to engage safely in practice as a physician assistant;
  (6) no licensure, certificate, or registration as a physician assistant under current discipline, revocation, suspension, probation, or investigation for cause resulting from the applicant's practice as a physician assistant;
  (7) good moral character;
  (8) submitted to the board any other information the board considers necessary to evaluate the applicant's qualifications;
  (9) appeared before a board member with his or her supervising physician and all original diplomas and certificates and demonstrated knowledge of the contents of this article;
  (10) successfully completed an examination administered by the committee on the statutes and regulations regarding physician assistant practice and supervision.
(B) A limited license is not renewable and is valid only until the results of a limited licensee's two consecutive NCCPA certifying examinations are reported to the board. When a limited licensee has failed two consecutive NCCPA certifying examinations, or fails one exam and does not take the NCCPA certifying examination at the next

opportunity or, after applying for a limited license, fails to register for the next offering of the examination, the limited license is immediately void and the applicant is no longer eligible to apply for further limited licensure.

(C) The supervising physician of a limited licensee must be physically present on the premises at all times when the limited licensee is performing any task. No on-the-job training, or task not listed on the application, may be approved for a limited license holder.

South Carolina PA Prac. Act sec. 40-47-950

SOUTH DAKOTA

Upon application and payment of a fifty dollar fee, the board may issue a temporary permit to practice as a physician assistant to an applicant who has successfully completed an approved program and the curriculum requirements pursuant to §§ 36-4A-12 and 36-4A-13 and has submitted evidence to the board that he is a candidate accepted to write the examination required by § 36-4A-8 or is awaiting the results of the first examination for which the applicant is eligible after graduation from an approved physician assistant program. A temporary permit may be issued only once and is effective for a term of not more than eight months. A temporary permit expires on the occurrence of the following:

(1) Issuance of a regular license;

(2) Failure to pass the licensing examination; or

(3) Expiration of the term for which the temporary permit was issued.

South Dakota Codified Laws 36-4A-8.1

TENNESSEE

(1) A graduate of an accredited P.A. educational program who is awaiting an opportunity to take the licensure examination may practice as a P.A. upon issuance of a temporary license obtained pursuant to T.C.A. §63-19-105.

(2) Temporary licenses issued pursuant to T.C.A. §63-19-105(a) (2) are subject to the following restrictions:

(a) Initial issuance is valid for only the fifteen (15) month period immediately following graduation from an accredited P.A. educational program.

(b) If a person attempts but fails the first licensure examination and cannot take the examination again during the time remaining on the initially issued temporary license, that license may be extended for an additional one (1) year period from the date of expiration of the initial license upon proof of examination failure.

(c) Temporary licenses are valid only for those who are attempting to take the licensure examination and shall expire if the person fails to take every scheduled examination until successful completion.

(d) Temporary Licenses shall become invalid upon the holder obtaining permanent licensure from the Committee and Board or on the last day of the fifteenth (15th) month after graduation unless extended in which case the license shall become invalid on the last day of the twenty-seventh (27th) month after graduation. In any case, the temporary license expires upon failure to take a scheduled examination.

(e) Persons holding temporary licenses shall be subject to discipline up to and including revocation for the same causes and pursuant to the same procedures as persons holding permanent licenses.

TENNESSEE RRT SEC. 0880-3-14

TEXAS

(a) The board, or its designee may issue a temporary license to an applicant who:

(1) meets all the qualifications for a license under the Physician Assistant Licensing Act but is waiting for the next scheduled meeting of the board for the license to be issued;

(2) seeks to temporarily substitute for a licensed physician assistant during the licensee's absence, if the applicant:

(A) is licensed or registered in good standing in another state, territory, or the District of Columbia;

(B) submits an application on a form prescribed by the board; and

(C) pays the appropriate fee prescribed by the board; or

(3) has graduated from an educational program for physician assistants or surgeon assistants accredited by the Commission on Accreditation of Allied Health Education Programs or by the committee's predecessor or successor entities no later than six months previous to the application for temporary licensure and is waiting for examination results from the National Commission on Certification of Physician Assistants.

(b) A temporary license may be valid for not more than one year from the date issued.

TEXAS CODE ANN. SEC. 185.7

UTAH

(1) An applicant for licensure as a physician assistant who has met all qualifications for licensure except passing an examination component as required in Section 58-70a-302, may apply for and be granted a temporary license to practice under Subsection (2).

(2) (a) The applicant shall submit to the division evidence of completion of a physician assistant program as defined in Subsection 58-70a-302(4).

(b) The temporary license shall be issued for a period ending on the earlier of the date of the next succeeding physician assistant examination, if the applicant does not take that examination, or ten days after the date examination results of the next succeeding physician assistant examination are available to those taking the examination.

(c) A physician assistant holding a temporary license may work only under the direct supervision of an approved supervising or substitute supervising physician in accordance with a delegation of services agreement, and all patient charts shall be reviewed and countersigned by the supervising or substitute supervising physician.

UTAH CODE ANN. SEC. 58-70A-306

VERMONT

(a) The applicant may be issued a temporary certification if:

(1) The applicant is applying for certification for the first time in this state; and

(2) The applicant has graduated from a board-approved school for physician assistants, or has completed a board-approved apprenticeship program; and

(3) Either (A) the applicant is eligible and has applied to sit for the first NCCPA examination (B) the applicant is a graduate of a Board-approved apprenticeship program and has applied to sit for the first Board-approved evaluation available after completion of the application process; and

(4) The required fee is paid,

(5) If the applicant fails the first examination or evaluation, the applicant may sit for the next scheduled examination or evaluation. If the applicant fails the examination or evaluation after the second sitting, the applicant must obtain additional training before sitting again for the examination or evaluation. Temporary certification is not valid during training periods.

In no case shall a temporary certificate be valid for longer than two-years.

VERMONT RULES OF THE BD. OF MED. SEC. II.5.6

VIRGINIA

Pending the outcome of the next examination administered by the NCCPA, an applicant who has met all other requirements of 18VAC85-50-50 at the time his initial application is submitted may be granted provisional licensure by the board. The provisional licensure shall be valid until the applicant takes the next subsequent NCCPA examination and its results are reported, but this period of validity shall not exceed 30 days following the reporting of the examination scores, after which the provisional license shall be invalid.

18 VIRGINIA ADMIN. CODE SEC. 85-50-55

WASHINGTON

(1) The commission shall adopt rules fixing the qualifications and the educational and training requirements for licensure as a physician assistant or for those enrolled in any physician assistant training program. The requirements shall include completion of an accredited physician assistant training program approved by the commission and within one year successfully take and pass an examination approved by the commission, if the examination tests subjects substantially equivalent to the curriculum of an accredited physician assistant training program. An interim permit may be granted by the department of health for one year provided the applicant meets all other requirements. Physician assistants licensed by the board of medical examiners, or the medical quality assurance commission as of July 1, 1999, shall continue to be licensed.

(2) (a) The commission shall adopt rules governing the extent to which:

    (i) Physician assistant students may practice medicine during training; and

    (ii) Physician assistants may practice after successful completion of a physician assistant training course.

(b) Such rules shall provide:

    (i) That the practice of a physician assistant shall be limited to the performance of those services for which he or she is trained; and

    (ii) That each physician assistant shall practice medicine only under the supervision and control of a physician licensed in this state, but such supervision and control shall not be construed to necessarily require the personal presence of the supervising physician or physicians at the place where services are rendered.

(3) Applicants for licensure shall file an application with the commission on a form prepared by the secretary with the approval of the commission, detailing the education, training, and experience of the physician assistant and such other information as the commission may require. The application shall be accompanied by a fee determined by the secretary as provided in RCW 43.70.250 and 43.70.280. A surcharge of twenty-five dollars per year shall be charged on each license renewal or issuance of a new license to be collected by the department and deposited into the impaired physician account for physician assistant participation in the impaired physician program. Each applicant shall furnish proof satisfactory to the commission of the following:

(a) That the applicant has completed an accredited physician assistant program approved by the commission and is eligible to take the examination approved by the commission;

(b) That the applicant is of good moral character: and

(c) That the applicant is physically and mentally capable of practicing medicine as a physician assistant with reasonable skill and safety. The commission may require an applicant to submit to such examination or examinations as it deems necessary to determine an applicant's physical or mental capability, or both, to safely practice as a physician assistant.

(4) The commission may approve, deny, or take other disciplinary action upon the application for license as provided in the Uniform Disciplinary Act, chapter 18.130 RCW.

REV. CODE WASHINGTON SEC. 18.71A.020

Osteopathic

No Provision

WEST VIRGINIA

4.1. An application completed by the applicant and a job description signed by the supervising physician listing in numerical order the duties which will be performed by the physician assistant must be in the office of the Board of Medicine, 101 Dee Drive, Charleston, West Virginia 25311, thirty (30) days prior to a Board meeting. Meetings are held bimonthly or as needed, beginning in January.

The filing of an application and job description does not entitle a physician assistant to licensure. The Board is the only legal authority for approval and licensure.

4.2. Applications for licensure and the proposed job description shall be accompanied by proof of qualifications as follows:

a. documentation that the applicant graduated from an approved program,

b. documentation that the applicant attained a baccalaureate or masters degree,

c. the required fee,

d. documentation that the applicant has unencumbered licensure or certification status in all states where he or she was previously licensed or certified, and

e. documentation that the applicant passed the NCCPA examination. Noncertified physician assistants who are issued a temporary license under W. Va. Code §30-3-16 (f) shall sit for and obtain a passing score on the examination next offered following graduation from an approved program. No applicant shall receive a temporary license who, following graduation from an approved program, has sat for and not obtained a passing score on the NCCPA examination.

4.3. The Board may provide interim approval to a physician to supervise a currently licensed physician assistant provided that:

a. A completed application and proposed job description has been received at the office of the Board of Medicine;

b. The skills and training of the prospective supervising physician are appropriate to supervise the range of medical services provided for in both the proposed and previously approved job descriptions;

c. The physician assistant is limited to performing those medical services provided for in the previously approved job description, until the Board has approved the proposed job description; and

d. The licenses of the prospective supervising physician and the physician assistant are in good standing.

4.4. Application for changes to the standard approved job description as provided for in subdivision 13.1. of this rule or a previously approved job description shall be made by the physician assistant or supervising physician thirty (30) days prior to a Board meeting. The proposed job description shall be signed by the supervising physician and physician assistant.

WEST VIRGINIA RULES SEC. 11-1B-4

Osteopathic

A graduate of an approved program submits a job description and an application for an Osteopathic PA Certificate to the board; the board issues a temporary certificate good for one year. The temporary certificate may be renewed for one year at the request of the supervising physician. A PA who has not been certified by the NCCPA is restricted to working under the direct supervision of a physician.

http://www.aapa.org/grandp/temprov.html

WISCONSIN

(1) An applicant for licensure may apply to the board for a temporary license to practice as a physician assistant if the applicant:
   (a) Remits the fee specified in s. 440.05 (6), Stats.
   (b) Is a graduate of an approved school and is scheduled to take the examination for physician assistants required by s. Med 8.05
      (1) or has taken the examination and is awaiting the results; or
   (c) Submits proof of successful completion of the examination required by s. Med 8.05 (1) and applies for a temporary license no later than 30 days prior to the date scheduled for the next oral examination.
(2) (a) Except as specified in par. (b), a temporary license expires on the date the board grants or denies an applicant permanent licensure. Permanent licensure to practice as a physician assistant is deemed denied by the board on the date the applicant is sent notice from the board that he or she has failed the examination required by s. Med 8.05 (1) (c).
   (b) A temporary license expires on the first day of the next regularly scheduled oral examination for permanent licensure if the applicant is required to take, but failed to apply for, the examination.
(3) A temporary license may not be renewed.
(4) An applicant holding a temporary license may apply for one transfer of supervising physician and location during the term of the temporary license.

WISCONSIN ADMIN. CODE SEC. 8.06

WYOMING

The board may issue a temporary license to any person who successfully completes a CAAHEP or other board-approved program for the education and training of a physician assistant but has not passed a certification examination. To allow the opportunity to take the next available certification examination, any temporary license issued pursuant to this subsection shall be issued for a period not to exceed one (1) year and under conditions as the board determines pursuant to W.S. 33-26-505.

WYOMING STAT. ANN. SEC. 33-26-504

State-by-State Continuing Medical Education Requirements

ALABAMA

(a) Effective January 1, 2003, every physician assistant licensed by the Board shall earn or receive not less than twenty-four (24) hours of Category I continuing medical education within the preceding twenty-four (24) month period ending December 31st as a condition precedent to receiving his or her annual renewal of license.

(b) For the purposes of this Chapter, Category I Continuing Medical Education shall mean those programs of continuing medical education designated as Category I which are sponsored or conducted by those organizations or entities accredited by the Council on Medical Education of the Medical Association of the State of Alabama or by the Accreditation Council for Continuing Medical Education (ACCME) to sponsor or conduct Category I Continuing Medical Education Programs or by the Education Council of the American Academy of Physicians Assistants.

(c) Every physician assistant subject to the minimum continuing medical education requirement established under these rules shall maintain records of attendance or certificates of completion demonstrating compliance with the minimum continuing medical education requirement. Documentation adequate to demonstrate compliance with the minimum continuing medical education requirements of these rules shall consist of certificates of attendance, completion certificates, proof of registration, or similar documentation issued by the organization or entity sponsoring or conducting the continuing medical education program. The records must be maintained by the physician assistant for a period of three (3) years following the year in which the continuing medical education credits were earned and shall be subject to examination by representatives of the State Board of Medical Examiners upon request. Every physician assistant subject to the continuing medical education requirements of these rules must, upon request, submit a copy of such records to the State Board of Medical Examiners for verification.

(d) Every physician assistant shall certify annually that he or she has met the minimum annual continuing medical education requirement established pursuant to these rules. This certification will be made on a form provided on the annual renewal of license application required to be submitted by every physician assistant on or before December 31st of each year.

(e) A physician assistant who is unable to meet the minimum continuing medical education requirement by reason of illness, disability or other circumstances beyond his or her control may apply to the Board for a waiver of the requirement for the calendar year in which such illness, disability or other hardship condition existed. Such waiver may be granted or denied within the sole discretion of the Board and the decision of the Board shall not be considered a contested case and shall not be subject to judicial review under the Alabama Administrative Procedure Act.

ALABAMA ADMIN. CODE R. 540-X-7-.29

ALASKA

Documented evidence that the applicant has met the continuing medical education and recertification requirements of the NCCPA, including the NCCPA recertification examination, and is currently certified by NCCPA;

12 ALASKA ADMIN. CODE 40.470(2)

ARIZONA

Each holder of a regular license shall renew the license on or before June 1 of each year by paying the prescribed renewal fee and supplying the board with information it deems necessary including proof of having completed twenty hours of category I continuing medical education approved by the American Academy of Physician Assistants, the American Medical Association, the American Osteopathic Association or other accrediting organization acceptable to the board within the previous renewal year of July 1 through June 30.

ARIZONA REV. STAT. ANN. SEC. 32-2523(A)

ARKANSAS

Maintain current NCCPA certification.

ARKANSAS CODE 17-105-(110-13)

CALIFORNIA

Training to Perform Additional Medical Services.

A physician assistant may be trained to perform medical services which augment his or her current areas of competency in the following settings:

(a) In the physical presence of an approved supervising physician who is directly in attendance and assisting the physician assistant in the performance of the procedure;

(b) In an approved program;

(c) In a medical school approved by the Division of Licensing under Section 1314;

(d) In a residency or fellowship program approved by the Division of Licensing under Section 1321;

(e) In a facility or clinic operated by the Federal government;

(f) In a training program which leads to licensure in a healing arts profession or is approved as Category I continuing medical education.

CALIFORNIA CODE OF REGS. TIT. 16 SEC. 1399.543

COLORADO

No Provision

CONNECTICUT

Satisfy the mandatory continuing medical education requirements of the national commission for current certification by such commission and has passed any examination or continued competency assessment the passage of which may be required by the national commission for maintenance of current certification by such commission.

CONNECTICUT GEN. STATUTE SEC. 20-12(A)4

DELAWARE

Completion of required renewal form, and submission of documentation of one hundred (100) hours of Continuing Medical Education (CME), forty (40) hours of which shall be of the Category I type as outlined within the AMA Physician's Recognition Award as adopted by the AAPA.

DELAWARE PA REGS. 25.2.2

DISTRICT OF COLUMBIA

An applicant for renewal of a license to practice as a physician assistant shall submit proof pursuant to § 4906.7 of having completed during the two-year (2) period preceding the date the license expires approved continuing medical education as follows:

(a) Forty (40) hours of credit in continuing medical education meeting the requirements of Category 1, as specified in § 4907.2; and

(b) Sixty (60) hours of credit in continuing medical education meeting the requirements of either Category 1 or Category 2

TIT. 17 D.C. MUN. REGS. SEC. 4906

FLORIDA

Each licensed physician assistant shall biennially complete 100 hours of continuing medical education or shall hold a current certificate issued by the National Commission on Certification of Physician Assistants.

The physician assistant must file with the department, before commencing to prescribe, evidence that he or she has completed a continuing medical education course of at least 3 classroom hours in prescriptive practice, conducted by an accredited program approved by the boards, which course covers the limitations, responsibilities, and privileges involved in prescribing medicinal drugs, or evidence that he or she has received education comparable to the continuing education course as part of an accredited physician assistant training program.

The physician assistant must file with the department, before commencing to prescribe, evidence that the physician assistant has a minimum of 3 months of clinical experience in the specialty area of the supervising physician.

The physician assistant must file with the department a signed affidavit that he or she has completed a minimum of 10 continuing medical education hours in the specialty practice in which the physician assistant has prescriptive privileges with each licensure renewal application.

FLORIDA STAT. CH. 458.347 (3-5)

GEORGIA

(1) Physician's Assistants certified to practice pursuant to O.C.G.A. 43-34-101 shall complete Board-approved continuing medical education of not less than (40) hours biennially. Physician's Assistants who are authorized to carry out prescription drug orders shall be required as a part of the number of hours of continuing medical

education required herein, to complete minimum of (3) hours in practice specific pharmaceuticals in which the Physician's Assistant has prescription order privileges. This rule shall not apply to the following persons:

(a) Physician's assistants who are initially certified by the Board and who have not renewed their certification for the first time;

(b) Physician's assistants whose certifications are not active, such as those who are inactive or revoked. Physician's assistants who are suspended or in some way disciplined by the Board must meet the requirement unless otherwise stipulated by Board order;

(c) Physician's assistants specifically exempted from this requirement by Board Order due to cases of hardship, disability, illness, service in the United States Congress, military service or other circumstances as the Board deems appropriate if supported by adequate documentation acceptable to the Board.

(2) The Board accepts the A.M.A. (American Medical Association) Category 1, the A.O.A. (American Osteopathic Association) Category 1, A.A.A.A. (American Academy of Anesthesiologist's Assistants) Category 1, and the A.A.P.A. (American Academy of Physician's Assistants) Category 1 credit as meeting its requirement for Board approval. It is the responsibility of the physician's assistant to verify approval with the source of the program, not with the Board, and the physician's assistant should verify approval before taking the course.

(3) Physician's assistants who must meet the requirement of this Chapter must document the completion of Board-approved continuing education of not less than 40 hours from January 1 of odd numbered years and ending December 31 of even numbered years. This time period constitutes the biennial renewal cycle pursuant to Rule 360-5-.06(1).

(4) Each certified physician's assistant who must meet these requirements must maintain records of attendance and supporting documents for continuing education for a period of 5 years from the date of attendance. At a minimum, the following must be kept: (a) Name of Provider; (b) Date of completion; (c) Evidence of A.M.A. Category 1 credit; A.O.A. Category 1 credit; A.A.P.A. Category 1 credit; or A.A.A.A. Category 1 credit.

GEORGIA COMP. R. AND REGS. R. 360-5.10

HAWAII

Evidence of current NCCPA certification.

HAWAII ADMIN. R SEC. 16-85-46

IDAHO

CONTINUING EDUCATION REQUIREMENTS

Continuing Competence. A physician assistant may be required by the Board at any time to demonstrate continuing competence in the performance of any of the tasks for which he has been previously approved.

Requirements For Renewal. Every other year, and prior to renewal of license for that year, physician assistants will be required to present evidence of having received one hundred (100) hours of continuing medical education over a two-year period. The courses and credits shall be subject to approval of the Board.

IDAHO ADMIN. CODE SEC. 22.01.03.029

ILLINOIS

Certification from the National Commission on Certification of Physician Assistants

ILLINOIS ADMIN. CODE TIT. 68 SEC. 1350.40

INDIANA

"Physician assistant" means an individual who has:
(1) graduated from an approved physician assistant or surgeon assistant program; and
(2) passed the certifying examination and maintains certification by the NCCPA.

INDIANA ADMIN. CODE TIT. 844 R. 2.2-1-5

IOWA

Provide a copy of the initial certification from NCCPA, or its successor agency, sent directly to the board from the NCCPA, or its successor agency. Additionally, provide one of the following documents:
a. Copy of current certification from the NCCPA, or its successor agency, sent directly to the board from the NCCPA, or its successor agency; or
b. Proof of completion of 100 CME hours for each biennium since initial certification.

IOWA ADMIN. CODE R. 645-326.4(4)

KANSAS

On and after February 1, 2001, each physician assistant shall submit with a renewal application one of the following:

(1) Evidence of satisfactory completion of a minimum of 50 continuing education credit hours during the preceding year. A minimum of 20 continuing education credit hours shall be acquired from category I if 50 hours are submitted with the renewal application; or

(2) 100 continuing education credit hours during the preceding two-year period. A minimum of 40 continuing education credit hours shall be acquired from category I if 100 continuing education credit hours are submitted with the renewal application.

(a) A continuing education credit hour shall be 50 minutes of instruction or its equivalent. Meals and exhibit breaks shall not be included in the calculation of continuing education credit hours.

(b) Any applicant that does not meet the requirements for license renewal in subsection (a) may request an extension from the board. The request shall include a plan for completion of the continuing education requirements within the requested extension period. An extension of up to six months may be granted by the board if documented circumstances make it impossible or extremely difficult for the individual to reasonably obtain the required continuing education hours.

(c) Any physician assistant initially licensed within one year of a renewal registration date shall be exempt from the continuing education required by subsection (a) for that first renewal period.

(d) The categories of continuing education credit shall be the following:

(1) Category I: attendance at an educational presentation approved by the board. Courses accepted by the American Academy of Physician Assistants shall be approved by the board; and

(2) Category II: participating in or attending an educational activity that does not meet the criterion specified in paragraph (e)(1) but that is approved by the board. Category II continuing education may include self-study or group activities.

(e) Evidence of satisfactory completion of continuing education shall be submitted to the board as follows:

(1) Documented evidence of attendance at or participation in category I and II activities; and

(2) verification, on a form provided by the board, of self-study from reading professional literature or other self-study activities.

KANSAS ADMIN. REGS. 100-28A-5

KENTUCKY

The holder shall provide evidence of completion during the previous two (2) years of a minimum of one hundred (100) hours of continuing education approved by the American Medical Association, the American Osteopathic Association, the American Academy of Family Physicians, the American Academy of Physician Assistants, or by another entity approved by the board;

The holder shall provide evidence of completion of a continuing education course on the human immunodeficiency virus and acquired immunodeficiency syndrome in the previous ten (10) years that meets the requirements of KRS 214.610; and

The holder shall provide proof of current certification with the National Commission on Certification of Physician Assistants.

KENTUCKY REV. STAT. SEC. 311.844

LOUISIANA

Satisfactory documentation of current certification by the National Commission on Certificate of Physicians Assistants.

LOUISIANA ADMIN. CODE SEC. 1517

MAINE

CONTINUING MEDICAL EDUCATION (CME) REQUIREMENTS
A. Beginning with the biennial licensure renewal in 1996, each physician assistant licensed with this Board shall provide the Board with evidence of having completed one hundred (100) hours of continuing medical education during the preceding twenty-four months. If the time of the first renewal is less than 15 months from initial licensure, continuing medical education requirements will be prorated.
   1. Although the total one hundred (100) hours may be in Category 1, at least forty (40) hours must be in Category 1.
   2. No more than sixty (60) credit hours may be in Category 2.
B. Definitions of Continuing Medical Education Categories:

Category I activities are those planned CME programs sponsored or co-sponsored by an organization or institution and that have been accredited by one or more of the following agencies: American Academy of Physician Assistants; the American Medical Association Council on Medical Education; the Accreditation Council for Continuing Medical Education, and/or the American Academy of Family Practice.

All Category I CME programs must be properly identified as such by the approved sponsoring or co-sponsoring organization.

One credit hour may be claimed for each clock hour of participation.

Each full academic year of post-graduate education and training in a health-related discipline may be claimed as fifty (50) hours of Category 1 credit.

Category 2 activities include CME programs with non-accredited sponsorship, medical teaching, papers, publications, books, presentations or exhibits, non-supervised individual CME activities, staff meetings and other meritorious learning experiences. Category 2 credit hour accrual will be as follows:

1. CME programs with non-accredited sponsorship are those medical meetings and CME programs not within the definition of Category 1. One credit hour is earned for each hour of participation.

2. Medical teaching includes teaching of physician assistant students, medical students, interns, residents, practicing physicians and other health professionals. One credit hour is earned for each hour of participation.

3. Papers, publications, books, as described below are creditable. Credit may be claimed only for the first time the materials are presented and should be claimed as of the date materials were presented or published. Twenty (20) credit hours are earned for each presentation or publication:
   a. a paper published in a recognized medical journal.
   b. each chapter of a book that is written by the physician assistant and published.
   c. presentations or exhibits offered to a professional audience, including allied health professionals.

4. Non supervised individual CME activities. Value: one credit for each hour of participation:
   a. self-instructions such as the reading of medical publications, the use of audio tapes, videotapes, slides, programmed instructions or computer assisted instructions;
   b. self-assessment programs: Peer review activities; e.g., medical audit, utilization review, participation of PRO or its equivalent;
   c. other meritorious learning experiences as individually approved by the Board.

Each full academic year of postgraduate education training in a health-related discipline may be claimed as fifty (50) hours of Category 1 credits.

Code Maine R. sec. 02 373 13

MARYLAND

The supervising physician shall:

A. Delegate the authority to write medication orders; and

B. Ensure that the delegation agreement includes:

   (1) A statement describing whether controlled dangerous substances, noncontrolled substances, and nonprescription medications may be ordered by the physician assistant;

   (2) Evidence of:

   (a) Certification by the National Commission on Certification of Physician Assistants, Inc. within the previous 2 years, or

   (b) Successful completion of 8 Category I hours in pharmacology education within the previous 2 years; and

   (3) An attestation that the physician assistant will comply with:

   (a) State and federal laws governing the prescribing of medications, and

   (b) The protocols established by the hospital, public health facility, correctional facility, or detention center where the physician assistant is requesting permission to write medication orders.

MARYLAND REGS. CODE TIT. 10. SEC. 32.03.07

MASSACHUSETTS

As a condition for renewal of said registration, each registered physician assistant must certify, under the pains and penalties of perjury, that he or she has completed at least 100 hours of continuing education in courses or programs approved by the American Academy of Physician Assistants, the American Medical Association, or like accrediting body approved by the Board, since the date of his or her last registration. At least 40 hours of such continuing education must be in courses or programs which meet the criteria for Category I courses or programs established by the American Medical Association or the American Academy of Physician Assistants. The Board reserves the right to require any registered physician assistant to submit written documentation satisfactory to the Board of his or her completion of all or any part of such continuing education.

CODE MASSACHUSETTS REGS. TIT. 263 SEC. 3.05

MICHIGAN

An applicant for relicensure pursuant to section 16201(4) of the code shall submit a completed application on a form provided by the department, together with the requisite fee. In addition to meeting the other requirements of the code, the applicant shall establish that he or she has passed either the certifying or recertifying examination conducted and scored by the national commission on certification of physicians' assistants within the 6-year period immediately preceding the date of the application.

MICHIGAN ADMIN. CODE R. 338.6308

MINNESOTA

Current certification from the National Commission on Certification of Physician Assistants, or its successor agency as approved by the board;

MINNESOTA STAT. ANN. SEC. 147A.02

MISSISSIPPI

Current NCCPA certification and on or after December 31, 2004, applicants for physician assistant licensure must have obtained a minimum of a master's degree in a health-related or science field.

MISSISSIPPI CODE ANN. SEC. 573-26-3

Each licensed Physician Assistant must show proof of completing 50 hours of CME each year, 20 hours of which must be Category I, as defined by the Accreditation Council for Continuing Medical Education (ACCME). Physician Assistants who are certified by the NCCPA may meet this requirement by providing evidence of current NCCPA certification.

MISSISSIPPI RULES CH. XXII SEC. 4(J)

MISSOURI

All applicants shall have verification of active certification submitted to the board directly from the National Commission on Certification of Physician Assistants.

MISSOURI CODE OF REGS. TIT. 4 SEC. 150-7.125

MONTANA

Must hold a current certificate from the National Commission on Certification of Physician Assistants.

MONTANA CODE ANN. SEC. 37-20-402

NEBRASKA

50 hours Category 1 biennial

http://www.hhs.state.ne.us/crl/msh.htm

NEVADA

1. The Board shall, as a prerequisite for the:
    (a) Renewal of a license as a physician assistant; or
    (b) Biennial registration of the holder of a license to practice medicine, require each holder to comply with the requirements for continuing education adopted by the Board.
2. These requirements:
    (a) May provide for the completion of one or more courses of instruction relating to risk management in the performance of medical services.
    (b) Must provide for the completion of a course of instruction, within 2 years after initial licensure, relating to the medical consequences of an act of terrorism that involves the use of a weapon of mass destruction. The course must provide at least 4 hours of instruction that includes instruction in the following subjects:
        (1) An overview of acts of terrorism and weapons of mass destruction;
        (2) Personal protective equipment required for acts of terrorism;
        (3) Common symptoms and methods of treatment associated with exposure to, or injuries caused by, chemical, biological, radioactive and nuclear agents;
        (4) Syndromic surveillance and reporting procedures for acts of terrorism that involve biological agents; and
        (5) An overview of the information available on, and the use of, the Health Alert Network.
            The Board may thereafter determine whether to include in a program of continuing education additional courses of instruction relating to the medical consequences of an act of terrorism that involves the use of a weapon of mass destruction.
3. The Board shall encourage each holder of a license who treats or cares for persons who are more than 60 years of age to receive, as a portion of their continuing education, education in geriatrics and gerontology, including such topics as:
    (a) The skills and knowledge that the licensee needs to address aging issues;
    (b) Approaches to providing health care to older persons, including both didactic and clinical approaches;
    (c) The biological, behavioral, social and emotional aspects of the aging process; and

(d) The importance of maintenance of function and independence for older persons.

NEVADA REV. STAT. SEC. 630.253

1. The license of a physician assistant may be renewed biennially. The application must be filed with the board not less than 30 days before the expiration of the license. The license will not be renewed unless the physician assistant provides satisfactory proof:
   (a) Of current certification by the National Commission on Certification of Physician Assistants; and
   (b) That he has completed the following number of hours of continuing medical education as defined by the American Academy of Physician Assistants:
      (1) If licensed during the first 6 months of the biennial period of registration, 40 hours.
      (2) If licensed during the second 6 months of the biennial period of registration, 30 hours.
      (3) If licensed during the third 6 months of the biennial period of registration, 20 hours.
      (4) If licensed during the fourth 6 months of the biennial period of registration, 10 hours.
2. A physician assistant shall notify the board within 10 days if his certification by the National Commission on Certification of Physician Assistants is withdrawn.
3. To allow for the renewal of a license to practice as a physician assistant by each person to whom a license was issued or renewed in the preceding renewal period, the board will make such reasonable attempts as are practicable to:
   (a) Mail a renewal notice at least 60 days before the expiration of a license to practice as a physician assistant; and
   (b) Send a renewal application to a licensee at the last known address of the licensee on record with the board.
4. If a licensee fails to pay the fee for biennial registration after it becomes due, his license to practice in this state is automatically suspended. Within 2 years after the date his license is suspended, the holder may be reinstated to practice as a physician assistant if he:
   (a) Pays twice the amount of the current fee for biennial registration to the secretary-treasurer of the board; and
   (b) Is found to be in good standing and qualified pursuant to chapter 630 of NAC.

NEVADA ADMIN. CODE SEC. 630.350

NEW HAMPSHIRE

Certified copy of current national certification issued by the NCCPA.

NEW HAMPSHIRE CODE ADMIN. R. ANN. (MED) SEC. 608.01

NEW JERSEY

The board, or the committee if so delegated by the board, shall:

(1) approve only such continuing professional education programs as are available to all physician assistants in this State on a reasonable nondiscriminatory basis. Programs may be held within or without this State, but shall be held so as to enable physician assistants in all areas of the State to attend;

(2) establish standards for continuing professional education programs, including the specific subject matter and content of courses of study and the selection of instructors;

(3) accredit educational programs offering credits towards the continuing professional education requirements; and

(4) establish the number of credits of continuing professional education required of each applicant for license renewal. Each credit shall represent or be equivalent to one hour of actual course attendance, or in the case of those electing an alternative method of satisfying the requirements of this act, shall be approved by the board and certified pursuant to procedures established for that purpose.

   a. The board may, at its discretion:

   (1) waive the requirements of paragraph (2) of subsection b. of section 4 of this Act 1 for due cause; and

   (2) accredit courses with non-hourly attendance, including home study courses, with appropriate procedures for the issuance of credit upon satisfactory proof of the completion of such courses.

   b. If any applicant for renewal of registration completes a number of credit hours in excess of the number established pursuant to paragraph (4) of subsection a. of this section, the excess credit may, at the discretion of the board, be applicable to the continuing education requirement for the following biennial renewal period but shall not be applicable thereafter.

NEW JERSEY STAT. ANN. SEC. 45: 9-27.25

NEW MEXICO

A physician assistant shall biennially submit proof of current certification by the national Commission on Certification of Physician

Assistants and shall renew the license and registration of supervision of the physician assistant with the board. Applications for licensure or registration of supervision shall include the applicant's name, current address, the name and office address of the supervising licensed physician and other additional information as the board deems necessary.

NEW MEXICO STAT. ANN. SEC. 61-6-7

NEW YORK

Physician assistants must complete course work or training appropriate to their practice regarding infection control and barrier precautions, including engineering and work controls to prevent the transmission of human immunodeficiency virus (HIV) and the hepatitis b virus (HBV) in the course of professional practice. Coursework must be completed **no later than 90 days** after initial licensure/registration and every four years thereafter. You must attest compliance to the State Education Department at the time of each registration.

If you graduated from a New York State program after September 1, 1993, you are automatically credited with having completed the initial requirement as part of your coursework.

http://www.op.nysed.gov/rpa.htm#educ

No other provisions

NORTH CAROLINA

(a) In order to maintain physician assistant licensure, documentation must be maintained by the physician assistant of 100 hours of continuing medical education (CME) completed for every two year period, at least 40 hours of which must be American Academy of Physician Assistants Category I CME or the equivalent. CME documentation must be available for inspection by the Board or an agent of the Board upon request.

(b) Any physician assistant who prescribes controlled substances shall complete at least three hours of CME every two years on the medical and social effects of the misuse and abuse of alcohol, nicotine, prescription drugs (including controlled substances), and illicit drugs.

21 NORTH CAROLINA ANN. CODE 32 SEC. .0106

NORTH DAKOTA

Every second year after the initial licensure of a physician assistant, the assistant's license renewal application must be accompanied with evidence of the successful completion of one hundred hours of continued education for physician assistants. Every sixth year, the applicant must demonstrate that the applicant has successfully passed reexamination by the national commission on certification of physician assistants or other certifying reexamination approved by the board.

NORTH DAKOTA ADMIN. CODE SEC. 50-03-01-14

OHIO

To be eligible for renewal, a physician assistant must certify to the board both of the following:

(1) That the physician assistant has maintained certification by the national commission on certification of physician assistants or a successor organization that is recognized by the board by meeting the standards to hold current certification from the commission or its successor, including completion of continuing medical education requirements and passing periodic recertification examinations;

(2) Except as provided in division (D) of this section, that the physician assistant has completed during the current registration period not less than one hundred hours of continuing medical education acceptable to the board. The board shall adopt rules in accordance with Chapter 119. of the Revised Code specifying the types of continuing medical education that must be completed to fulfill the board's requirements. The board shall not adopt rules that require a physician assistant to complete in any registration period more than one hundred hours of continuing medical education acceptable to the board. In fulfilling the board's requirements, a physician assistant may use continuing medical education courses or programs completed to maintain certification by the National Commission on Certification of Physician Assistants or a successor organization that is recognized by the board if the standards for acceptable courses and programs of the commission or its successor are at least equivalent to the standards established by the board.

OHIO REV. CODE SEC. 4730.12(B)

OKLAHOMA

Licenses issued to physician assistants shall be renewed annually on a date determined by the State Board of Medical Licensure and Supervision. Each application for renewal shall document that the physician assistant has earned at least twenty (20) hours of continuing medical education during the preceding calendar year.

OKLOUISIANA STAT. ANN. TIT. 59 SEC. 519.8

(a) Applicants initially licensed as a physician assistant will be exempt from reporting Continuing Medical Education (CME) credits until one year after licensure, thereafter each applicant for renewal must provide evidence that he or she has successfully earned at least twenty (20) hours of Category I CME hours.

(b) At least one (1) hour of Category I CME shall be earned each calendar year concerning the topic of substance abuse.

(c) The CME hours shall be logged and reported to the Board on an annual basis by the Oklahoma Academy of Physician Assistants, Inc. The applicant shall bear the cost of this requirement.

OKLAHOMA ADMIN. CODE SEC. 435:15-3-17

OREGON

Maintain NCCPA Certification.

OREGON ADMIN. RULES SEC. 847-050-0015

PENNSYLVANIA

To be eligible for renewal of physician assistant certification, the physician assistant shall maintain his National certification by completing current recertification mechanisms available to the profession and recognized by the Board.

PENNSYLVANIA ADMIN. CODE SEC. 18.145

RHODE ISLAND

Pursuant to section 5-54-12.1 of the Rhode Island General Laws, as amended, every physician assistant licensed to practice within the state shall be required to have satisfactorily completed ten (10) hours of approved continuing medical education annually.

The annual period for accumulation of continuing medical education hours shall commence on the first day of July and run through the thirty-first day of June. Beginning with the annual renewal period commencing the first day of July 1997, the Administrator shall not renew the certificate of licensure until satisfactory evidence of completion of the required continuing medical education has been provided to the Division.

Course descriptions, proof of attendance, or other documentation of completion shall be retained by the licensee for a minimum of four (4) years and is subject to random audit by the Board.

RHODE ISLAND R5-54-PA-7.0

SOUTH CAROLINA

A physician assistant's license must be renewed on or before the first of January of each licensure period. Upon payment of the nonrefundable renewal fee provided for in Section 40-47-1015 and submission of documentation that the physician assistant certificate with the National Commission on Certification of Physician Assistants, Inc., or its successor, is active and current, the board shall renew the physician assistant's license.

SOUTH CAROLINA PA PRAC. ACT SEC. 40-47-1010

SOUTH DAKOTA

A renewal request shall be accompanied by the prescribed fee together with evidence satisfactory to the board of the completion during the preceding twelve months of at least thirty hours of post-graduate studies in family medicine approved by the board.

SOUTH DAKOTA CODIFIED LAWS 36-4A-32

TENNESSEE

(1) Continuing Education—Hours Required
  (a) All physician assistants must, within a two (2) year period prior to the application for license renewal, complete one hundred (100) hours of continuing medical education satisfactory to the Committee. The division of hours between Category I and Category II continuing medical education must be consistent with the requirements of the N.C.C.P.A. as described on the most current N.C.C.P.A. "Continuing Medical Education Logging Form."
  (b) The Committee approves a course for only the number of hours contained in the course. The approved hours of any individual course will not be counted more than once in a calendar year toward the required hourly total regardless of the number of times the course is attended or completed by any individual.
  (c) The committee may waive or otherwise modify the requirements of this rule in cases where there is retirement or an illness, disability or other undue hardship which prevents a physician assistant from obtaining the requisite number of continuing education hours required for renewal. Requests for waivers or modification must be sent in writing to the Committee prior to the expiration of the renewal period in which the continuing education is due.

(2) Continuing Education—Proof of Compliance

   (a) All physician assistants must indicate, by their signature on the license renewal form, that they have completed the required number of continuing medical education hours, during whichever of the following two (2) year periods applies to the applicant:

      1. For those certified by the N.C.C.P.A.; the most recent two (2) year period (depending upon the year of initial certification of the applicant by the N.C.C.P.A.) utilized by N.C.C.P.A. to determine whether that person has obtained sufficient continuing medical education hours to maintain his or her professional certification.

      2. For those not certified by the N.C.C.P.A.; the most recent two (2) year period (depending upon the year of birth of the licensee rather than the year of initial certification by the N.C.C.P.A.), which if utilized by the N.C.C.P.A. would determine whether that person would have (had he or she been nationally certified) obtained sufficient continuing medical education hours to maintain his or her professional certification.

   (b) All physician assistants must retain independent documentation of completion of all continuing education hours. This documentation must be retained for a period of four (4) years from the end of the renewal period in which the continuing education was acquired. This documentation must be produced for inspection and verification, if requested in writing by the Committee during its verification process.

      1. Certificates verifying the licensed individual's completion of the continuing education program(s) consist of any one or more of the following:

         (i) The National Commission on the Certification of Physician Assistants' "Continuing Medical Education Logging Certificate."

         (ii) Certificates must include the following: Continuing education program's sponsor, date, length in minutes awarded (continuing education units must be converted to clock hours), program title, licensed individual's name, license number and social security number.

         (iii) An original letter on official stationery from the continuing education program's sponsor indicating date, length in minutes awarded (continuing education units must be converted to clock hours), program title, licensed individual's name, license number and social security number.

(c) If a person submits documentation for training that is not clearly identifiable as appropriate continuing education, the Committee will request a written description of the training and how it applies to the practice as a physician assistant. If the Committee determines that the training cannot be considered appropriate continuing education, the individual will be given 90 days to replace the hours not allowed. Those hours will be considered replacement hours and cannot be counted during the next renewal period.

(3) Acceptable continuing education—To be utilized for satisfaction of the continuing education requirements of this rule, the continuing education program must be approved in content, structure and format by the A.M.A., the A.A.P.A., or the N.C.C.P.A.

(4) Violations

(a) Any physician assistant who falsely attests to completion of the required hours of continuing education may be subject to disciplinary action pursuant to Rule 0880-3-.15.

(b) Any physician assistant who fails to obtain the required continuing education hours may be subject to disciplinary action pursuant to Rule 0880-3-.15 and may not be allowed to renew licensure.

(c) Education hours obtained as a result of compliance with the terms of a Committee or Board order in any disciplinary action shall not be credited toward the continuing education hours required to be obtained in any renewal period.

TENNESSEE RRT SEC. 0880-3-12

TEXAS

(1) Continuing Medical Education. As a prerequisite to the annual registration of a physician assistant's license, 40 hours of continuing medical education (CME) are required to be completed in the following categories:

(A) at least one-half of the hours are to be from formal courses that are designated for Category I credit by a CME sponsor approved by the American Academy of Physician Assistants.

(B) The remaining hours may be from Category II composed of informal self-study, attendance at hospital lectures, grand rounds, case conferences, or by providing volunteer medical services at a site serving a medically underserved population, other than at a site that is the primary practice site of the license holder, and shall be recorded in a manner that can be easily transmitted to the board upon request.

(2) A physician assistant must report on the annual registration form if she or he has completed the required continuing medical education during the previous year. A licensee may carry forward CME credit hours earned prior to annual registration which are in excess of the 40 hour annual requirement and such excess hours may be applied to the following years' requirements. A maximum of 80 total excess credit hours may be carried forward and shall be reported according to whether the hours are Category I and/ or Category II. Excess CME credit hours of any type may not be carried forward or applied to an annual report of CME more than two years beyond the date of the annual registration following the period during which the hours were earned.

(3) A physician assistant may request in writing an exemption for the following reasons:

(A) catastrophic illness;

(B) military service of longer than one year's duration outside the United States;

(C) residence of longer than one year's duration outside the United States; or

(D) good cause shown on written application of the licensee that gives satisfactory evidence to the board that the licensee is unable to comply with the requirement for continuing medical education.

(4) Exemptions are subject to the approval of the licensure committee of the board.

(5) A temporary exception under paragraph (3) of this subsection may not exceed one year but may be renewed annually, subject to the approval of the board.

(6) This section does not prevent the board from taking disciplinary action with respect to a licensee or an applicant for a license by requiring additional hours of continuing medical education or of specific course subjects.

(7) The board may require written verification of both formal and informal credits from any licensee within 30 days of request. Failure to provide such verification may result in disciplinary action by the board.

(8) Unless exempted under the terms of this section, a physician assistant licensee's apparent failure to obtain and timely report the 40 hours of CME as required and provided for in this section shall result in nonrenewal of the license until such time as the

physician assistant obtains and reports the required CME hours; however, the executive director of the board may issue to such a physician assistant a temporary license numbered so as to correspond to the nonrenewed license. Such a temporary license shall be issued at the direction of the executive director for a period of no longer than 90 days. A temporary license issued pursuant to this subsection may be issued to allow the physician assistant who has not obtained or timely reported the required number of hours an opportunity to correct any deficiency so as not to require termination of ongoing patient care.

TEXAS CODE ANN. SEC. 185.6

UTAH

In accordance with Subsection 58-70a-304(1)(a), the requirements for qualified continuing professional education (CPE) are as follows:

(1) CPE shall consist of 40 hours in category 1 offerings as established by the Accreditation Council for Continuing Medical Education (ACCME) in each preceding two year licensure cycle.

(2) Offerings or courses must be approved by institutions accredited by the ACCME to approve continuing medical education.

(3) If requested, the licensee shall provide documentation of completed qualified continuing professional education by any of the following means:

(a) certificates from sponsoring agencies;

(b) transcripts of participation on applicable institutions letterhead; or

(c) copy of current national certification by NCCPA.

(4) Continuing professional education for licensees who have not been licensed for the entire two year period will be prorated from the date of licensure.

(5) A licensee shall be responsible for maintaining competent records of completed continuing professional education for a period of four years after close of the two-year period to which the records pertain. It is the responsibility of the licensee to maintain such information with respect to continuing professional education and to demonstrate it meets the requirements under this section.

UTAH ADMIN. CODE SEC. R156-70A-304

VERMONT

As evidence of continued competence in the knowledge and skills of a physician assistant, all physician assistants shall complete a continuing medical education program of 100 approved credit hours every two years. A minimum of 40 credit hours shall be from category 1. Proof of completion shall be submitted to the Board with the application for renewal of certification. Certification or recertification by the NCCPA at any time during a two-year licensure period may be accepted in lieu of 100 hours continuing medical education credits for that 2-year period.

VERMONT RULES OF THE BD. OF MED. SEC. II.8.1

VIRGINIA

A. Every licensed physician assistant intending to continue to practice shall biennially renew the license in each odd numbered year in the licensee's birth month by:
   1. Returning the renewal form and fee as prescribed by the board; and
   2. Verifying compliance with continuing medical education standards established by the NCCPA.
B. Any physician assistant who allows his NCCPA certification to lapse shall be considered not licensed by the board. Any such assistant who proposes to resume his practice shall make a new application for licensure.

18 VIRGINIA ADMIN. CODE SEC. 85-50-56

WASHINGTON

(1) Licensed physician assistants must complete one hundred hours of continuing education every two years as required in chapter 246-12 WAC, Part 7.
(2) In lieu of one hundred hours of continuing medical education the commission will accept a current certification with the National Commission for Certification of Physician Assistants and will consider approval of other programs as they are developed.
(3) The commission approves the following categories of creditable continuing medical education. A minimum of forty credit hours must be earned in Category I.
   Category I Continuing medical education activities with accredited sponsorship.
   Category II Continuing medical education activities with nonaccredited sponsorship and other meritorious learning experience.
(4) The commission adopts the standards approved by the American Academy of Physician Assistants for the evaluation of continuing medical education requirements in determining the acceptance and category of any continuing medical education experience.

(5) It will not be necessary to inquire into the prior approval of any continuing medical education. The commission will accept any continuing medical education that reasonably falls within these regulations and relies upon each licensee's integrity in complying with this requirement.

(6) Continuing medical education sponsors need not apply for nor expect to receive prior commission approval for a formal continuing medical education program. The continuing medical education category will depend solely upon the accredited status of the organization or institution. The number of hours may be determined by counting the contact hours of instruction and rounding to the nearest quarter hour. The commission relies upon the integrity of the program sponsors to present continuing medical education for licensees that constitutes a meritorious learning experience.

WASHINGTON ANN. CODE SEC. 246-918-180

WEST VIRGINIA

Beginning the first day of April, 1993, each physician assistant, as a condition of his or her biennial renewal of physician assistant license, shall provide to the Board written documentation of participation in and successful completion during the preceding two (2) year period of a minimum of fifty (50) hours of continuing education designated as Category I by either the American Medical Association, American Academy of Physician Assistants or the Academy of Family Physicians, and fifty (50) hours of continuing education designated as Category II by the association or either academy. The written documentation may consist of a current NCCPA certificate.

For those individuals who are not NCCPA certified, written documentation shall consist of original certificates from the entities named in subdivision 15.1., of this rule, evidencing participation in and successful completion of the fifty (50) hours and the fifty (50) hours both as described in subdivision 15.1 of this rule.

A physician assistant shall submit all written documentation to the Board, with the completed biennial renewal form, so that the completed biennial renewal form and all written documentation is received prior to the first day of April of the year of renewal of the physician assistant license.

The Board shall automatically suspend the license of a physician assistant who fails to timely submit written documentation as set forth in subdivision 15.3. of this rule until such time as the written documentation is submitted to and approved by the Board.

WEST VIRGINIA RULES SEC. 11-1B-15

WISCONSIN

Proof that the applicant is currently certified by the National Commission on Certification of Physician Assistants or its successor agency.

Wisconsin Admin. Code sec. 8.05

WYOMING

Certification by the National Commission on Certification of Physician Assistants.

Wyoming Stat. Ann. sec. 33-26-504

CHAPTER 4

Prescriptive Authority

Preparation for Prescribing • Controlled Substances • DEA Registration • Medication Errors • Prescription Writing • Practices to Avoid When Writing Prescriptions • Practices That Reduce Medication Errors • Dispensing • Samples • Licensure Violations • **Appendix 4** Prescriptive Privileges State-by-State

State laws and regulations have been enacted in 48 states, the District of Columbia, and Guam that allow supervising physicians to delegate prescriptive authority to physician assistants. PAs do not have prescriptive authority in Indiana or Ohio. Supervising physicians can delegate prescriptive authority to write for controlled substances in 43 states. (See Table 4-1.)

Table 4-1 Authority to Prescribe Controlled Substances

State/Territory	Controlled Substances
Alabama	Formulary, no authority to prescribe controlled substances
Alaska	Schedule III–V
Arizona	Schedule II–III (14-day supply with board prescribing certification, 72 hours without), Schedule IV–V (no more than 5 times in a 6-month period per patient)
Arkansas	Schedule III–V
California	Schedule II–V
Colorado	Schedule II–V
Connecticut	Schedule IV–V, Schedule II–III in hospital, long-term care facilities
Delaware	Schedule II–V
District of Columbia	No authority to prescribe controlled substances
Florida	Formulary of prohibited drugs, no authority
Georgia	Formulary, Schedule III–V
Guam	Schedule III–V

State/Territory	Controlled Substances
Hawaii	Schedule III–V
Idaho	Schedule II–V
Illinois	Schedule III–V
Indiana	No prescriptive authority
Iowa	Schedule III–V, Schedule II (except stimulants and depressants)
Kansas	Schedule II–V
Kentucky	No authority to prescribe controlled substances
Louisiana	Schedule III–V (pending adoption of rules by the Medical Board)
Maine	Schedule III–V, board may approve Schedule II for individual PAs
Maryland	Schedule II–V
Massachusetts	Schedule II–V
Michigan	Schedule III–V, Schedule II for 7-day supply at discharge
Minnesota	Formulary, Schedule II–V
Mississippi	Schedules II–V
Missouri	No authority to prescribe controlled substances
Montana	Schedule II–V (Schedule II with 34-day supply limit)
Nebraska	Schedule II–V
Nevada	Schedule II–V
New Hampshire	Schedule II–V
New Jersey	No authority to prescribe controlled substances
New Mexico	Formulary, Schedule II–V
New York	Schedule III–V
North Carolina	Schedule II–V (Schedule II–III with 30-day supply limit)
North Dakota	Schedule III–V
Ohio	No prescriptive authority
Oklahoma	Formulary, Schedule III–V
Oregon	Schedule II–V
Pennsylvania	Formulary, Schedule III–V (30-day supply limit, unless for a chronic condition)
Rhode Island	Schedule II–V
South Carolina	Formulary, Schedule V
South Dakota	Schedule II–V, Schedule II with 48-hour supply limit
Tennessee	Schedule II–V

State/Territory	Controlled Substances
Texas	Schedule III–V (in specific practice locations, 30-day supply limit)
Utah	Schedule II–V
Vermont	Formulary, Schedule II–V
Virginia	Schedule III–V
Washington	Schedule II–V
West Virginia	Formulary, Schedule III–V (Schedule III with 72-hour supply limit)
Wisconsin	Schedule II–V
Wyoming	Schedule II–V

Source: http://www.aapa.org; accessed October 2004.

In 2004 PAs were responsible for 206 million patient visits and recommended or prescribed an estimated 250 million pharmaceutical products.[1]

PREPARATION FOR PRESCRIBING

All physician assistant programs have pharmacology courses, which are usually taught by doctors of pharmacy and/or clinical pharmacists. A PA student receives approximately 78 hours (national mean) of formal classroom instruction in pharmacology. Instruction in pharmacology focuses on pharmacokinetics, drug interactions, adverse effects, contraindications, indications, risk and benefit ratios, and dosages. PAs receive a mean of 308.6 hours of clinical experience, which includes additional pharmacology exposure (based on national data).[2] During clinical experiences PA students focus on patient evaluation and management and gain supplementary pharmacologic training under the supervision of physicians, PAs, and other mid-level practioners. All PA educational programs must meet the same set of national standards for accreditation, which address pharmacological instruction. The National Commission on the Certification of Physician Assistants (NCCPA) covers clinical therapeutics on both the initial certification exam that all PAs must pass to obtain licensure in all states and on the recertification exams that all PAs must pass every 6 years in order to maintain certification. PAs continue to expand their knowledge base through continuing education programs and through the everyday work they do under the direction of their supervising physician.

CONTROLLED SUBSTANCES

Controlled substances are medications regulated by provisions in state and federal law because of their potential for abuse and dependence. These medications are grouped into five "Schedules" based on their potential for abuse. Scheduled medications are an integral part of medical care and are widely used. Scheduled medications are used to control coughs, diarrhea, depression, anxiety, and pain caused by injuries, surgery, and terminal illness. "Controlled substances have legitimate clinical usefulness and the prescriber should not hesitate to consider prescribing them when they are indicated for the comfort and well-being of patients."[3]

Schedule I

Schedule I substances have a high potential for abuse and have no acceptable medical use in the United States.

Examples according to federal law include heroin, LSD, marijuana, mescaline, methaqualone, and peyote.

Schedule II

Schedule II substances have a high abuse potential and can lead to severe psychological and physical dependence. This schedule contains certain narcotics, stimulants, and depressants. In general these substances have therapeutic utility.
Examples include:
    Narcotics: codeine, fentanyl, hydromorphone (Dilaudid), levorphanol, meperidine (Demerol), and morphine
    Stimulants: amphetamine
    Depressants: pentobarbital

Schedule III

Schedule III substances are stimulants and depressants that have less potential of abuse and dependence than those in Schedules II and I. This schedule contains compounds that include limited quantities of certain narcotic and nonnarcotic drugs.
Examples include:
    Codeine (Tylenol with codeine); mixtures of amobarbital, pentobarbital, or secobarbital with other noncontrolled medications; paregoric and anabolic steroids

Schedule IV

Schedule IV substances include stimulants and depressants with less abuse potential than those in Schedule III.
Examples include:
    Depressants: alprazolam, clonazepam, diazepam, and flurazepam
    Stimulants: phentermine, and pentazocine (Talwin-NX)

Schedule V

Schedule V substances include narcotics and stimulants not listed in another schedule and have an abuse potential less than substances in Schedule IV. These drugs are preparations containing limited quantities of narcotic and stimulant drugs for antitussive, antidiarrheal, and analgesic purposes.

Further Information

A comprehensive list of substances controlled under the Controlled Substance Act is located in Title 21, Code of Federal Regulations, Part 1300 to end, or can be found at the federal Drug Enforcement Administration's Web site at www.deadiversion.usdoj.gov/schedules/schedules.htm. Many prescribing references provide the class of each drug in its description.

State laws and regulations that allow supervising physicians to delegate the ability to prescribe controlled medications to PAs benefit the physician as well as the patient. PAs who can prescribe controlled substances are not forced to continually interrupt their supervising physician in order to obtain a prescription, allowing the physician more time to spend with more complex patients. Patients in rural and underserved areas who are treated by PAs also benefit when PAs have the authority to prescribe controlled substances. Unnecessary visits to emergency departments and follow-up appointments by patients who have to return to be seen when a physician is available can be decreased, saving health care dollars by lowering costs to patients and physicians. PAs have been prescribing controlled substances in some states for over 20 years. No state has ever rescinded its laws allowing supervising physicians to delegate prescriptive authority to PAs. Liability or malpractice claims have not significantly increased as a result of PAs prescribing controlled substances. Liability insurance premiums do not increase if the authority to prescribe controlled substances is given to a PA.[4]

DEA REGISTRATION

The federal government through the Drug Enforcement Administration (DEA) oversees the prescribing of controlled substances. DEA registration is used to track health care providers' controlled substances prescribing practices and to control the unauthorized prescribing of controlled substances. A prescription for a controlled substance that does not have an authorized DEA number on the prescription will not be filled.

If a state requires a separate controlled substance license, that should be obtained first and should be included in the federal application. If the state does not authorize a supervising physician to delegate authority to a PA to write prescriptions for controlled substances, the DEA will not issue a DEA number to the PA.

The cost of a DEA registration or renewal registration is $390 for 3 years. As of 2003 there were over a million practitioners registered with the DEA; 24,077 were PAs.[5]

DEA Registration Requirements for Physician Assistants, Nurse Practitioners, and Nurse Midwives

DEA regulations prohibit a physician from delegating the use of his or her signature and DEA registration to another person. Consequently, if the mid-level practitioner is delegated authority to prescribe controlled substances, in order for the prescription to be acceptable under DEA regulations the mid-level practitioner must be registered with the DEA. Therefore, the DEA requires that all physicians assistants, nurse practitioners, and nurse midwives who prescribe controlled substances via delegation from a physician prescriber obtain a DEA mid-level controlled substances registration.[6]

PAs must use their DEA number on prescriptions for controlled substances. It is important that they protect their DEA number to prevent unauthorized use.

- Only include a DEA number on prescriptions where it is required.
- Do not have a DEA number printed on prescription pads.
- PAs should always carry their prescription pad with them.
- PAs should not leave prescription pads in exam rooms, in unlocked drawers, or in unsecured areas of the office, at home, or in a vehicle.
- PAs should keep track of the number of printed prescription pads in the office so that they will be able to identify whether any of the pads are missing.
- Do not use a DEA number as a provider identifier at pharmacies, suppliers, insurance companies, or to obtain journals online.
- Keep all DEA certificates in a secure location and limit the number of office staff who have access to DEA numbers.[7]

Applicants for a DEA mid-level registration may visit the DEA application Web site at www.deadiversion.usdoj.gov/online_forms.htm to obtain the necessary form or call the DEA Registration Unit at (800) 882-9539. Request a DEA application, mid-level practitioner addendum form, and a mid-level practitioner-prescribing manual.

MEDICATION ERRORS

Medication errors kill up to 98,000 patients per year. A study of inpatients found that adverse drug events occurred at a rate of 6.5 per 100 admissions. Of these events, 42% were serious or life threatening and nearly half of these events were preventable.

Common medication errors occur when practitioners choose the wrong medication or fail to monitor side effects. Many preventable medication errors occur when patients are prescribed a medication that they are allergic to. In one study antibiotics were associated with nearly 40% of prescribing errors, partially as a result of undocumented drug allergies and cross-reactions. Ampicillin, amoxicillin, penicillin, and piperacillin are drugs that commonly cross-react.[8]

Before prescribing a medication a PA should be sure to:

- Research the indications, contraindications, appropriate doses, routes of administration, and drug–drug interactions.
- Ask the patient if she is pregnant or breast-feeding, or if he or she has any medication allergies, or has had any adverse drug reactions.
- Ask if the patient has any chronic medical conditions, especially kidney or liver disease.

- Ask if the patient has ever taken this medication before, whether it was effective, and if he or she had any side effects while on the medication.
- Educate the patient on the potential side effects of the medication, the proper dosing schedule, and the importance of compliance with the medical plan.
- Ask if the patient takes any over-the-counter medication, vitamins, supplements, or alternative medicines.

Once the PA has decided on the medication, be sure that:

- The prescription is written legibly.
- Treatment options are discussed with the patient, the patient's decision and involvement in the treatment plan are documented as well as the patient's willingness to accept the potential side effects of the medication chosen.
- The PA has followed any practice- or facility-wide guidelines or has adhered to the standard of care by referring to the *Physician's Desk Reference.*
- The PA has addressed any cross-sensitivities.
- The correct dosage is prescribed.
- The PA has informed the patient to call, return to the office, or seek medical attention at the emergency department if the patient's condition worsens or any adverse side effects develop.

PRESCRIPTION WRITING

Up to one third of all outpatient prescriptions contain errors. It is important that a PA provide all the required information when writing a prescription. Be sure to include the following:

- The date the prescription was written.
- The prescriber's information including the name and title of the prescriber, the address and telephone number of the practice or institution, and the DEA number when prescribing controlled substances
- Patient identification including the patient's legal name (not a nickname), address, age or date of birth, and for pediatric patients include the patient's weight.

When writing a prescription keep the following in mind:

- Preprinted prescription pads should have the name of the PA along with the PA's license, certification, or registration number and the supervising and alternate physicians' names and their license numbers.
- The inscription identifies the name and strength of the medication. Indicate tablets or liquid, and avoid abbreviating the name of the medication.
- The subscription provides information on the dosage form and the number of units or dosages to dispense in order to complete the treatment.
- The signa or sig provides specific information on how the patient should take the medication including the route, any special instructions, and the indication for the medication, which is especially important if the medication is being dosed PRN.

- Refill information up to one year.
- Whether the prescription should be dispensed as written or whether a generic form of the drug is acceptable for substitution.
- Specify any warning labels that should be attached to the medication.
- A legible practitioner's signature.
- When writing a prescription for a controlled medication, write out the quantity to be dispensed numerically as well as spell out the number in order to prevent tampering with the prescription.
- Many states require prescriptions to be dispensed in childproof containers. If the patient will have a difficult time opening a childproof container, write for the script to be dispensed in a nonchildproof container.[9]

PRACTICES TO AVOID WHEN WRITING PRESCRIPTIONS

- Avoid using > and <, as they are often mistaken for the opposite of what was intended. Instead, write out *greater than* or *less than*.
- Avoid using slash marks to separate doses because they are often mistaken as the number 1 (*35 units/10 units* read as *35 units and 110 units*).
- Avoid running names, letters, and dose numbers together (*Inderal40 mg* incorrectly read as *Inderal 140 mg*).
- Avoid abbreviations. (See Table 4-2.)

Table 4-2 Dangerous Abbreviations

Abbreviation	Anticipated Interpretation	Misinterpretation
AU, AS, AD	both ears, left ear, right ear	OU (both eyes); OS (left eye); OD (right eye)
BT	bedtime	BID (twice daily)
cc	cubic centimeter	U (units)
D/C	discontinue or discharge	improper discontinuation of medications
HS	half strength	hour of sleep
IU	international unit	IV (intervenous)
MS, MSO_4, $MGSO_4$		confused for one another
od	every day	OD (right eye)
per os	orally	OS (left eye)
qd or QD	every day	QID (4x/day)
qhs or qn	nightly	qh (every hour)
qod or QOD	every other day	QID (4x/day)
q6PM	every day at 6 p.m.	every 6 hours
SC or SQ	subcutaneous	SL (sublingual); q (every) or 5 every

Abbreviation	Anticipated Interpretation	Misinterpretation
ss	sliding scale	55
TWI	three times a week	twice weekly or three times a day
U	unit	0, 4, or "cc"
Ug or ugm	microgram	mg
x 3 d		may be interpreted as doses or days

Source: Sullivan, D.D., & Mattingly, L.J. (2004). *Documentation for physician assistants.* Philadelphia: F.A. Davis. 156
ISMP List of Error-Prone Abbreviations, Symbols and Dose Designations. (2005). ISMP Medication Safety Alert, *8*(24). Retrieved January 2005, from http://www.ismp.org/PDF/ErrorProne.pdf.
Doherty, K., & McKinney, P.G. (2004). The 10 most common prescribing errors: Tips on avoiding the pit falls. *Consultant, 44*(2). 176

- Avoid using trailing zeros; use leading zeros:

Incorrect	Misread as	Correct
1.0 mg	10 mg	1 mg
.5 mg	5 mg	0.5 mg

PRACTICES THAT REDUCE MEDICATION ERRORS

- Keep a flow sheet in front of the chart that lists all of the patient's medications, refill history, adverse drug events, and allergies.
- Document prescriptions called in to the pharmacy in the patient's chart.
- Always document the drug name, amount given, the dose, and frequency in the patient's chart.
- When calling in a prescription to the pharmacy, have the person taking the order repeat back the information and have them spell out the drug names.
- Use electronic prescriptions.
- Give legible written instructions to older individuals and recommend a pillbox.
- Be sure to adequately monitor drug therapies with appropriate lab work.
- Patients on anticoagulants have a disproportionately high rate of adverse events; refer patients to anticoagulation clinics for monitoring whenever possible.
- Pay close attention to patients with declining renal function and respond quickly to signs of drug toxicity.
- Develop a protocol for follow-up contact with patients after the initiation of a new drug therapy in order to identify potential problems early.
- Cardiovascular medications are the most frequent class of drugs associated with adverse drug reactions; carefully document all cardiovascular medications the patient is on.
- Ask the patient to bring his or her prescriptions, over-the-counter medications,

and alternative medications to the office every few months in order to maintain an updated drug list on his or her chart.

- If there is a question of adherence or drug-seeking behavior, a call to the patient's pharmacist can provide the patient's prescription profile.

DISPENSING

Twenty-eight jurisdictions allow supervising physicians to delegate the authority to dispense drugs to physician assistants. Certain states restrict the ability to dispense by location, facility, and quantity of drug.[10]

SAMPLES

In 1987, Congress enacted the Prescription Drug Marketing Act (Public Law 100-293), which regulates the distribution of drug samples to health care providers. The law allows affiliated practitioners who are licensed by a state and have independent or delegated prescriptive authority to request and sign for prescription drug samples. Pharmaceutical companies have combined the request and receipt for drug samples into one form for ease of record keeping. Since only a prescriber may request samples, only PAs who have prescriptive authority can request and sign for samples. Some states have specific legislation or rules that govern the authority of PAs to request, sign for, and distribute samples. PAs may only request a sample of a medication that they have the authority to prescribe. PAs who work in states that do not allow the delegation of the authority to write for controlled substances could not request or sign for a sample of a controlled medication. Similarly, if a PA works in a state that limits PAs' prescription-writing authority to those medications listed in a formulary or specified in an agreement with his or her supervising physician, a PA may only request and sign for drugs included in the formulary or specified in the agreement. [10]

LICENSURE VIOLATIONS

A state may refuse to renew, limit, suspend, revoke, or take other disciplinary action against a license if the licensee signs a blank, undated, or predated prescription or prescribes, sells, administers, or distributes any drug legally classified as a prescription drug other than for the proper medical purpose that the drug was intended. A physician assistant who uses a prescription pad pre-signed by his or her supervising physician may also be subject to disciplinary action.

REFERENCES

1. The American Academy of Physician Assistants. Number of patient visits made to physician assistants, number of medications prescribed or recommended by physician assistants in 2004. Available at http://www.aapa.org/research/04-visits-rx.pdf. Accessed March 2005.

2. American Academy of Physician Assistants. Issue Brief, PA prescribing education and delegation. Available at http://www.aapa.org/gandp/issuebrief/prescrib.pdf. Accessed March 2005.

3. Drug Enforcement Administration. (1993). *Mid-level practioner's manual.* Washington, DC: DEA.

4. American Academy of Physician Assistants. (2001). *Physician assistants as prescribers of controlled medications.* Alexandria, VA: AAPA.

5. Pennsylvania Society of Physician Assistants. (Winter 2003). DEA registration costs increase. *PSPA News.*

6. U.S. Department of Justice. Drug Enforcement Administration. Available at http://www.deadiversion.usdoj.gov/drugreg/offices/index.html. Accessed March 2005.

7. Sullivan, D.D., & Mattingly, L.J. (2004). *Documentation for physician assistants.* Philadelphia: F.A. Davis, pp. 162–169.

8. Doherty, K., & McKinney P.G. (2004). The 10 most common prescribing errors: Tips on avoiding the pitfalls. *Consultant, 44*(2): 173–182.

9. Sullivan, D.D., & Mattingly, L.J. (2004). *Documentation for physician assistants.* Philadelphia: F.A. Davis, pp. 153–156.

10. American Academy of Physician Assistants. (2004). *From program to practice: A guide to the physician assistant profession.* Alexandria, VA: AAPA, p. 34.

Prescriptive Privileges State-by-State

ALABAMA

(1) A physician assistant may prescribe a legend drug to a patient subject to both of the following conditions being met:
    (a) The drug type, dosage, quantity prescribed, and number of refills are authorized in the job description which is signed by the supervising physician to whom the physician assistant is currently registered and which is approved by the Board;
    (b) The drug is included in the formulary approved under the guidelines established by the Board for governing the prescription practices of physician assistants.

(2) A physician assistant shall not prescribe any drug, substance or compound which is listed in Schedules I through V of the Alabama Uniform Controlled Substances Act.

(3) The supervising physician and the physician assistant shall adhere to and follow all requirements and procedures stated in written guidelines established by the Board to govern the prescribing practices of physician assistants.

(4) A physician assistant may not initiate a call-in prescription in the name of the supervising physician for any drug which the assistant is not authorized to prescribe unless the drug is specifically ordered for the patient by the supervising physician either in writing or by a verbal order reduced to writing and signed by the physician within the time specified in the guidelines established by the Board.

(5) For any drug which the physician assistant is authorized to prescribe, a written prescription signed by the physician assistant and entered into the patient's chart may be called-in to a pharmacy.

(6) Whenever a physician assistant calls in a prescription to a pharmacy, the physician assistant shall identify his or her supervising physician.

(7) A physician assistant may administer any legend drug which the assistant is authorized to prescribe.

(8) For hospitalized patients, physician assistants may enter verbal admission orders and verbal subsequent orders for medications from the physician. All such orders must be validated by the ordering physician within 24 hours or within the time period specified in the hospital bylaws or policies.

(9) When prescribing legend drugs a physician assistant shall use a prescription form which includes all of the following:

(a) The name, medical practice site address and telephone number of the physician supervising the physician assistant;

(b) The physician assistant's name printed below or to the side of the physician's name;

(c) The medical practice site address and telephone number of the physician assistant, if different from the address of the supervising physician;

(d) The physician assistant's license number assigned by the Board;

(e) The words "Product Selection Permitted" printed on one side of the prescription form directly underneath a signature line;

(f) The words "Dispense as written" printed on one side of the prescription form directly underneath a signature line.

ALABAMA ADMIN. CODE R. 540-X-7-.28

ALASKA

(a) A physician assistant who prescribes, orders, administers, or dispenses controlled substances must have a current Drug Enforcement Administration (DEA) registration number, valid for that handling of that controlled substance on file with the department.

(b) A physician assistant may not write a prescription for a schedule I or II controlled substance.

(c) A physician assistant with a valid DEA registration number may write a prescription for a schedule III, IV, or V controlled substance only with the authorization of the physician assistant's primary collaborating physician.

The authorization must be documented in the physician assistant's current plan of collaboration approved under 12 AAC 40.980.

(d) A physician assistant with a valid DEA registration number may order, administer, and dispense a schedule II controlled substance only with the authorization of the physician assistant's primary collaborating physician. The authorization must be documented in the physician assistant's current plan of collaboration approved under 12 AAC 40.980. For purposes of this subsection, the primary collaborating physician's current DEA registration number, reflecting the physician level of authority to handle controlled substances, must be included in the physician assistant's current plan of collaboration approved under 12 AAC 40.980;

(e) A physician assistant may use the physician assistant's own DEA registration number to request, receive, order, or procure a controlled substance sample from a pharmaceutical distributor, warehouse, or other entity only with the explicit authorization of the physician assistant's primary collaborating physician. The authorization must be documented in the physician assistant's current plan of collaboration approved under 12 AAC 40.980.

(f) A physician assistant may prescribe, order, administer, or dispense a medication that is not a controlled substance only with the authorization of the physician assistant's primary collaborating physician. The authorization must be documented in the physician assistant's current plan of collaboration approved under 12 AAC 40.980.

(g) A graduate physician assistant licensed under this chapter may not prescribe, order, administer, or dispense a controlled substance.

(h) Termination of a collaborative relationship terminates a physician assistant's authority to prescribe, order, administer, and dispense medication under that relationship.

(i) A prescription written under this section by a physician assistant must include the
(1) primary collaborating physician's name;
(2) primary collaborating physician's DEA registration number;
(3) physician assistant's name; and
(4) physician assistant's DEA registration number.

(j) In this section,
(1) "order" means writing instructions on an order sheet to dispense a medication to a patient from an on-site pharmacy or drug storage area; for purposes of this paragraph, "on-site pharmacy" means a secured area that provides for the storage and dispensing of controlled substances and other drugs and is located in the facility where the physician assistant is practicing;
(2) "prescription" means a written document regarding a medication, prepared for transmittal to a licensed pharmacy for the dispensing of the medication;

(3) "schedule" used in conjunction with a controlled substance, means the relevant schedule of controlled substances under 21 U.S.C. 812 (Sec. 202, Federal Controlled Substances Act).

12 ALASKA ADMIN. CODE 40.450

ARIZONA

A. Except as provided in subsection F of this section, a physician assistant shall not prescribe, dispense or administer:
   1. A schedule II or schedule III controlled substance as defined in the federal controlled substances act of 1970 (P.L. 91-513; 84 Stat. 1242; 21 United States Code section 802) without delegation by the supervising physician, board approval and drug enforcement administration registration.
   2. A schedule IV or schedule V controlled substance as defined in the federal controlled substances act of 1970 without drug enforcement administration registration and delegation by the supervising physician.
   3. Prescription-only medication without delegation by the supervising physician.
B. All prescription orders issued by a physician assistant shall contain the name, address and telephone number of the supervising physician. A physician assistant shall issue prescription orders for controlled substances under the physician assistant's own drug enforcement administration registration number.
C. Unless certified for fourteen day prescription privileges pursuant to section 32-2504, subsection A, a physician assistant shall not prescribe a schedule II or III controlled substance for a period exceeding seventy-two hours. For each schedule IV or schedule V controlled substance, a physician assistant may not prescribe the controlled substance more than five times in a six month period for each patient.
D. A prescription for a schedule II or III controlled substance is not refillable without the written consent of the supervising physician.
E. Prescription-only drugs shall not be dispensed, prescribed or refillable for a period exceeding one year.
F. Except in an emergency, a physician assistant may dispense schedule II or schedule III controlled substances for a period of use not to exceed seventy-two hours with board approval or any other controlled substance for a period of use not to exceed thirty-four days and may administer controlled substances without board approval if it is medically indicated in an emergency dealing with potential loss of life or limb or major acute traumatic pain.

G. Except for samples provided by manufacturers, all drugs dispensed by a physician assistant shall be:
   1. Prepackaged in a unit-of-use package by the supervising physician or a pharmacist acting on a written order of the supervising physician.
   2. Labeled to show the name of the supervising physician and physician assistant.
H. A physician assistant shall not obtain a drug from any source other than the supervising physician or a pharmacist acting on a written order of the supervising physician. A physician assistant may receive manufacturers' samples if allowed to do so by the supervising physician.
I. If a physician assistant is approved by the board to prescribe, administer or dispense schedule II and schedule III controlled substances, the physician assistant shall maintain an up-to-date and complete log of all schedule II and schedule III controlled substances he administers or dispenses.
J. The board shall advise the state board of pharmacy and the United States Drug Enforcement Administration of all physician assistants who are authorized to prescribe or dispense drugs and any modification of their authority.
K. The state board of pharmacy shall notify all pharmacies at least quarterly of physician assistants who are authorized to prescribe or dispense drugs.

Arizona Rev. Stat. Ann. sec. 32-2532

ARKANSAS

(a) Physicians supervising physician assistants may delegate prescriptive authority to physician assistants to include prescribing, ordering, and administering Schedule III through V controlled substances as described in the Uniform Controlled Substances Act, §§ 5-64-101–5-64-608, and 21 C.F.R. Part 1300, all legend drugs, and all nonschedule prescription medications and medical devices. All prescriptions and orders issued by a physician assistant shall also identify his or her supervising physician.
(b) At no time shall a physician assistant's level of prescriptive authority exceed that of the supervising physician.
(c) Physician assistants who prescribe controlled substances must register with the Drug Enforcement Administration as part of the Drug Enforcement Administration's Mid-Level Practitioner registry, 21 C.F.R. Part 1300, 58 FR 31171-31175, and the Federal Controlled Substances Act.

Arkansas Code 17-105-108

CALIFORNIA

A supervising physician and surgeon who delegates authority to issue a drug order to a physician assistant may limit this authority by specifying the manner in which the physician assistant may issue delegated prescriptions.

(2) Each supervising physician and surgeon who delegates the authority to issue a drug order to a physician assistant shall first prepare and adopt, or adopt, a written, practice-specific formulary and protocols that specify all criteria for the use of a particular drug or device, and any contraindications for the selection. The drugs listed shall constitute the formulary and shall include only drugs that are appropriate for use in the type of practice engaged in by the supervising physician and surgeon. When issuing a drug order, the physician assistant is acting on behalf of and as an agent for a supervising physician and surgeon.

(a) "Drug order" for purposes of this section means an order for medication which is dispensed to or for a patient, issued and signed by a physician assistant acting as an individual practitioner within the meaning of Section 1306.02 of Title 21 of the Code of Federal Regulations. Notwithstanding any other provision of law,

  (1) a drug order issued pursuant to this section shall be treated in the same manner as a prescription or order of the supervising physician,

  (2) all references to "prescription" in this code and the Health and Safety Code shall include drug orders issued by physician assistants pursuant to authority granted by their supervising physicians, and

  (3) the signature of a physician assistant on a drug order shall be deemed to be the signature of a prescriber for purposes of this code and the Health and Safety Code.

(b) A drug order for any patient cared for by the physician assistant that is issued by the physician assistant shall either be based on the protocols described in subdivision (a) or shall be approved by the supervising physician before it is filled or carried out.

  (1) A physician assistant shall not administer or provide a drug or issue a drug order for a drug other than for a drug listed in the formulary without advance approval from a supervising physician and surgeon for the particular patient. At the direction and under the supervision of a physician and surgeon, a physician assistant may hand

to a patient of the supervising physician and surgeon a properly labeled prescription drug prepackaged by a physician and surgeon, manufacturer as defined in the Pharmacy Law, or a pharmacist.

(2) A physician assistant may not administer, provide or issue a drug order for Schedule II through Schedule V controlled substances without advance approval by a supervising physician and surgeon for the particular patient.

(3) Any drug order issued by a physician assistant shall be subject to a reasonable quantitative limitation consistent with customary medical practice in the supervising physician and surgeon's practice.

(c) A written drug order issued pursuant to subdivision (a), except a written drug order in a patient's medical record in a health facility or medical practice, shall contain the printed name, address, and phone number of the supervising physician and surgeon, the printed or stamped name and license number of the physician assistant, and the signature of the physician assistant. Further, a written drug order for a controlled substance, except a written drug order in a patient's medical record in a health facility or a medical practice, shall include the federal controlled substances registration number of the physician assistant. The requirements of this subdivision may be met through stamping or otherwise imprinting on the supervising physician and surgeon's prescription blank to show the name, license number, and if applicable, the federal controlled substances number of the physician assistant, and shall be signed by the physician assistant. When using a drug order, the physician assistant is acting on behalf of and as the agent of a supervising physician and surgeon.

(d) The medical record of any patient cared for by a physician assistant for whom the supervising physician and surgeon's drug order has been issued or carried out shall be reviewed and countersigned and dated by a supervising physician and surgeon within seven days.

(e) All physician assistants who are authorized by their supervising physicians to issue drug orders for controlled substances shall register with the United States Drug Enforcement Administration.

CALIFORNIA BUS. & PROF. CODE SEC. 3502.1

COLORADO

I. A LICENSED physician assistant may issue a prescription order for any drug or controlled substance provided that:

   A. Each and every prescription and refill order is entered on the patient's chart.

   B. Each written prescription order shall be signed by the physician assistant and shall contain in legible form the name, address and telephone number of the supervising physician and the name of the physician assistant.

   C. Nothing in this Section 3 shall prohibit a physician supervisor from restricting the ability of a supervised physician assistant to prescribe drugs or controlled substances.

   D. A physician assistant may not issue a prescription order for any controlled substance unless the physician assistant has received a registration from the United States Drug Enforcement Administration.

II. Physician assistants shall not write or sign prescriptions or perform any services which the supervising physician for that particular patient is not qualified or authorized to prescribe or perform.

III. No drug which a physician assistant is authorized to prescribe, dispense, administer or deliver shall be obtained by said physician assistant from a source other than a supervising physician, pharmacist or pharmaceutical representative.

IV. No device which a physician assistant is authorized to prescribe, dispense, administer or deliver shall be obtained by said physician assistant from a source other than a supervising physician, pharmacist or pharmaceutical representative.

COLORADO CODE REGS. SEC. 400-3

CONNECTICUT

A physician assistant may, as delegated by the supervising physician within the scope of such physician's license,

(A) prescribe and administer drugs, including controlled substances in schedule IV or V in all settings,

(B) renew prescriptions for controlled substances in schedule II or III in outpatient settings, and

(C) prescribe and administer controlled substances in schedule II or III to an inpatient in a short-term hospital, chronic disease hospital, emergency room satellite of a general hospital, or after an admission evaluation by a physician, in a chronic and convalescent nursing home, as defined in the regulations of Connecticut state agencies and licensed pursuant to subsection (a) of section 19a-491, provided in all cases where the physician assistant prescribes a controlled substance in schedule II or III, the physician under whose supervision the physician assistant is prescribing shall cosign the order not later than twenty-four hours thereafter. The physician assistant may, as delegated by the supervising physician within the scope of such physician's license, dispense drugs, in the form of professional samples as defined in section 20-14c or when dispensing in an outpatient clinic as defined in the regulations of Connecticut state agencies and licensed pursuant to subsection (a) of section 19a-491 that operates on a not-for-profit basis, or when dispensing in a clinic operated by a state agency or municipality. Nothing in this subsection shall be construed to allow the physician assistant to dispense any drug the physician assistant is not authorized under this subsection to prescribe.

All prescription forms used by physician assistants shall contain the printed name, license number, address and telephone number of the physician under whose supervision the physician assistant is prescribing, in addition to the signature, name, address and license number of the physician assistant.

CONNECTICUT GEN. STATUTE 20-12D

DELAWARE

Prescriptive authority for the therapeutic drugs and treatments will include the following:

Prescriptive authority is a delegated medical service by the supervising physician.

Prescriptive authority will be practice specific of the supervising physician.

PAs may prescribe legend medication including Schedule II–V controlled substances (as defined in the Controlled Substance Act), parenteral medications, medical therapeutics, devices and diagnostics.

PAs will be assigned a provider identifier number as outlined by the Division of Professional Regulation.

Controlled Substances registration will be as follows:

PAs must register with the Drug Enforcement Agency (DEA) and use such DEA number for controlled substance prescriptions.

PAs must register biennially with the Secretary of the Department of Health and Social Services in accordance with 16 Del.C. §4732(a).

Prescriptions must include the printed or legibly handwritten names of both the PA and the supervising physician. Controlled prescriptions may not be written for amounts to exceed a three month supply and non-controlled prescriptions to exceed a six month supply. The supervising physician must reevaluate the continued therapeutic needs of such patients before a new supply can be issued.

PAs' prescriptions must include the Division of Professional Regulation provider identifier number.

PA prescriptions for a controlled substance must include the PA's DEA number, as well as Professional Regulation provider identifier number.

Prescription container labels must bear the name of the PA and the supervising physician.

As a delegated medical/surgical practice PAs may request and issue professional samples of legend and over-the-counter medications and must be labeled in compliance with 24 Del.C. §2536(c).

DELAWARE PA REGS. 25.3

DISTRICT OF COLUMBIA

All prescription orders issued by a physician assistant shall be written on a prescription pad that bears the printed names of the physician assistant and the supervising physician. A physician assistant may sign the prescription order.

A physician assistant shall not dispense drugs unless they are as follows:

(a) Packaged by the manufacturer as a sample; or

(b) Prepackaged in a unit of use package by a supervising physician.

All drugs dispensed by a physician assistant shall be labeled to show the following:

(a) The name and address of the physician assistant;

(b) The name of the supervising physician;

(c) The name of the patient;

(d) The date dispensed;

(e) The name and strength of the drug;

(f) Directions for use;

(g) Cautionary statements, if appropriate;

(h) The lot and control number; and

(i) The expiration date of the drug.

A physician assistant shall not dispense a drug from any source other than a supervising physician or a pharmacist acting on a written order of a supervising physician.

A physician assistant who administers, dispenses, or prescribes a prescription drug shall enter a progress note in the patient's chart on the date of the transaction which shall include the following information:

(a) Each prescription that a physician assistant orders; and

(b) The name, strength, and quantity of each drug that a physician assistant dispenses or administers.

A physician assistant shall not dispense or prescribe controlled substances, except that a physician assistant may advise a patient of the availability of over-the-counter drugs that are listed in Schedule V.

Tit. 17 D. C. Mun. Regs. sec. 4912

FLORIDA

The physician assistant must file with the department, before commencing to prescribe, evidence that he or she has completed a continuing medical education course of at least 3 classroom hours in prescriptive practice, conducted by an accredited program approved by the boards, which course covers the limitations, responsibilities, and privileges involved in prescribing medicinal drugs, or evidence that he or she has received education comparable to the continuing education course as part of an accredited physician assistant training program.

The physician assistant must file with the department, before commencing to prescribe, evidence that the physician assistant has a minimum of 3 months of clinical experience in the specialty area of the supervising physician.

The physician assistant must file with the department a signed affidavit that he or she has completed a minimum of 10 continuing medical education hours in the specialty practice in which the physician assistant has prescriptive privileges with each licensure renewal application.

The department shall issue a license and a prescriber number to the physician assistant granting authority for the prescribing of medicinal drugs authorized within this paragraph upon completion of the foregoing requirements.

The prescription must be written in a form that complies with chapter 499 and must contain, in addition to the supervisory physician's name, address, and telephone number, the physician assistant's prescriber number. Unless it is a drug sample dispensed by the physician assistant, the prescription must be filled in a pharmacy permitted under chapter 465 and must be dispensed in that pharmacy by a pharmacist licensed under chapter 465. The appearance of the prescriber number creates a presumption that the physician assistant is authorized to prescribe the medicinal drug and the prescription is valid.

The physician assistant must note the prescription in the appropriate medical record, and the supervisory physician must review and sign each notation. For dispensing purposes only, the failure of the supervisory physician to comply with these requirements does not affect the validity of the prescription.

This paragraph does not prohibit a supervisory physician from delegating to a physician assistant the authority to order medication for a hospitalized patient of the supervisory physician.

This paragraph does not apply to facilities licensed pursuant to chapter 395.

The council shall establish a formulary of medicinal drugs that a fully licensed physician assistant, licensed under this section or s. 459.022, may not prescribe. The formulary must include controlled substances as defined in chapter 893, antipsychotics, general anesthetics and radiographic contrast materials, and all parenteral preparations except insulin and epinephrine.

In establishing the formulary, the council shall consult with a pharmacist licensed under chapter 465, but not licensed under this chapter or chapter 459, who shall be selected by the Secretary of Health.

Only the council shall add to, delete from, or modify the formulary. Any person who requests an addition, deletion, or modification of a medicinal drug listed on such formulary has the burden of proof to show cause why such addition, deletion, or modification should be made.

The boards shall adopt the formulary required by this paragraph, and each addition, deletion, or modification to the formulary, by rule. Notwithstanding any provision of chapter 120 to the contrary, the formulary rule shall be effective 60 days after the date it is filed with the Secretary of State. Upon adoption of the formulary, the department shall mail a copy of such formulary to each fully licensed physician assistant, licensed under this section or s. 459.022, and to each pharmacy licensed by the state. The boards shall establish, by rule, a fee not to exceed $200 to fund the provisions of this paragraph and paragraph (e).

FLORIDA STAT. CH. 458.347

GEORGIA

(1) A Physician's Assistant may carry out a prescription drug or device order in any authorized health care setting provided that:
   (a) The supervising physician delegates the authority to carry out a prescription drug or device order in the Physician Assistant's approved job description and the prescription drug or device is one which the supervising physician routinely prescribes in his/her practice.
   (b) The Physician Assistant shall not carry out a prescription drug

or device order for more than a thirty (30) day supply, except in cases of chronic illnesses where a ninety (90) day supply may be ordered. The Physician Assistant may authorize refills up to (6) months from the date of the original prescription drug or device order, provided, however, that refills may be authorized up to (12) months from the date of the original prescription drug or device order for oral contraceptives or other drugs or devices approved by the Board.

(c) The Physician Assistant's supervising physician shall personally reevaluate, at least every three (3) months, any patient receiving controlled substances, or at least six (6) months any patient receiving other prescription drugs or devices.

(d) The Physician Assistant shall inform and document in the medical records that the patient has the right to see the physician prior to any prescription drug or device order being carried out by the Physician Assistant.

(2) A Physician Assistant may be authorized to carry a prescription drug order or orders for any device, as defined in O.C.G.A. 26-4-2.

(a) A Physician Assistant may be authorized to carry out a prescription drug order or orders for any device included in the formulary approved by the Board.

(b) The formulary approved by the Board shall include any dangerous drug as defined in O.C.G.A. 16-13-71, or any Schedule III, IV or V controlled substances as defined in O.C.G.A. 16-13-21.

(3) A prescription drug or device order shall be issued on a form which contains the following:

(a) The name, address, and telephone number of the prescribing supervising physician, the name and address of the patient, the drug or device prescribed, the number of refills and directions to the patient with regard to taking and dosage of the drug.

(b) The form shall be signed by the Physician Assistant using the following language:

This prescription authorized through (the prescribing supervising physician) (M.D. or D.O.) by (the Physician Assistant).

(4) In addition to the copy of the prescription drug or device order delivered to the patient, a record of such prescription shall be maintained in the office of the prescribing physician in the following manner:

(a) A copy of the prescription drug or device order shall be maintained in the patient's medical file; and a copy, as described in

360-5-.12(4)(a), shall mean a duplicate prescription or a photo-copy, and

(b) The supervising physician shall countersign the prescription drug or device order copy or the medical record entry for each prescription or drug device order within a reasonable time, not to exceed seven (7) working days, unless the countersignature is required sooner by a specific regulation, policy or requirement.

(5) Procedures to evaluate a job description containing the authority to carry out a prescription drug or device order shall be in compliance with 360-5-.03(c)(2).

GEORGIA COMP. R. AND REGS. R. 360-05-.12

A physician assistant may order medication for institutionalized or hospitalized patients as outlined in the approved job description. All such orders by a physician assistant are subject to approval by the supervising physician.

(a) A physician assistant may order/select a drug, including a dangerous drug or a controlled substance, or order medical treatment, or diagnostic study in any health care setting, provided that:

1. The supervising physician delegates this authority in accordance with an approved job description.

2. Controlled substances are selected from a formulary of such drugs approved by the Board. For the purpose of this rule the formulary of controlled substances shall include any controlled substance defined in Code Section 16-31-21, except any Schedule I controlled substance listed in Code Section 16-13-25.

3. Ordering/Selecting of a drug under such delegation in accordance with an approved job description may include writing, telephoning or otherwise orally communicating such order, except that oral orders for Schedule II controlled substances shall be authorized only in emergency situations and thereafter shall be promptly reduced to writing as a prescription signed by the supervising physician; ordering/selecting of a drug under such delegation shall not be construed to authorize prescribing, which act can only be performed by the supervising physician; nor shall such ordering/selecting of a drug be construed to authorize the issuance of a written prescription by the physician assistant. Provided, however, that nothing contained herein shall be construed as precluding the physician assistant from preparing a written prescription, the issuance of which has been authorized by the supervising physician, so long as

such written prescription is signed by the supervising physician on the date when issued, and so long as the prescription is not signed in blank.

(b) A physician assistant may dispense one or more doses of a dangerous drug, except a controlled substance, in a suitable container with appropriate labeling for subsequent administration to, or use by, a patient under the authority of an order issued in conformity with an approved job description, provided that:

1. The physician assistant is an agent or employee of:

    (i) The Division of Public Health of the Department of Human Resources.

    (ii) Any county board of health; or

    (iii) Any organization which is exempt from federal taxes pursuant to Section 501 (c)(3) of the Internal Revenue Code other than an organization which is a hospital, preferred provider organization, health maintenance organization, or similar organization; or is established under the authority of or receiving funds pursuant to 42 U.S.C. Section 254b or 254c of the United States Public Health Service Act; or is an outpatient clinic which is owned or operated by a licensed hospital, and whose services are primarily provided to the medically disadvantaged and which provides such drugs free of charge to the patient based solely upon the patient's ability to pay;

2. The supervising physician delegates this authority in accordance with an approved job description;

3. In the case of dispensing of dangerous drugs, the dispensing is in accordance with a dispensing procedure for dangerous drugs which shall include a written document signed by a licensed pharmacist and a licensed physician which document establishes the appropriate manner under which drugs may be dispensed and the dispensing of dangerous drugs is performed in compliance with applicable Georgia Law, including Code Section 26-4-4, and the Rules of the State Board of Pharmacy, Chapters 480-28, Practitioner Dispensing of Drugs and 480-30, Dispensing of Drugs Under Authority of Job Description or Nurse Protocol.

The physician(s) who apply for or utilize a Physician Assistant shall be responsible for any violation of the above enumerated limitations on the practice of a Physician Assistant.

A physician assistant may gather data based on a new patient or an established patient with a new problem and then shall transmit this information to the supervising physician.

Except in life threatening situations, the supervising physician shall be readily available for personal supervision and shall be responsible for follow up care.

GEORGIA COMP. R. AND REGS. R. 360-05-.07(8)

HAWAII

A supervising physician must be authorized to allow the physician assistant to prescribe, dispense, and administer medications and medical devices to the extent delegated by the supervising physician and subject to the following requirements:

(A) Prescribing and dispensing of medications may include Schedule III through V and all legend medications. No physician assistant may prescribe Schedule II medications;

(B) A physician assistant who has been delegated the authority to prescribe Schedule III through V medications shall register with the Drug Enforcement Administration (DEA);

(C) Each prescription written by a physician assistant shall include the name, address, and phone number of the supervising physician and physician assistant. The printed name of the supervising physician shall be on one side of the form and the printed name of the physician assistant shall be on the other side. A physician assistant who has been delegated the authority to prescribe shall sign the prescription next to the printed name of the physician assistant;

(D) A physician assistant employed or extended privileges by a hospital or extended care facility may, if allowed under the bylaws, rules, and regulations of the hospital or extended care facility, write orders for medications Schedule II through V, for inpatients under the care of the supervising physician;

(E) The board of medical examiners shall notify the pharmacy board in writing, at least annually or more frequently if required by changes, of each physician assistant authorized to prescribe;

(F) A physician assistant may request, receive, and sign for professional samples and may distribute professional samples to patients; and

(G) All dispensing activities shall comply with appropriate federal and state regulations.

(b) The supervising physician or physicians and the physician assistant shall notify the board within ten days of severance of supervision or employment of the physician assistant.

HAWAII ADMIN. R. SEC. 16-85-49(8)

IDAHO

Approval And Authorization Required. A physician assistant may issue written or oral prescriptions for legend drugs and controlled drugs, Schedule II through V only in accordance with approval and authorization granted by the Board and in accordance with the current delegation of services agreement and shall be consistent with the regular prescriptive practice of the supervising physician.

Application. A physician assistant who wishes to apply for prescription writing authority shall submit an application for such purpose to the Board of Medicine. In addition to the information contained in the general application for physician assistant approval, the application for prescription writing authority shall include the following information:

Documentation of all pharmacology course content completed, the length and whether a passing grade was achieved (at least thirty (30) hours).

A statement of the frequency with which the supervising physician will review prescriptions written.

A signed statement from the supervising physician certifying that, in the opinion of the supervising physician, the physician assistant is qualified to prescribe the drugs for which the physician assistant is seeking approval and authorization.

The physician assistant to be authorized to prescribe Schedule II through V drugs shall be registered with the Federal Drug Enforcement Administration and the Idaho Board of Pharmacy.

Prescription Forms. Prescription forms used by the physician assistant must be printed with the name, address, and telephone number of the physician assistant and of the supervising physician.

Record Keeping. The physician assistant shall maintain accurate records, accounting for all prescriptions written and medication delivered.

Delivery of Medication.

Pre-Dispensed Medication. The physician assistant may legally provide a patient with more than one (1) dose of a medication at sites or at times when a pharmacist is not available. The pre-dispensed medications shall be for an emergency period to be determined on the basis of individual circumstances, but the emergency period will extend only until a prescription can be obtained from a pharmacy.

Consultant Pharmacist. The physician assistant shall have a consultant pharmacist responsible for providing the physician assistant with pre-dispensed medication in accordance with federal and state statutes for packaging, labeling, and storage.

Limitation Of Items. The pre-dispensed medication shall be limited to only those categories of drug identified in the delegation of services agreement, except a physician assistant may provide other necessary emergency medication to the patient as directed by a physician.

Exception From Emergency Period. Physician assistant in agencies, clinics or both, providing family planning, communicable disease and chronic disease services under government contract or grant may provide pre-dispensed medication for these specific services and shall be exempt from the emergency period. Agencies, clinics or both, in remote sites without pharmacies shall be exempt from the emergency period, providing that they must submit an application and obtain formal approval from the Board of Medicine.

IDAHO ADMIN. CODE SEC. 22.01.03.042-3

ILLINOIS

a) A supervising physician may delegate limited prescriptive author- ity to a physician assistant. This authority may, but is not required to, include prescription and dispensing of legend drugs and leg- end controlled substances categorized as Schedule III, IV, or V con- trolled substances, as defined in Article II of the Illinois Controlled Substances Act, as delegated in the written guidelines required by the Physician Assistant Practice Act of 1987. To prescribe Schedule III, IV, or V controlled substances under this Section, a physician assistant must obtain a mid-level practitioner controlled substances license. Medication orders issued by a physician assis- tant shall be reviewed periodically by the supervising physician. The supervising physician shall file with the Department notice of delegation of prescriptive authority to a physician assistant and termination of delegation, specifying the authority delegated or terminated. Upon receipt of this notice delegating authority to prescribe Schedule III, IV, or V controlled substances, the physi- cian assistant shall be eligible to register for a mid-level practi- tioner controlled substances license under Section 303.05 of the Illinois Controlled Substances Act. Nothing in this Act shall be construed to limit the delegation of tasks or duties by the supervis- ing physician to a nurse or other appropriately trained personnel. (Section 7.5 of the Act)

b) Written Guidelines.

1) If the supervising physician has delegated prescriptive author- ity to the physician assistant, the written guidelines shall include a statement indicating that the supervising physician has delegated prescriptive authority for legend drugs and any

schedule of controlled substances. The delegation must be appropriate to the physician's practice and within the scope of the physician assistant's training.

2) The written guidelines shall be signed by both the physician and the physician assistant and a copy maintained at each location where the physician assistant practices along with the physician assistant's state controlled substance license number and the Drug Enforcement Administration (DEA) registration number.

c) A physician assistant may only prescribe or dispense prescriptions or orders for drugs and medical supplies within the scope of practice of the supervising physician or alternate supervising physician.

d) The name of the supervising physician shall appear on any prescription written by the physician assistant.

ILLINOIS ADMIN. CODE TIT. 68 SEC. 1350.55

INDIANA

No Prescriptive Privileges

IOWA

Prescribe drugs and medical devices under the following conditions:

(1) The physician assistant shall have passed the national certifying examination conducted by the National Commission on Certification of Physician Assistants or its successor examination approved by the board. Physician assistants with a temporary license may order drugs and medical devices only with the prior approval and direction of a supervising physician. Prior approval may include discussion of the specific medical problems with a supervising physician prior to the patient's being seen by the physician assistant.

(2) The physician assistant may not prescribe Schedule II controlled substances which are listed as stimulants or depressants in Iowa Code chapter 124. The physician assistant may order Schedule II controlled substances which are listed as stimulants or depressants in Iowa Code chapter 124 only with the prior approval and direction of a physician. Prior approval may include discussion of the specific medical problems with a supervising physician prior to the patient's being seen by the physician assistant.

(3) The physician assistant shall inform the board of any limitation on the prescriptive authority of the physician assistant in addition to the limitations set out in 327.1(1)"s"(2).

(4) A physician assistant shall not prescribe substances that the supervising physician does not have the authority to prescribe except as allowed in 327.1(1)"n."

(5) The physician assistant may prescribe, supply and administer drugs and medical devices in all settings including, but not limited to, hospitals, health care facilities, health care institutions, clinics, offices, health maintenance organizations, and outpatient and emergency care settings except as limited by 327.1(1)"s"(2).

(6) A physician assistant who is an authorized prescriber may request, receive, and supply sample drugs and medical devices except as limited by 327.1(1)"s"(2).

(7) The board of physician assistant examiners shall be the only board to regulate the practice of physician assistants relating to prescribing and supplying prescription drugs, controlled substances and medical devices.

Supply properly packaged and labeled prescription drugs, controlled substances or medical devices when pharmacist services are not reasonably available or when it is in the best interests of the patient as delegated by a supervising physician.

(1) When the physician assistant is the prescriber of the medications under 327.1(1)"s," these medications shall be supplied for the purpose of accommodating the patient and shall not be sold for more than the cost of the drug and reasonable overhead costs as they relate to supplying prescription drugs to the patient and not at a profit to the physician or physician assistant.

(2) When a physician assistant supplies medication on the direct order of a physician, subparagraph (1) does not apply.

(3) A nurse or staff assistant may assist the physician assistant in supplying medications when prescriptive drug supplying authority is delegated by a supervising physician to the physician assistant under 327.1(1)"s."

When a physician assistant supplies medications as delegated by a supervising physician in a remote site, the physician assistant shall secure the regular advice and consultation of a pharmacist regarding the distribution, storage and appropriate use of prescription drugs, controlled substances, and medical devices.

IOWA ADMIN. CODE R. 645-327.1 (S-U)

KANSAS

The responsible physician request form to be presented to the board pursuant to K.S.A. 2000 Supp. 65-28a03, and amendments thereto, shall contain the following information:

(a) the date and signatures of the responsible physician and the physician assistant;

(b) the license numbers of the responsible physician and the physician assistant;

(c) a description of the physician's practice and the way in which the physician assistant is to be utilized;

(d) a statement that the responsible physician will always be available for communication with the physician assistant within 30 minutes of the performance of patient service by the physician assistant;

(e) a completed drug prescription protocol on a form provided by the board specifying categories of drugs, medicines, and pharmaceuticals that the physician assistant will be allowed to prescribe, and the drugs within any category that the physician assistant will not be allowed to supply, prescribe, receive, or distribute;

(f) the name and address of each practice location, including hospitals, where the physician assistant will routinely perform acts that constitute the practice of medicine and surgery;

(g) signatures of all designated physicians who routinely provide direction and supervision to the physician assistant in the temporary absence of the responsible physician, and a description of the procedures to be followed to notify a designated physician in the responsible physician's absence;

(h) an acknowledgment that failure to adequately direct and supervise the physician assistant in accordance with K.S.A. 2000 Supp. 65-28a01 through K.S.A. 65-28a09, and amendments thereto, or regulations adopted under these statutes by the board, shall constitute grounds for revocation, suspension, limitation, or censure of the responsible physician's license to practice medicine and surgery in the state of Kansas;

(i) a statement that a current copy of the form will be maintained at each practice location of the responsible physician and the physician assistant and that any changes to the form will be provided to the board within 10 days; and

(j) an acknowledgment that the responsible physician has established and implemented a method for initial and periodic evaluation of the professional competency of the physician assistant and that evaluations will be performed at least annually.

KANSAS ADMIN. REGS. 100-28A-9

(a) A physician assistant may prescribe a prescription-only drug or administer or supply a prescription-only drug as authorized by the drug prescription protocol required by K.A.R.100-28a-9 and as authorized by this regulation.

(b) As used in this regulation, "emergency situation" shall have the meaning ascribed to it in K.A.R. 68-20-19(a)(5).

(c) A physician assistant may directly administer a prescription-only drug as follows:

    (1) If directly ordered or authorized by the responsible or designated physician;

    (2) if authorized by a written drug prescription protocol between the responsible physician and the physician assistant; or

    (3) if an emergency situation exists.

(d) (1) A physician assistant may prescribe a schedule II controlled substance in the same manner as that in which the physician assistant may perform acts that constitute the practice of medicine and surgery as specified in K.A.R. 100-28a-6. Except as specified in paragraph (d)(2), each prescription for a schedule II controlled substance shall be in writing.

(2) A physician assistant may, by oral or telephonic communication, prescribe a schedule II controlled substance in an emergency situation. Within seven days after authorizing an emergency prescription order, the physician assistant shall cause a written prescription, completed in accordance with appropriate federal and state laws, to be delivered to the dispenser of the drug.

(e) A physician assistant may orally, telephonically, or in writing prescribe a controlled substance listed in schedule III, IV, or V, or a prescription-only drug not listed in any schedule as a controlled substance in the same manner as that in which the physician assistant may perform acts that constitute the practice of medicine and surgery as specified in K.A.R. 100-28a-6.

(f) Each written prescription order by a physician assistant shall meet the following requirements:

    (1) Contain the name, address, and telephone number of the responsible physician;

    (2) contain the name, address, and telephone number of the physician assistant;

    (3) be signed by the physician assistant with the letters "P.A." following the signature;

    (4) contain any DEA registration number issued to the physician assistant if a controlled substance is prescribed; and

    (5) indicate whether the prescription order is being transmitted by direct order of the responsible or designated physician,

pursuant to a written protocol, or because of an emergency situation.

(g) A physician assistant may supply a prescription-only drug to a patient only if all of the following conditions are met:

   (1) If the drug is supplied under the same conditions as those in which a physician assistant may directly administer a prescription-only drug, as described in subsection (b) above;

   (2) if the drug has been provided to the physician assistant or the physician assistant's responsible physician or employer at no cost;

   (3) if the drug is commercially labeled and is supplied to the patient in the original prepackaged unit-dose container; and

   (4) if the drug is supplied to the patient at no cost.

(h) A physician assistant shall not administer, supply, or prescribe a prescription-only drug for any quantity or strength in excess of the normal and customary practice of the responsible physician.

KANSAS ADMIN. REGS. 100-28A-13

KENTUCKY

A physician assistant may prescribe and administer all nonscheduled legend drugs and medical devices as delegated by the supervising physician. A physician assistant who is delegated prescribing authority may request, receive, and distribute professional sample drugs to patients.

KENTUCKY REV. STAT. SEC. 311.858

LOUISIANA

Prescriptive privileges effective August 15, 2004, including Schedule III-V controlled medications. The medical board must adopt rules prior to PAs actually writing scripts.

LEGISLATIVE WATCH. AMERICAN ACADEMY OF PHYSICIAN ASSISTANTS,
ALEXANDRIA, VA, MAY 12, 2004

MAINE

The prescribing and dispensing of drugs and medical devices to the extent permitted by state and federal law. Prescribing and dispensing drugs may include Schedule III through V substances and all legend drugs. A Physician Assistant and primary supervising physician may together request individual consideration for authorization to prescribe schedule II drugs under specific individual guidelines detailed by the Board. Physician assistants may request, receive, and sign for professional samples and may distribute professional samples to patients.

CODE MAINE R. SEC. 02 373 6

MARYLAND

The supervising physician shall:
A. Delegate the authority to write medication orders; and
B. Ensure that the delegation agreement includes:
   (1) A statement describing whether controlled dangerous substances, noncontrolled substances, and nonprescription medications may be ordered by the physician assistant;
   (2) Evidence of:
       (a) Certification by the National Commission on Certification of Physician Assistants, Inc. within the previous 2 years, or
       (b) Successful completion of 8 Category I hours in pharmacology education within the previous 2 years; and
   (3) An attestation that the physician assistant will comply with:
       (a) State and federal laws governing the prescribing of medications, and
       (b) The protocols established by the hospital, public health facility, correctional facility, or detention center where the physician assistant is requesting permission to write medication orders.

MARYLAND REGS. CODE TIT. 10. SEC. 32.03.07

The supervising physician shall delegate prescriptive authority and ensure that the delegation agreement includes:
A. A statement describing whether the physician intends to delegate prescribing of controlled dangerous substances, prescription drugs, or medical devices;
B. An attestation that all prescribing activities of the physician assistant will comply with applicable federal and State regulations;
C. An attestation that all medical charts and records:
   (1) Contain a notation of any prescriptions written by a physician assistant, and
   (2) Be reviewed and cosigned by the supervising physician in accordance with Health Occupations Article, §15-302.2, Annotated Code of Maryland;
D. An attestation that all prescriptions written include the physician assistant's name and the supervising physician's name, business address, and business telephone number legibly written or printed;
E. Evidence demonstrating:

(1) Passage of the physician assistant national certification exam administered by the National Commission on Certification of Physician Assistants, Inc. within the previous 2 years, or

(2) Successful completion of 8 Category I hours of pharmacology education within the previous 2 years; and

F. Evidence demonstrating:

(1) A bachelor's degree or its equivalent,

(2) 2 years of work experience as a physician assistant, or

(3) Prior approval by the Board of a job description, including approval for writing medication orders.

MARYLAND REGS. CODE TIT. 10. SEC. 32.03.08

MASSACHUSETTS

(1) Any physician assistant who holds a full certificate of registration, issued by the Board pursuant to 263 CMR 3.02, may issue written or oral prescriptions or medication orders for a patient, provided that he or she does so in accordance with all applicable state and federal laws and regulations, including but not limited to M.G.L. c. 112, § 9E; M.G.L. c. 94C, §§ 7, 9 and 20; 105 CMR 700.000 and 263 CMR 5.07(1).

(2) A physician assistant who holds a temporary certificate of registration, issued by the Board pursuant to 263 CMR 3.04, may prepare a written or oral prescription or medication order for a patient, provided that:

(a) Any such written prescription or medication order is signed by his or her supervising physician, or by another licensed physician who has been designated to assume temporary supervisory responsibilities with respect to that physician assistant pursuant to 263 CMR 5.05(4)(g), prior to the issuance of said prescription or medication order to the patient;

(b) Any such oral prescription or medication order is approved, in writing, by his or her supervising physician, or by another licensed physician who has been designated to assume temporary supervisory responsibilities with respect to that physician assistant pursuant to 263 CMR 5.05(4)(g), prior to the issuance of that oral prescription or medication order; and

(c) All such oral or written prescriptions or medication orders are issued in the name of the supervising physician, and are otherwise issued in accordance with all applicable state and federal laws and regulations, including but not limited to M.G.L. c. 112, § 9E; M.G.L. c. 94C, §§ 7, 9 and 20; 105 CMR 700.000; and 263 CMR 5.07(2).

(3) Any prescription or medication order issued by a physician assistant for a Schedule II controlled substance, as defined in 105 CMR 700.002, shall be reviewed by his or her supervising physician, or by a temporary supervising physician designated pursuant to 263 CMR 5.05(4)(g), within 96 hours after its issuance.

(4) All physician assistants shall issue prescriptions or medication orders in accordance with written guidelines governing the prescription of medication which are mutually developed and agreed upon by the physician assistant and his or her supervising physician(s).

    (a) Such guidelines shall address, but need not be limited to, the following issues:

       1. Identification of the supervising physician(s) for that work setting;

       2. Frequency of medication reviews by the physician assistant and his or her supervising physician;

       3. Types and classes of medications to be prescribed by the physician assistant;

       4. The initiation and/or renewal of prescriptions for medications which are not within the ordinary scope of practice for the specific work setting in question, but which may be needed to provide appropriate medical care;

       5. The quantity of any medication to be prescribed by a physician assistant, including initial dosage limits and refills;

       6. The types and quantities of Schedule VI medications which may be ordered by the physician assistant from a drug wholesaler, manufacturer, laboratory or distributor for use in the practice setting in question;

       7. Review of initial prescriptions or changes in medication; and

       8. Procedures for initiating intravenous solutions.

    (b) Such guidelines shall be available for review by any duly authorized representative of the Board, the Massachusetts Board of Registration in Medicine, the Massachusetts Department of Public Health, and such other state or federal government agencies as may be reasonably necessary and appropriate to ensure compliance with all applicable state or federal laws and regulations. Copies of such guidelines, however, need not be filed with those agencies.

    (c) All such guidelines must be in writing and must be signed by both the supervising physician and the physician assistant. Such guidelines shall be reviewed annually and dated and initialed by both the supervising physician and the physician assistant at the time of each such review. The physician assistant and his/her supervising physician may alter such guidelines at any time and any such changes shall be initialed by both parties and dated.

(5) All prescriptions or medication orders issued by a physician assistant shall be issued in a manner which is consistent with the scope of practice of the physician assistant, the guidelines developed pursuant to 263 CMR 5.07(4), and accepted standards of good medical practice for licensed physicians with respect to prescription practices.

(6) At least four hours of the continuing medical education which a physician assistant is required to obtain pursuant to 263 CMR 3.05(3) as a condition for license renewal shall be in the field of pharmacology and/or pharmacokinetics.

(7) All prescriptions written by a physician assistant shall be written in accordance with the regulations of the Massachusetts Department of Public Health at 105 CMR 721.000.

(8) A physician assistant may order only Schedule VI controlled substances from a drug wholesaler, manufacturer, distributor or laboratory, and only in accordance with the written guidelines developed with his/her supervising physician pursuant to 263 CMR 5.07(4). A physician assistant may sign only for sample Schedule VI controlled substances received by or sent to the practice setting by a pharmaceutical representative.

(9) The use of pre-signed prescription blanks or forms is prohibited.

(10) A physician assistant shall not prescribe controlled substances in Schedules II, III and IV for his or her own use. Except in an emergency, a physician assistant shall not prescribe Schedule II controlled substances for a member of his or her immediate family, including a parent, spouse or equivalent, child, sibling, parent-in-law, son/daughter-in-law, brother/sister-in-law, step-parent, step-child, step-sibling, or other relative permanently residing in the same residence as the physician assistant.

(11) The physician assistant and the supervising physician for that work setting shall be jointly responsible for all prescriptions or medication orders issued by the physician assistant in that work setting.

CODE MASSACHUSETTS REGS. TIT. 263. SEC. 5.07

MICHIGAN

(1) A physician who supervises a physician assistant under sections 17048 and 17049 of the code may delegate the prescription of controlled substances listed in schedules 3 to 5 to a physician assistant if the delegating physician establishes a written authorization that contains all of the following information:

    (a) The name, license number, and signature of the supervising physician.

    (b) The name, license number, and signature of the physician assistant.

    (c) The limitations or exceptions to the delegation.

    (d) The effective date of the delegation.

(2) A delegating physician shall review and update a written authorization on an annual basis from the original date or the date of amendment, if amended. A delegating physician shall note the review date on the written authorization.

(3) A delegating physician shall maintain a written authorization in each separate location of the physician's office where the delegation occurs.

(4) A delegating physician shall ensure that an amendment to the written authorization is in compliance with subrule (1)(a) to (d) of this rule.

(5) A delegating physician may delegate the prescription of schedule 2 controlled substances only if all of the following conditions are met:

    (a) The supervising physician and physician assistant are practicing within a health facility as defined in section 20106(d), (g), or (i) of the code; specifically, freestanding surgical outpatient facilities, hospitals, and hospices.

    (b) The patient is located within the facility described in subdivision (a) of this subrule.

    (c) The delegation is in compliance with this rule.

(6) A delegating physician may not delegate the prescription of schedule 2 controlled substances issued for the discharge of a patient for a quantity for more than a 7-day period.

(7) A delegating physician shall not delegate the prescription of a drug or device individually, in combination, or in succession for a woman known to be pregnant with the intention of causing either a miscarriage or fetal death.

MICHIGAN ADMIN. CODE R. SEC. 338.2304(4)

Requirements for a Controlled Substance Prescription Written By Mid-Level Practioners in Michigan

Prescriptions for controlled substances written by Physician Assistants, Nurse Practitioners, and Certified Nurse Midwives in Michigan must contain the name of the delegating physician, the physician's DEA number and the mid-level practitioner's DEA registration number.

Applicant's whose practice is in a hospital setting, free standing surgical suite and those in oncology/hospice/palliative care are eligible to apply for Schedules II–V. All others are eligible to apply for Schedules III–V.

Although the application and other required documents are sent to the DEA in Washington D.C., to expedite your application process, you may wish to submit a copy of your State of Michigan Physician's Assistant/Nurse Practitioner or Midwife license/certification and a copy of the Delegation of Prescriptive Authority Agreement signed by your supervising physician to:

DEA
Rick Finley Building
431 Howard Street
Detroit, MI 48226
Attn: Annie Witherspoon or Fax copies to the above DEA office at (313) 234-4149

Source: DEA ALERT NO. 012403

MINNESOTA

(a) A supervising physician may delegate to a physician assistant who is registered with the board, certified by the National Commission on Certification of Physician Assistants or successor agency approved by the board, and who is under the supervising physician's supervision, the authority to prescribe, dispense, and administer legend drugs, medical devices, and controlled substances subject to the requirements in this section. The authority to dispense includes, but is not limited to, the authority to request, receive, and dispense sample drugs. This authority to dispense extends only to those drugs described in the written agreement developed under paragraph (b).

(b) The agreement between the physician assistant and supervising physician and any alternate supervising physicians must include a statement by the supervising physician regarding delegation or nondelegation of the functions of prescribing, dispensing, and administering of legend drugs and medical devices to the physician assistant. The statement must include a protocol indicating categories of drugs for which the supervising physician delegates prescriptive and dispensing authority. The delegation must be appropriate to the physician assistant's practice and within the scope of the physician assistant's training. Physician assistants who have been delegated the authority to prescribe, dispense, and administer legend drugs and medical devices shall provide evidence of current certification by the National Commission on Certification of Physician Assistants or its successor agency when registering or reregistering as physician assistants. Physician assistants who have been delegated the authority to prescribe controlled substances must present evidence of the certification and hold a valid DEA certificate. Supervising physicians shall retrospectively review the prescribing, dispensing, and administering of legend and controlled drugs and medical devices by physician assistants, when this authority has been delegated to the physician assistant as part of the delegation agreement between the physician and the physician assistant. This review must take place at least weekly. The process and schedule for the review must be outlined in the delegation agreement.

(c) The board may establish by rule:

(1) a system of identifying physician assistants eligible to prescribe, administer, and dispense legend drugs and medical devices;

(2) a system of identifying physician assistants eligible to prescribe, administer, and dispense controlled substances;

(3) a method of determining the categories of legend and controlled drugs and medical devices that each physician assistant is allowed to prescribe, administer, and dispense; and

(4) a system of transmitting to pharmacies a listing of physician assistants eligible to prescribe legend and controlled drugs and medical devices.

Subd. 2. Termination and reinstatement of prescribing authority.

(a) The authority of a physician assistant to prescribe, dispense, and administer legend drugs and medical devices shall end immediately when:

(1) the agreement is terminated;

(2) the authority to prescribe, dispense, and administer is terminated or withdrawn by the supervising physician; or

(3) the physician assistant reverts to inactive status, loses National Commission on Certification of Physician Assistants

or successor agency certification, or loses or terminates registration status.

(b) The physician assistant must notify the board in writing within ten days of the occurrence of any of the circumstances listed in paragraph (a).

(c) Physician assistants whose authority to prescribe, dispense, and administer has been terminated shall reapply for reinstatement of prescribing authority under this section and meet any requirements established by the board prior to reinstatement of the prescribing, dispensing, and administering authority.

Subd. 3. Other requirements and restrictions.

(a) The supervising physician and the physician assistant must complete, sign, and date an internal protocol which lists each category of drug or medical device, or controlled substance the physician assistant may prescribe, dispense, and administer. The supervising physician and physician assistant shall submit the internal protocol to the board upon request. The supervising physician may amend the internal protocol as necessary, within the limits of the completed delegation form in subdivision 5. The supervising physician and physician assistant must sign and date any amendments to the internal protocol. Any amendments resulting in a change to an addition or deletion to categories delegated in the delegation form in subdivision 5 must be submitted to the board according to this chapter, along with the fee required.

(b) The supervising physician and physician assistant shall review delegation of prescribing, dispensing, and administering authority on an annual basis at the time of reregistration. The internal protocol must be signed and dated by the supervising physician and physician assistant after review. Any amendments to the internal protocol resulting in changes to the delegation form in subdivision 5 must be submitted to the board according to this chapter, along with the fee required.

(c) Each prescription initiated by a physician assistant shall indicate the following:

(1) the date of issue;

(2) the name and address of the patient;

(3) the name and quantity of the drug prescribed;

(4) directions for use; and

(5) the name, address, and telephone number of the prescribing physician assistant and of the physician serving as supervisor.

(d) In prescribing, dispensing, and administering legend drugs and medical devices, including controlled substances as defined in section 152.01, subdivision 4, a physician assistant must conform with the agreement, chapter 151, and this chapter.

Subd. 4. Notification of pharmacies.

(a) The board shall annually provide to the Board of Pharmacy and to registered pharmacies within the state a list of those physician assistants who are authorized to prescribe, administer, and dispense legend drugs and medical devices, or controlled substances.

(b) The board shall provide to the Board of Pharmacy a list of physician assistants authorized to prescribe legend drugs and medical devices every two months if additional physician assistants are authorized to prescribe or if physician assistants have authorization to prescribe withdrawn.

(c) The list must include the name, address, telephone number, and Minnesota registration number of the physician assistant, and the name, address, telephone number, and Minnesota license number of the supervising physician.

(d) The board shall provide the form in subdivision 5 to pharmacies upon request.

(e) The board shall make available prototype forms of the physician-physician assistant agreement, the internal protocol, the delegation form, and the addendum form.

Subd. 5. Delegation form for physician assistant prescribing.

The delegation form for physician assistant prescribing must contain a listing by drug category of the legend drugs and controlled substances for which prescribing authority has been delegated to the physician assistant.

Minnesota Stat. Ann. sec. 147.18

MISSISSIPPI

1. Physician Assistants shall practice according to a Board-approved protocol which has been mutually agreed upon by the Physician Assistant and the supervising physician. Each protocol shall be prepared taking into consideration the specialty of the supervising physician, and must outline diagnostic and therapeutic procedures and categories of pharmacologic agents which may be ordered, administered, dispensed and/or prescribed for patients

with diagnoses identified by the Physician Assistant. Each protocol shall contain a detailed description of back-up coverage if the supervising physician is away from the primary office. Although licensed, no Physician Assistant Mississippi State Board of Medical Licensure shall practice until a duly executed protocol has been approved by the Board.

MISSISSIPPI RULES CH. XXII SEC. 4(D)

Regulations to authorize physicians to delegate prescriptive authority for controlled substances (Schedules II–V) became effective on October 17, 2004.

LEGISLATIVE WATCH OCTOBER 15, 2004, AAPA

MISSOURI

Physician assistants shall not prescribe nor dispense any drug, medicine, device or therapy independent of consultation with the supervising physician, nor prescribe lenses, prisms or contact lenses for the aid, relief or correction of vision or the measurement of visual power or visual efficiency of the human eye, nor administer or monitor general or regional block anesthesia during diagnostic tests, surgery or obstetric procedures. Prescribing and dispensing of drugs, medications, devices or therapies by a physician assistant shall be pursuant to a physician assistant supervision agreement which is specific to the clinical conditions treated by the supervising physician and the physician assistant shall be subject to the following:

(1) A physician assistant shall not prescribe controlled substances;

(2) The types of drugs, medications, devices or therapies prescribed or dispensed by a physician assistant shall be consistent with the scopes of practice of the physician assistant and the supervising physician;

(3) All prescriptions shall conform with state and federal laws and regulations and shall include the name, address and telephone number of the physician assistant and the supervising physician;

(4) A physician assistant or advanced practice nurse as defined in section 335.016, RSMo, may request, receive and sign for non-controlled professional samples and may distribute professional samples to patients;

(5) A physician assistant shall not prescribe any drugs, medicines, devices or therapies the supervising physician is not qualified or authorized to prescribe; and

(6) A physician assistant may only dispense starter doses of medication to cover a period of time for seventy-two hours or less.

MISSOURI REV. STAT. SEC. 334.75.3

MONTANA

(1) A physician assistant-certified may prescribe, dispense, and administer drugs to the extent authorized by the board by rule, by the utilization plan, or both. The prescribing, dispensing, and administration of drugs are also subject to the authority of the supervising physician, and the supervising physician may impose additional limitations on the prescribing and dispensing authority granted by the board.

(2) All dispensing activities allowed by this section must comply with 37-2-104 and with packaging and labeling guidelines developed by the board of pharmacy under Title 37, chapter 7.

(3) The prescribing and dispensing authority granted a physician assistant-certified may include the following:

   (a) Prescribing, dispensing, and administration of Schedule III drugs listed in 50-32-226, Schedule IV drugs listed in 50-32-229, and Schedule V drugs listed in 50-32-232 is authorized.

   (b) Prescribing, dispensing, and administration of Schedule II drugs listed in 50-32-224 may be authorized for limited periods not to exceed 34 days.

   (c) Records on the dispensing and administration of scheduled drugs must be kept.

   (d) A physician assistant-certified shall maintain registration with the federal drug enforcement administration.

   (e) Prescriptions written by physician assistants-certified must comply with regulations relating to prescription requirements adopted by the board of pharmacy.

   (f) The board shall adopt rules regarding the refilling of prescriptions written by physician assistants-certified.

MONTANA CODE ANN. SEC. 37-20-404

NEBRASKA

Physician assistants; prescribe drugs and devices; restrictions. A physician assistant may prescribe drugs and devices as delegated to do so by a supervising physician. A supervising physician may delegate to a physician assistant the authority to prescribe all drugs and devices, except that Schedule II controlled substances may only be prescribed for a seventy-two-hour period for the relief of pain and such prescription shall not be renewable by the physician assistant. All prescriptions and prescription container labels shall bear the name of the supervising physician and the physician assistant. A physician assistant to whom has been delegated the authority to prescribe controlled substances shall obtain a federal Drug Enforcement Administration registration number. When prescribing Schedule II controlled substances, the prescription container label shall bear all information required by the federal Controlled Substances Act of 1970.

NEBRASKA REV. STAT. SEC. 71-1.107.30

NEVADA

Contents of license The license issued by the board must contain:
1. The name of the physician assistant;
2. The name of each supervising physician;
3. The duration of the license;
4. The kinds and amounts of controlled substances, poisons, dangerous drugs or devices which the physician assistant may prescribe, possess, administer or dispense;
5. The area in which the physician assistant may possess those controlled substances, poisons, dangerous drugs and devices; and
   Any other limitations or requirements which the board prescribes.

NEVADA ADMIN. CODE SEC. 630.330

NEW HAMPSHIRE

Jurisprudence Examination.

(a) Any physician assistant requesting the authority to issue prescriptions for legend drugs shall successfully complete the jurisprudence examination administered by the board of pharmacy.

(b) The jurisprudence examination shall evaluate the physician assistant's knowledge of current state and federal laws governing the possession, storage and prescription of controlled and other legend drugs, namely RSA 318, RSA 318-B and 21 CFR 1300 et seq.

(c) The minimum passing score for the jurisprudence examination shall be 75.

(d) The jurisprudence examination shall be administered by appointment only at the offices of the New Hampshire board of pharmacy. Upon receipt of a license from the board, the physician assistant shall contact the board of pharmacy and arrange to sit for the next examination.

(e) Failure to sit for or pass the jurisprudence examination shall preclude the physician assistant from exercising any prescriptive privileges, regardless of the scope of practice established by his or her written protocol.

NEW HAMPSHIRE CODE ADMIN. R. ANN. (MED) SEC. 6012.01

Re-examination.

(a) Any physician assistant who failed to attain the minimum passing score on jurisprudence examination as required by Med 608.01(e) may elect to be re-examined within 30 days.

(b) Re-examination shall be scheduled by the board of pharmacy upon the request of the physician assistant.

NEW HAMPSHIRE CODE ADMIN. R. ANN. (MED) SEC. 6012.02

Examination Fees.

All candidates for the jurisprudence examination and re-examination shall pay an examination fee as determined by the board of pharmacy.

NEW HAMPSHIRE CODE ADMIN. R. ANN. (MED) SEC. 6012.03

Scope of Prescriptive Practice.

(a) Physician assistants who have passed the jurisprudence examination shall transmit prescriptions for any patient only in accordance with a delegation agreement, or a patient specific order of the RSP or ARSP, and in compliance with all requirements of RSA 318 and RSA 318-B.

(b) Physician assistants, acting in accordance with a delegation agreement as the agent of the RSP or ARSP, may dispense samples of prescription drugs as necessary and appropriate for patient care.

(c) Physician assistants shall not engage in the act of prescribing controlled substances unless they have obtained the proper registration from the US Drug Enforcement Administration.

(d) A licensed physician assistant may prescribe, dispense and administer drugs and medical devices to the extent delegated by the supervising physician in compliance with RSA 318 and RSA 318-B.

(e) Physician assistants may request, receive, and sign for professional samples and may distribute professional samples to patients.

NEW HAMPSHIRE CODE ADMIN. R. ANN. (MED) SEC. 6012.04

NEW JERSEY

Ordering of medications in inpatient setting

A physician assistant treating a patient in an inpatient or outpatient setting may order or prescribe medications, subject to the following conditions:

a. no controlled dangerous substances may be ordered;
b. the order or prescription is administered in accordance with pro-
    tocols or specific physician direction pursuant to subsection b. of
    section 7 of this act;
c. the prescription states whether it is written pursuant to protocol or
    specific physician direction; and
d. the physician assistant signs his own name, prints his name and
    license number and prints the supervising physicians name.

NEW JERSEY STAT. ANN. SEC. 45: 9-27.19

Authority of temporary licensed physician assistant to write order for medication; countersignature of physician.

A temporary licensed physician assistant may write an order for medications; however, the order may not be executed without the immediate countersignature of a physician or licensed physician assistant.
When the countersignature is provided by a licensed physician assistant, the order must also be countersigned by a physician within 24
hours of its entry by the temporary licensed physician assistant. Any
limitation on the authority of a temporary licensed physician assistant
to order medications as provided in this section shall be in addition to
any such limitation on a licensed physician assistant pursuant to the
"Physician Assistant Licensing Act."

NEW JERSEY STAT. ANN. SEC. 45: 9-27.19A

NEW MEXICO

Physician assistants may prescribe, administer and distribute dangerous drugs other than controlled substances in Schedule I of the
Controlled Substances Act pursuant to rules adopted by the board
after consultation with the board of pharmacy if the prescribing,
administering and distributing are done under the direction of a
supervising licensed physician and within the parameters of a board
approved formulary and guidelines established under Subsection
C of Section 61-6-9 NMSA 1978. The distribution process shall comply with state laws concerning prescription packaging, labeling and
record keeping requirements. Physician assistants shall not otherwise
dispense dangerous drugs or controlled substances.

NEW MEXICO STAT. ANN. SEC. 61-6-7

NEW YORK

If delegated by the physician, physician assistants may write medical orders and prescriptions. In an inpatient setting, the physician

assistant may prescribe all medications including Schedule III-V controlled substances, with physician's counter-signature required within 24 hours. Counter signature is not required prior to execution of the order.

In the outpatient setting, the PA may prescribe all medications including Schedule III-V (excluding schedule II) controlled substances if delegated by the supervising physician. PAs may apply to the DEA to obtain their own, individual registration numbers as "mid-level practitioners." Once duly registered by the DEA, they may write Schedules III, IV and V drugs subject to any limitations imposed by the supervising physician and/or clinic or hospital where such prescribing activity may occur. Such prescriptions are to be written on the supervising physician's prescriptions form. The prescription form must include: the imprinted name of the of the PA; the imprinted name of the supervising physician; the practice address and phone number; the PA's signature followed by the designated RPA; the PA's New York State Registration number; the physician's license number.

PAs may also prescribe Schedule III-V controlled substances which require the use of New York State official prescription forms provided these are written on forms issues to the PA. PAs are not authorized to issue prescriptions for Schedule II controlled substances at any time.

NEW YORK STATE DEPT. OF HEALTH OFFICE OF PROFESSIONAL
MEDICAL CONDUCT EASY REFERENCE INFORMATION REGARDING
THE REGISTERED PA, N.Y. STATE DEPT. OF HEALTH SEC. F

NORTH CAROLINA

Physician assistants are authorized to write prescriptions for drugs under the following conditions:

(1) The North Carolina Medical Board has adopted regulations governing the approval of individual physician assistants to write prescriptions with such limitations as the Board may determine to be in the best interest of patient health and safety.

(2) The physician assistant holds a current license issued by the Board.

(3) The North Carolina Medical Board has assigned an identification number to the physician assistant which is shown on the written prescription.

(4) The supervising physician has provided to the physician assistant written instructions about indications and contraindications for prescribing drugs and a written policy for periodic review by the physician of the drugs prescribed.

    (a) Physician assistants are authorized to compound and dispense drugs under the following conditions:

(1) The function is performed under the supervision of a licensed pharmacist.

(2) Rules and regulations of the North Carolina Board of Pharmacy governing this function are complied with.

(3) The physician assistant holds a current license issued by the Board.

(b) Physician assistants are authorized to order medications, tests and treatments in hospitals, clinics, nursing homes, and other health facilities under the following conditions:

(1) The North Carolina Medical Board has adopted regulations governing the approval of individual physician assistants to order medications, tests, and treatments with such limitations as the Board may determine to be in the best interest of patient health and safety.

(2) The physician assistant holds a current license issued by the Board.

(3) The supervising physician has provided to the physician assistant written instructions about ordering medications, tests, and treatments, and when appropriate, specific oral or written instructions for an individual patient, with provision for review by the physician of the order within a reasonable time, as determined by the Board, after the medication, test, or treatment is ordered.

(4) The hospital or other health facility has adopted a written policy, approved by the medical staff after consultation with the nursing administration, about ordering medications, tests, and treatments, including procedures for verification of the physician assistants' orders by nurses and other facility employees and such other procedures as are in the interest of patient health and safety.

(c) Any prescription written by a physician assistant or order given by a physician assistant for medications, tests, or treatments shall be deemed to have been authorized by the physician approved by the Board as the supervisor of the physician assistant and the supervising physician shall be responsible for authorizing the prescription or order.

(d) Any registered nurse or licensed practical nurse who receives an order from a physician assistant for medications, tests, or treatments is authorized to perform that order in the same manner as if it were received from a licensed physician.

NORTH CAROLINA GEN. STAT. SEC. 90-18.1(B)

A physician assistant is authorized to prescribe, order, procure, dispense and administer drugs and medical devices subject to the following conditions:

(1) The physician assistant and the supervising physician(s) shall acknowledge that each is familiar with the laws and rules regarding prescribing and shall agree to comply with these laws and rules by incorporating the laws and rules into the written prescribing instructions required for each approved practice site; and

(2) The physician assistant has received from the supervising physician written instructions for prescribing, ordering, and administering drugs and medical devices and a written policy for periodic review by the physician of these instructions and policy; and

(3) In order to compound and dispense drugs, the physician assistant must obtain approval from the Board of Pharmacy and must carry out the functions of compounding and dispensing by current Board of Pharmacy rules and any applicable federal guidelines; and

(4) In order to prescribe controlled substances, both the physician assistant and the supervising physician must have a valid DEA registration and the physician assistant shall prescribe in accordance with information provided by the Medical Board and the DEA. All prescriptions for substances falling within schedules II, IIN, III, and IIIN, as defined in the federal Controlled Substances Act, shall not exceed a legitimate 30 day supply; and

(5) Each prescription issued by the physician assistant shall contain, in addition to other information required by law, the following:

   (a) the physician assistant's name, practice address, telephone number; and

   (b) the physician's assistant's license number and, if applicable, the physician assistant's DEA number for controlled substances prescription; and

   (c) the responsible supervising physician's (primary or back-up) name and telephone number; and

(6) Documentation of each prescription must be noted on the patient's record and must include the following information:

   (a) medication name and dosage, amount prescribed, directions for use, number of refills; and

   (b) signature of physician assistant with supervising physician's co-signature according to the site specific rule in 21 NCAC 32S .0110.

(7) Physician Assistants who request, receive, and dispense professional medication samples to patients must comply with all applicable state and federal regulations.

21 NORTH CAROLINA ANN. CODE 32 SEC. .0109

NORTH DAKOTA

A physician assistant may prescribe medications as delegated to do so by a supervising physician. This may include schedule III through V controlled substances; however, a physician assistant may not prescribe schedule II controlled substances. A physician assistant who is a delegated prescriber of controlled substances must register with the federal drug enforcement administration.

NORTH CAROLINA MED. PRAC. ACT SEC. 43-17-02.1

A physician assistant may dispense prepackaged medications prepared by a registered pharmacist acting on a physician's written order and labeled to show the name of the physician assistant and physician. The dispensation authorized shall be limited to controlled drugs of schedules four and five and non-scheduled drugs. The dispensation by the physician assistant must be authorized by, and within, the pre-established guidelines of the supervising physician

NORTH DAKOTA ADMIN. CODE SEC. 50-03-01-07

OHIO

No provision

OKLAHOMA

(a) A physician assistant may issue written and oral prescriptions and other orders for drugs and medical supplies, including controlled medications in Schedules III, IV, and V under 63 Okla. Stat. ss 2-312 as delegated by and within the established scope of practice of the supervising physician and as approved by the Board.

(b) A physician assistant may write an order for a Schedule II drug for immediate or ongoing administration on site. Prescriptions and orders for Schedule II drugs written by a physician assistant must be included on a written protocol determined by the supervising physician and approved by the medical staff committee of the facility or by direct verbal order of the supervising physician.

(c) Written prescriptions shall be issued in the format and in accordance with the Physician Assistant Drug Formulary, listed in Subchapter 11 of this Chapter, as established by the Board in consultation with the Oklahoma State Board of Pharmacy.

(d) All written prescriptions and orders for drugs shall be written on the prescription blank of the supervising physician and must bear the name and phone number of the physician, the printed name and license number of the physician assistant, the original signature of the physician assistant, and any other information the Board may require. If more than one physician name appears on the prescription blank, the physician assistant shall indicate which is the supervising physician.

(e) A physician assistant may not issue prescriptions or orders for drugs and medical supplies that the physician is not permitted to prescribe.

(f) A physician assistant may not dispense drugs but may request, receive and sign for professional samples and may distribute professional samples to patients.

Oklahoma Admin. Code sec. 435:15-5-10

OREGON

(1) A physician assistant may issue written or oral prescriptions for medications, Schedule III-V, which the supervising physician has determined the physician assistant is qualified to prescribe commensurate with the practice description and approved by the Board if the following conditions are met:

(a) The physician assistant has met the requirements of OAR 847-050-0020(1); or is an Oregon grandfathered physician assistant who has passed the Physician Assistant National Certifying Examination (PANCE) or other specialty examination approved by the Board prior to July 12, 1984;

(b) The applicant must document adequate training and/or experience in pharmacology commensurate with the practice description;

(c) The Board may require the applicant to pass a pharmacological examination which may be written, oral, practical, or any combination thereof based on the practice description.

(2) The prescribing physician assistant, to be authorized to issue prescriptions for Schedules III through V controlled substances, must be registered with the Federal Drug Enforcement Administration.

(3) Written prescriptions shall be on a blank which includes the printed or handwritten name, office address, and telephone number of the supervising physician and the printed or handwritten name of the physician assistant. The prescription shall also bear the name of the patient and the date on which the prescription was written. The physician assistant shall sign the prescription and the signature shall be followed by the letter "P.A." Also the physician assistant's Federal Drug Enforcement Administration number shall be shown on prescriptions for controlled substances.

(4) A licensed physician assistant may make application to the Board

for emergency administering and dispensing authority. The application must be submitted in writing to the Board by the supervising physician and must explain the need for the request, as follows:

(a) Location of the practice site;

(b) Accessibility to the nearest pharmacy, and

(c) Medical necessity for emergency administering or dispensing.

(5) The dispensed medication must be pre-packaged by a licensed pharmacist, manufacturing drug outlet or wholesale drug outlet authorized to do so under ORS 689 and the physician assistant shall maintain records of receipt and distribution.

Oregon Admin. Rules sec. 847-050-0041

PENNSYLVANIA

Administration of controlled substances and whole blood and blood components.

(a) The physician assistant may administer controlled substances and whole blood and blood components if the authority to administer these medications and fluids is expressly set forth in the written agreement and the administration of these medications and fluids is separately ordered by the physician assistant supervisor and the physician assistant supervisor specifies a named drug for a named patient.

(b) The physician assistant shall comply with the minimum standards for administering controlled substances specified in § 16.92 (relating to prescribing, administering and dispensing controlled substances).

Pennsylvania Admin. Code sec. 18.157

Prescribing and dispensing drugs.

(a) The Board adopts the American Hospital Formulary Service (AHFS) Pharmacologic-Therapeutic Classification to identify drugs which a physician assistant may prescribe and dispense subject to the restrictions specified in subsection (c).

(1) Categories from which a physician assistant may prescribe and dispense without limitation are as follows:

(i) Antihistamines.

(ii) Anti-infective agents.

(iii) Cardiovascular drugs.

(iv) Contraceptives—for example, foams and devices.

      (v)   Diagnostic agents.

      (vi) Disinfectants—for agents used on objects other than skin.

    (vii) Electrolytic, caloric and water balance.

   (viii) Enzymes.

     (ix) Antitussives, expectorants and mucolytic agents.

      (x) Gastrointestinal drugs.

     (xi) Local anesthetics.

    (xii) Serums, toxoids and vaccines.

   (xiii) Skin and mucous membrane agents.

   (xiv) Smooth muscle relaxants.

    (xv) Vitamins.

(2) Categories from which a physician assistant may prescribe and dispense subject to exclusions and limitations listed:

      (i) *Autonomic drugs.* Drugs excluded under this category: Sympathomimetic (adrenergic) agents.

     (ii) *Blood formation and coagulation.* Drugs excluded under this category:

        (A) Anti-coagulants and coagulants.

        (B) Thrombolytic agents.

    (iii) *Central nervous system agents.* Drugs excluded under this category:

        (A) General anesthetics.

        (B) Monoamine oxidase inhibitors.

     (iv) *Eye, ear, nose and throat preparations.* Drugs limited under this category: Miotics and mydriatrics used as eye preparations require specific approval from the physician assistant supervisor for a named patient.

      (v) *Hormones and synthetic substitutes.* Drugs excluded under this category:

        (A) Pituitary hormones and synthetics.

        (B) Parathyroid hormones and synthetics.

(3) Categories from which a physician assistant may not prescribe or dispense are as follows:

      (i) Antineoplastic agents.

     (ii) Dental agents.

    (iii) Gold compounds.

    (iv) Heavy metal antagonists.

     (v) Oxytocics.

    (vi) Radioactive agents.

   (vii) Unclassified therapeutic agents.

  (viii) Devices.

    (ix) Pharmaceutical aids.

(4) New drugs and new uses for drugs will be considered approved for prescribing and dispensing purposes by physician assistants 90 days after approval by the Federal Drug Administration unless excluded in paragraphs (2) and (3).

(b) If the physician assistant supervisor intends to authorize a physician assistant to prescribe or dispense drugs, the supervisor shall:

(1) Establish a list of drugs, based on the categories listed in subsection (a), which the physician assistant may prescribe or dispense. The physician assistant supervisor shall assure that the physician assistant is able to competently prescribe or dispense those drugs.

(2) Submit the list of drugs to the Board, in duplicate, on a form supplied by the Board, and signed by both the physician assistant supervisor and the physician assistant. The list will become part of the physician assistant's written agreement if it is consistent with the approved classification.

(3) Notify the Board, in duplicate, on a form supplied by the Board, of an addition or deletion to the list of drugs. The amendment will become part of the physician assistant's written agreement if it is consistent with the approved classification.

(4) Assume full responsibility for every prescription issued and drug dispensed by a physician assistant under his supervision.

(5) Maintain a copy of the list of drugs submitted to the Board in his principal office and at all locations where the physician assistant practices under his supervision for review or inspection without prior notice by patients, the Board or its agents. The physician shall provide a pharmacy with a copy of the drug list upon request by the pharmacist.

(6) Immediately advise the patient, notify the physician assistant and, in the case of a written prescription, advise the pharmacy, if the physician assistant is prescribing or dispensing a drug inappropriately. The physician shall advise the patient and notify the physician assistant to discontinue using the drug, and in the case of a written prescription, shall notify the pharmacy to discontinue the prescription. The order to discontinue use of the drug or prescription shall be noted in the patient's medical record by the physician.

(c) Restrictions on a physician assistant's prescription and dispension practices are as follows:

(1) A physician assistant may only prescribe or dispense a drug approved by the Board from the categories specified in subsection (a).

(2) A physician assistant may only prescribe or dispense a drug for a patient who is under the care of the physician responsible for the supervision of the physician assistant and only in accordance with the physician's instructions and written agreement.

(3) A physician assistant shall comply with the minimum standards for prescribing and dispensing controlled substances specified in § 16.92 (relating to prescribing, administering and dispensing controlled substances) and the regulations of the Department of Health relating to Controlled Substances, Drugs, Devices and Cosmetics, 28 Pa. Code § § 25.51—25.58 (relating to prescriptions), and packaging and labeling dispensed drugs. See § § 16.93 and 16.94 (relating to packaging; and labeling of dispensed drugs) and 28 Pa. Code § § 25.91—25.95 (relating to labeling of drugs, devices and cosmetics).

(4) A physician assistant may not:

   (i) Prescribe or dispense a pure form or combination of drugs listed in subsection (a) unless the drug or class of drug is listed as permissible for prescription or dispension.

   (ii) Prescribe or dispense Schedule I or II controlled substances as defined by section 4 of the Controlled Substances, Drug, Device, and Cosmetic Act (35 P. S. § 780-104).

   (iii) Prescribe or dispense a drug for a use not permitted by the Food and Drug Administration.

   (iv) Prescribe or dispense a generic or branded preparation of a drug that has not been approved by the Food and Drug Administration.

   (v) Prescribe or dispense parenteral preparations other than insulin, emergency allergy kits and other approved drugs listed in subsection (a).

   (vi) Dispense a drug unless it is packaged in accordance with applicable Federal and State law pertaining to packaging by physicians. See § § 16.93 and 16.94.

   (vii) Compound ingredients when dispensing a drug, except for adding water.

   (viii) Issue a prescription for more than a 30-day supply, except in cases of chronic illnesses where a 90-day supply may be prescribed. The physician assistant may authorize refills up to 6 months from the date of the original prescription if not otherwise precluded by law.

(d) The requirements for prescription blanks are as follows:
  (1) Prescription blanks shall bear the certification number of the physician assistant and the name of the physician assistant in printed format at the heading of the blank, and a space for the entry of the Drug Enforcement Administration registration number as appropriate. The physician assistant supervisor shall also be identified as required in § 16.91 (relating to identifying information on prescriptions and orders for equipment and service).
  (2) The physician assistant supervisor is prohibited from presigning prescription blanks or allowing the physician assistant to use a device for affixing a signature copy on the prescription. The signature of a physician assistant shall be followed by the initials "PA-C" or similar designation to identify the signer as a physician assistant.
  (3) The physician assistant may use a prescription blank generated by a hospital if the information in paragraph (1) appears on the blank.
(e) Recordkeeping requirements are as follows:
  (1) When prescribing a drug, the physician assistant shall keep a copy of the prescription, including the number of refills, in a ready reference file, or record the name, amount and doses of the drug prescribed, the number of refills, the date of the prescription and the physician assistant's name in the patient's medical records.
  (2) When dispensing a drug, the physician assistant shall record his name, the name of the medication dispensed, the amount of medication dispensed, the dose of the medication dispensed and the date dispensed in the patient's medical records.
  (3) The physician assistant shall report, orally or in writing, to the physician assistant supervisor within 12 hours, a drug prescribed or medication dispensed by him while the physician assistant supervisor was not physically present, and the basis for each decision to prescribe or dispense.
  (4) The physician assistant supervisor shall countersign the prescription copy or medical record entry for each prescription or dispension within a reasonable time, not to exceed 3 days, unless countersignature is required sooner by regulation, policy within the medical care facility or the requirements of a third-party payor.
  (5) The physician assistant and the physician assistant supervisor shall provide immediate access to the written agreement to anyone seeking to confirm the physician assistant's authority to prescribe or dispense a drug.

PENNSYLVANIA ADMIN. CODE SEC. 18.158

Osteopathic

No provision

RHODE ISLAND

When employed by, or extended medical staff privileges by a licensed hospital or other licensed health care facility, a physician assistant may write medical orders for inpatients as delineated by the medical staff by-laws of the facility, as well as its credentialing process and applicable governing authority.

Hospitals and other licensed health care facilities shall have discretion to grant privileges to a physician assistant and to define the scope of privileges or services which a physician assistant may deliver in a facility. Hospitals or other licensed facilities shall not grant privileges to a physician assistant that would not be granted to the supervising physician.

Physician assistants employed directly by physicians, health maintenance organizations or other health care delivery organizations may prescribe legend medications, including schedules II, III, IV, and V medications under Title 21 Chapter 28 of the Rhode Island Uniform Controlled Substance Act, medical therapies, medical devices and medical diagnostics according to guidelines established by the employing physician, health maintenance organization, or other health care delivery organization.

Prescriptive privileges for physician assistants shall be granted for all legend medications, including controlled substances from schedules II, III, IV, and V, in accordance with the agreement developed by the supervising physician and the physician assistant cited in section 1.12 herein.

If a physician assistant does prescribe controlled substances from schedules II, III, IV, and V, under Title 21 of Chapter 28, he/she must obtain a state registration for prescribing controlled substances from the Board of Pharmacy, as well as a federal registration.

RHODE ISLAND R5-54-PA-6.4

SOUTH CAROLINA

(A) If the written scope of practice guidelines authorize the physician's assistant to prescribe drug therapy:
   (1) prescriptions for authorized drugs and devices shall comply with all applicable state and federal laws;
   (2) prescriptions must be limited to drugs and devices authorized by the supervising physician and set forth in the written scope of practice guidelines;

(3) prescriptions must be signed by the physician assistant and must bear the physician assistant's identification number as assigned by the board. The prescription form shall include the physician assistant's and physician's name, address, and phone number pre-printed on the form and shall comply with the provisions of Section 39-24-40;

(4) drugs or devices prescribed must be specifically documented in the patient record;

(5) the physician assistant may request, receive, and sign for professional samples, except for controlled substances in Schedules II through IV, and may distribute professional samples to patients in compliance with appropriate federal and state regulations.

(B) A physician assistant's prescriptive authorization may be terminated by the board if the physician assistant:

(1) practices outside the written scope of practice guidelines;

(2) violates any state or federal law or regulation applicable to prescriptions; or

(3) violates a state or federal law applicable to physician assistants.

SOUTH CAROLINA PA PRAC. ACT SEC. 40-47-965

SOUTH DAKOTA

Make a tentative medical diagnosis and institute therapy or referral; prescribe medications and provide drug samples or a limited supply of labeled medications, including controlled drugs or substances listed on Schedule II in chapter 34-20B for one period of not more than forty-eight hours, for symptoms and temporary pain relief; treat common childhood diseases; to assist in the follow-up treatment of geriatric and psychiatric disorders referred by the physicians. Medications or sample drugs provided to patients shall be accompanied with written administration instructions and appropriate documentation shall be entered in the patient's medical record;

SOUTH DAKOTA CODIFIED LAWS 36-4A-22

TENNESSEE

(1) Prescription writing shall be governed by T.C.A. § 63-19-107.

(2) A physician assistant authorized by his or her supervising physician to prescribe drugs shall complete a Notice of Authorization for Prescribing form, including the biographical information and formulary, and submit it to the following addresses:

Committee on Physician Assistants
First Floor, Cordell Hull Building
425 Fifth Avenue North
Nashville, TN 37247-1010

Tennessee Board of Pharmacy
Davy Crockett Tower
500 James Robertson Parkway, 2nd Floor
Nashville, TN 37243-1149

(3) As required by T.C.A. § 53-10-104, a physician assistant may not accept the delegated authority to issue a prescription or dispense any drug or medication whose sole purpose is to cause or perform an abortion.

RRT SEC. 0880-3-21

In accordance with rules adopted by the board and the committee, a supervising physician may delegate to a physician assistant working under the physician's supervision the authority to prescribe and/or issue legend drugs and controlled substances listed in Schedules II, III, IV, and V of title 39, chapter 17, part 4. The rules adopted prior to March 19, 1999, by the board and the committee governing the prescribing of legend drugs by physician assistants shall remain effective after March 19, 1999, and may be revised from time to time as deemed appropriate by the board and the committee. The board and the committee may adopt additional rules governing the prescribing of controlled substances by physician assistants. A physician assistant to whom is delegated the authority to prescribe and/or issue controlled substances must register and comply with all applicable requirements of the drug enforcement administration.

A physician assistant to whom the authority to prescribe legend drugs and controlled substances has been delegated by the supervising physician shall file a notice with the committee, containing the name of the physician assistant, the name of the licensed physician having supervision, control and responsibility for prescriptive services rendered by the physician assistant, and a copy of the formulary describing the categories of legend drugs and controlled substances to be prescribed and/or issued by the physician assistant. The physician assistant shall be responsible for updating this information.

The prescriptive practices of physician assistants, and the supervision by physicians under whom such physician assistants are rendering service, shall be monitored by the board and committee. As used in this section, "monitor" does not include the regulation of the practice of medicine or the regulation of the practice of a physician assistant, but may include site visits by members of the board and committee;

Any complaints against physician assistants and/or supervising physicians shall be reported to the director of the division of health related boards, the committee on physician assistants, and the board of medical examiners, as appropriate;

Every prescription issued by a physician assistant pursuant to this section shall be entered in the medical records of the patient and shall be written on a preprinted prescription pad bearing the name, address, and telephone number of the supervising physician and of the physician assistant, and the physician assistant shall sign each prescription so written. Where the preprinted prescription pad contains the names of more than one (1) physician, the physician assistant shall indicate on the prescription which of those physicians is the physician assistant's primary supervising physician by placing a checkmark beside or a circle around the name of that physician;

No drugs shall be dispensed by a physician assistant except under the supervision, control, and responsibility of the supervising physician.

TENNESSEE ANN. CODE SEC. 63-19-107

TEXAS

(a) In this section, "primary practice site" means:
   (1) the practice location of a physician at which the physician spends the majority of the physician's time;
   (2) a licensed hospital, a licensed long-term care facility, or a licensed adult care center where both the physician and the physician assistant or advanced practice nurse are authorized to practice;
   (3) a clinic operated by or for the benefit of a public school district to provide care to the students of that district and the siblings of those students, if consent to treatment at that clinic is obtained in a manner that complies with Chapter 32, Family Code;
   (4) the residence of an established patient; or
   (5) another location at which the physician is physically present with the physician assistant or advanced practice nurse.
(b) At a physician's primary practice site, a physician licensed by the board may delegate to a physician assistant or an advanced practice nurse acting under adequate physician supervision the act of administering, providing, or carrying out or signing a prescription drug order as authorized through a physician's order, a standing medical order, a standing delegation order, or another order or protocol as defined by the board.
(c) Physician supervision of the carrying out and signing of prescription drug orders must conform to what a reasonable, prudent physician would find consistent with sound medical judgment but may vary with the education and experience of the particular

advanced practice nurse or physician assistant. A physician shall provide continuous supervision, but the constant physical presence of the physician is not required.

(d) An alternate physician may provide appropriate supervision on a temporary basis as defined and established by board rule.

(e) A physician's authority to delegate the carrying out or signing of a prescription drug order is limited to:

    (1) three physician assistants or advanced practice nurses or their full-time equivalents practicing at the physician's primary practice site or at an alternate practice site under Section 157.0541; and

    (2) the patients with whom the physician has established or will establish a physician-patient relationship.

(f) For purposes of Subsection (e)(2), the physician is not required to see the patient within a specific period.

TEXAS MEDICAL PRACTICE ACT SEC. 157.053

Prescribing at facility-based practice sites.

(a) A physician licensed by the board may delegate, to one or more physician assistants or advanced practice nurses acting under adequate physician supervision whose practice is facility-based at a licensed hospital or licensed long-term care facility, the administration or provision of a drug and the carrying out or signing of a prescription drug order if the physician is:

    (1) the medical director or chief of medical staff of the facility in which the physician assistant or advanced practice nurse practices;

    (2) the chair of the facility's credentialing committee;

    (3) a department chair of a facility department in which the physician assistant or advanced practice nurse practices; or

    (4) a physician who consents to the request of the medical director or chief of medical staff to delegate the carrying out or signing of a prescription drug order at the facility in which the physician assistant or advanced practice nurse practices.

(b) A physician's authority to delegate under Subsection (a) is limited as follows:

    (1) the delegation must be made under a physician's order, standing medical order, standing delegation order, or another order or protocol developed in accordance with policies approved by the facility's medical staff or a committee of the facility's medical staff as provided by the facility bylaws;

    (2) the delegation must occur in the facility in which the physician

is the medical director, the chief of medical staff, the chair of the credentialing committee, or a department chair;

(3) the delegation may not permit the carrying out or signing of prescription drug orders for the care or treatment of the patients of any other physician without the prior consent of that physician;

(4) delegation in a long-term care facility must be by the medical director and is limited to the carrying out and signing of prescription drug orders to not more than three advanced practice nurses or physician assistants or their full-time equivalents; and

(5) a physician may not delegate at more than one licensed hospital or more than two long-term care facilities unless approved by the board.

(c) Physician supervision of the carrying out and signing of prescription drug orders must conform to what a reasonable, prudent physician would find consistent with sound medical judgment but may vary with the education and experience of the particular advanced practice nurse or physician assistant. A physician shall provide continuous supervision, but the constant physical presence of the physician is not required.

(d) An alternate physician may provide appropriate supervision on a temporary basis as defined and established by board rule.

TEXAS MEDICAL PRACTICE ACT SEC. 157.054

Prescribing at alternate sites.

(a) In this section, "alternate site" means a practice site:
(1) where services similar to the services provided at the delegating physician's primary practice site are provided; and
(2) located within 60 miles of the delegating physician's primary practice site.

(b) At an alternate site, a physician licensed by the board may delegate to an advanced practice nurse or physician assistant, acting under adequate physician supervision, the act of administering, providing, or carrying out or signing a prescription drug order as authorized through a physician's order, a standing medical order, a standing delegation order, or another order or protocol as defined by the board.

(c) Physician supervision is adequate for the purposes of this section if the delegating physician:
(1) is on-site with the advanced practice nurse or physician assistant at least 20 percent of the time;

(2) reviews at least 10 percent of the medical charts at the site; and

(3) is available through direct telecommunication for consultation, patient referral, or assistance with a medical emergency.

(d) An alternate physician may provide appropriate supervision to an advanced practice nurse or physician assistant under this section on a temporary basis as provided by board rule.

(e) The combined number of advanced practice nurses and physician assistants to whom a physician may delegate under this section and at a primary practice site under Section 157.053 may not exceed three physician assistants or advanced practice nurses or the full-time equivalent of three physician assistants or advanced practice nurses.

TEXAS MEDICAL PRACTICE ACT SEC. 157.0541

UTAH

(1) A physician assistant may provide any medical services that are not specifically prohibited under this chapter or rules adopted under this chapter, and that are:

(a) within the physician assistant's skills and scope of competence;

(b) within the usual scope of practice of the physician assistant's supervising physician; and

(c) provided under the supervision of a supervising physician and in accordance with a delegation of services agreement.

(2) A physician assistant, in accordance with a delegation of services agreement, may prescribe or administer an appropriate controlled substance if:

(a) the physician assistant holds a Utah controlled substance license and a DEA registration;

(b) the prescription or administration of the controlled substance is within the prescriptive practice of the supervising physician and also within the delegated prescribing stated in the delegation of services agreement; and

(c) the supervising physician cosigns any medical chart record of a prescription of a Schedule 2 or Schedule 3 controlled substance made by the physician assistant.

(3) A physician assistant shall, while practicing as a physician assistant, wear an identification badge showing his license classification as a practicing physician assistant.

(4) A physician assistant may not

(a) independently charge or bill a patient, or others on behalf of the patient, for services rendered;

   (b) identify himself to any person in connection with activities allowed under this chapter other than as a physician assistant; or

   (c) use the title "doctor" or "physician," or by any knowing act or omission lead or permit anyone to believe he is a physician.

UTAH CODE ANN. SEC. 58-70A-501

VERMONT

The certified physician assistant may prescribe only those drugs utilized by the primary supervising physician and permitted by the scope of practice submitted to and approved by the Board. The prescription form used by the PA must include:

(a) The printed name of the physician assistant;

(b) The printed name of the supervising physician;

(c) The practice address and telephone number;

(d) A space for the physician assistant's signature;

(e) A space for the physician assistant's DEA number.

Upon a pharmacist's request, the Board shall furnish a copy of the Board-approved scope of practice and a signature sample of the physician assistant.

VERMONT RULES OF THE BD. OF MED. SEC. II.7.4

VIRGINIA

Qualifications for approval of prescriptive authority.

An applicant for prescriptive authority shall meet the following requirements:

1. Hold a current, unrestricted license as a physician assistant in the Commonwealth;

2. Submit a protocol acceptable to the board prescribed in 18VAC85-50-101. This protocol must be approved by the board prior to issuance of prescriptive authority;

3. Submit evidence of successful passing of the NCCPA exam; and

4. Submit evidence of successful completion of a minimum of 35 hours of acceptable training to the board in pharmacology.

18 VIRGINIA ADMIN. CODE SEC. 85-50-130

Approved drugs and devices.

A. The approved drugs and devices which the physician assistant with prescriptive authority may prescribe, administer, or dispense manufacturer's professional samples shall be in accordance with provisions of §54.1-2952.1 of the Code of Virginia:

B. The physician assistant may prescribe only those categories of drugs and devices included in the practice agreement as submitted for authorization. The supervising physician retains the authority to restrict certain drugs within these approved categories.

C. The physician assistant, pursuant to §54.1-2952.1 of the Code of Virginia, shall only dispense manufacturer's professional samples or administer controlled substances in good faith for medical or therapeutic purposes within the course of his professional practice.

18 VIRGINIA ADMIN. CODE SEC. 85-50-140

Protocol regarding prescriptive authority.

A. A physician assistant with prescriptive authority may prescribe only within the scope of the written protocol as prescribed in 18VAC85-50-101.

B. A new protocol must be submitted with the initial application for prescriptive authority and with the application for each biennial renewal, if there have been any changes in supervision, authorization or scope of practice.

18 VIRGINIA ADMIN. CODE SEC. 85-50-150

WASHINGTON

A physician assistant may issue written or oral prescriptions as provided herein when approved by the commission and assigned by the supervising physician(s).

(1) A physician assistant may not prescribe controlled substances unless specifically approved by the commission or its designee. A physician assistant may issue prescriptions for legend drugs for a patient who is under the care of the physician(s) responsible for the supervision of the physician assistant.

   (a) Written prescriptions shall include the name, address, and telephone number of the physician or medical group; the name and address of the patient and the date on which the prescription was written.

   (b) The physician assistant shall sign such a prescription using his or her own name followed by the letters "PA."

   (c) Written prescriptions for schedule two through five must include the physician assistant's D.E.A. registration number, or, if none, the supervising physician's D.E.A. registration number, followed by the letters "PA." and the physician assistant's license number.

(2) A physician assistant employed or extended privileges by a hospital, nursing home or other health care institution may, if permissible under the bylaws, rules and regulations of the institution, order pharmaceutical agents for inpatients under the care of the physician(s) responsible for his or her supervision.

(3) The license of a physician assistant who issues a prescription in violation of these provisions shall be subject to revocation or suspension.

(4) Physician assistants may dispense medications the physician assistant has prescribed from office supplies. The physician assistant shall comply with the state laws concerning prescription labeling requirements

WASHINGTON ANN. CODE SEC. 246-918-030

A certified physician assistant may issue written or oral prescriptions as provided herein when approved by the commission or its designee.

(1) Written prescriptions shall include the name, address, and telephone number of the physician or medical group; the name and address of the patient and the date on which the prescription was written.

   (a) The certified physician assistant shall sign such a prescription using his or her own name followed by the letters "PA-C."

   (b) The written prescriptions for schedule two through five must include the physician assistant's D.E.A. registration number, or, if none, the sponsoring physician's D.E.A. registration number, followed by the letters "PA-C" and the physician assistant's license number.

(2) A certified physician assistant employed or extended privileges by a hospital, nursing home or other health care institution may, if permissible under the bylaws, rules and regulations of the institution, order pharmaceutical agents for inpatients under the care of the sponsoring physician(s).

(3) The license of a certified physician assistant who issues a prescription in violation of these provisions shall be subject to revocation or suspension.

(4) Certified physician assistants may dispense medications the certified physician assistant has prescribed from office supplies. The certified physician assistant shall comply with the state laws concerning prescription labeling requirements.

WASHINGTON ANN. CODE SEC. 246-918-035

WEST VIRGINIA

A physician assistant may be authorized by the Board to issue written or oral prescriptions for certain medicinal drugs at the direction of his or her supervising physician if all of the following conditions are met:

a. The physician assistant has performed patient care services for a minimum of two (2) years immediately preceding the submission to the Board of the job description requesting limited prescriptive privileges: Provided, that to meet this condition, the first year of patient care services may be as a student in an approved physician assistant program;

b. The physician assistant has successfully completed an accredited course of instruction in clinical pharmacology approved by the Board of not less than four (4) semester hours. The course of instruction may be completed within an approved undergraduate or graduate program for physician assistants. Physician assistants who have not met this requirement shall complete an additional course of study approved by the Board in which fifteen (15) contact hours equals one (1) semester hour. The Board may, at its discretion, grant up to fifteen (15) contact hours for two or more years of prescribing experience in other jurisdictions;

c. The physician assistant obtains Board approval of his or her job description which includes the categories of drugs the physician assistant proposes to prescribe at the direction of his or her supervising physician; and

d. The physician assistant continues to maintain national certification as a physician assistant, and in meeting the national certification requirements, completes a minimum of ten (10) hours of continuing education in rational drug therapy in each certification period.

Evidence of completion of all conditions for the granting of limited prescriptive privileges shall be included with the physician assistant's biennial renewal application and report to the Board.

The Board is responsible for approving a formulary classifying pharmacologic categories of all drugs which may be prescribed by a physician assistant authorized by the Board to prescribe drugs. The formulary shall exclude Schedules I and II of the Uniform Controlled Substances Act, anticoagulants, antineoplastics, radio-pharmaceuticals, general anesthetics and radiographic contrast materials. The formulary may be revised annually, and shall include the following designated sections:

a. Section a.—A choice of drugs commonly used in primary care outpatient settings to be prescribable by physician assistants who have completed an accredited course of study in clinical pharmacology approved by the Board.

b. Section b.—Additional drugs used less commonly in primary care outpatient settings to be prescribable by physician assistants who have satisfied the requirements to prescribe Section a. drugs set forth under paragraph 14.3.a., of this rule. In addition, Section b. drugs may be prescribed by physician assistants only in the following limited situations:

1. On a direct order from the supervising physician to the physician assistant during consultation at the time of the patient's examination by the physician assistant, which is specifically noted in the patient's chart; or

2. On a refill prescription for a previously diagnosed and stable patient whose prescription was initiated by the supervising physician.

A prescription drug not included in the approved formulary shall not be contained in the job description of any physician assistant.

Prescriptions issued by a physician assistant shall be issued consistent with the supervising physician's directions or treatment protocol provided to his or her physician assistant. The maximum dosage shall be indicated in the protocol and in no case may the dosage exceed the manufacturer's recommended average therapeutic dose for that drug.

Each prescription and subsequent refills given by the physician assistant shall be entered on the patient's chart.

The prescription form utilized by a physician assistant approved for limited prescriptive privileges shall be imprinted with the name of the supervising physician, the name of the approved physician assistant, the address of the health care facility, the telephone number of the health care facility, the categories of drugs or drugs within a category which the assistant may prescribe and the statement, "Physician Assistant Prescription—it is a violation of state law to dispense drugs not imprinted on this prescription." The physician assistant shall write the name of the patient, the patient's address and the date on each prescription form. The physician assistant shall sign his or her name to each prescription followed by the letters "PA-C." The supervising physician shall provide the Board with a copy of the prescription form used by his or her physician assistant prior to its use. A copy of this prescription form shall be provided by the physician assistant to area pharmacies where the physician assistant may issue a prescription by word of mouth, telephone or other means of communication in his or her name at the direction of the supervising physician.

Physician assistants authorized to issue prescriptions for Schedules III through V controlled substances shall write on the prescription form the Federal Drug Enforcement Administration number issued to that physician assistant. Prescriptions written for Schedule III drugs shall be limited to a seventy-two (72) hour supply and may not authorize a refill. The maximum amount of Schedule IV or Schedule V drugs shall be no more than ninety (90) dosage units or a thirty (30) day supply, whichever is less.

Prescriptions for other legend drugs shall not be prescribed or refillable for a period exceeding six (6) months.

The Board of Medicine shall provide the Board of Pharmacy with a list of physician assistants with limited prescriptive privileges and shall update the list within ten (10) days after additions or deletions are made.

Nothing in this rule shall be construed to permit any physician assistant to independently prescribe or dispense drugs.

Physician assistants given limited prescriptive privileges under this subsection may accept professional samples as defined in Board of Medicine Rules for Dispensing of Legend Drugs by Physicians and Podiatrists, 11 CSR 5 2.10., on behalf of their respective supervising physician.

WEST VIRGINIA RULES SEC. 11-1B-14

WISCONSIN

(1) A physician assistant may not prescribe or dispense any drug independently.

(2) A physician assistant may issue a prescription order only if all the following conditions apply:

(a) The physician assistant issues the prescription order only in patient situations specified and described in established written guidelines. The guidelines shall be reviewed at least annually by the physician assistant and his or her supervising physician.

(b) The supervising physician and physician assistant determine by mutual agreement that the physician assistant is qualified through training and experience to issue a prescription order as specified in the established written guidelines.

(c) The supervising physician is available for consultation as specified in s. Med 8.10 (3).

(d) The prescription orders prepared under procedures in this section contain all information required under s. 450.11 (1), Stats.

(e) The supervising physician either:

1. Reviews and countersigns the prescription order prepared by the physician assistant, or
2. Reviews and countersigns within 72 hours the patient record prepared by the physician assistant practicing in the office of the supervising physician or at a facility or a hospital in which the supervising physician has staff privileges, or
3. Reviews by telephone or other means, as soon as practicable but within a 72-hour period, and countersigns within one week, the patient record prepared by the physician assistant who practices in an office facility other than the supervising physician's main office of a facility or hospital in which the supervising physician has staff privileges.

WISCONSIN ADMIN. CODE SEC. 8.08

WYOMING

A physician assistant may prescribe medications only as an agent of the supervising physician. A physician assistant may not prescribe schedule I drugs as defined by W.S. 35-7-1013 through 35-7-1014. The supervising physician may delegate authority to the physician assistant to dispense prepackaged medications in rural clinics when pharmacy services are not physically available. The board shall, after consultation with the state board of pharmacy, promulgate rules and regulations governing the prescription of medications by a physician assistant.

WYOMING STAT. ANN. SEC. 33-26-510

CHAPTER 5

Employment Issues

Employment Outlook • Preparing a Resume or Curriculum Vitae • Interviewing • Interview Questions • Questions a PA Should Ask a Potential Employer • PA–Physician Team • Licensure • Should I Get a Written Contract? • Malpractice Insurance • Independent Contractor Status • Federal Regulation That May Affect PAs' Ownership in Medical Entities • Hospital Practice • Required Identification • Credentialing Service • **Appendix 5-A** Sample Cover Letters, Curricula Vitae and Resumes, and Thank-You Letters • **Appendix 5-B** Contract Checklist • **Appendix 5-C** Sample Practice Privilege Checklist and Guidelines • **Appendix 5-D** Credentialing Information

The majority of physician assistants are employed by single- or multispecialty physician group practices (43%). Hospitals are the next largest employers of PAs (22%), followed by solo physicians (14%), and governmental agencies (10%).[1] Although many PAs practice without the benefit of a contract and are "at-will employees," contracts are being offered to PAs on a more consistent basis. It is important to be prepared for a job interview as well as for the negotiation process. A PA should understand the protections a contract can offer as well as the restrictions contracts may place upon a PA. The first step in the employment process is for a PA to effectively market herself/himself.

EMPLOYMENT OUTLOOK

The number of PA jobs is expected to grow much faster than the average for all occupations through the year 2012 due to the expansion of the health care industry and the focus on cost containment. Job opportunities in areas that have a difficult time attracting physicians, such as rural areas and inner cities, will continue to offer excellent employment opportunities to PAs. PAs will also be utilized more frequently in states that have imposed legal limitations on the number of hours worked by physician residents to supply some of the services previously provided by physician residents.[2]

PREPARING A RESUME OR CURRICULUM VITAE

The resume is a short document (one to two pages) detailing your education, employment history, teaching experience, licensure (certification/registration), professional memberships, and knowledge of foreign language. Fluency in Spanish is especially important for practitioners in practices with large Spanish-speaking populations. A resume should include relevant volunteer and community service, summer jobs, and unpaid internships in the field. Your name, address, and phone number should appear at the top of the page, followed by your employment history, starting with your current employment. The employment history should include the dates of your employment, your job titles, and responsibilities. It is important to tailor your resume to the position so that you do not appear over- or underqualified. Employers (Table 5-1) are particularly interested in your experience as a PA. Highlight areas where your experience will be beneficial to the employer or practice.

Table 5-1 Employers

Self-employed	2.8%
Solo physician practice	14.2%
Single-specialty physician group	29.9%
Multispecialty physician group	13.2%
University hospital	7.1%
Other hospital	14.8%
Freestanding urgent care center	1.9%
Nursing home	0.3%
Health maintenance organization	1.0%
Community health center	2.7%
Medical staffing agency	0.3%
Management service	1.5%
Integrated health system	1.0%
Correctional system	1.0%
Other	3.6%

Source: AAPA 2004 Census Report.

The curriculum vitae (CV) is a more in-depth document detailing a publishing, public speaking, and research history. (See Appendix 5-A for sample cover letters, resumes and CVs, and thank-you letters.)

Along with your resume or CV you should include a cover letter. The cover letter should be short and include a statement why the employer interests you and why you are the best candidate for the position. Highlight your strengths without repeating what is in the resume or CV. Explain any gaps in your employment history. In the first paragraph explain why you are writing and where you heard about the position. Mention the person who referred you to the organization and why your background makes you a suitable candidate for the position. In the second paragraph emphasize the contributions you would make to the employer's practice or how the organization would benefit from hiring you. Be sure that the cover letter is no longer than one page. Always have someone proofread your resume or CV and cover letter. Avoid cover letters and resumes that are too long. Be sure that there aren't any misspellings or typographical errors. Do not include unimportant information, photos, binders, or calligraphy.

INTERVIEWING

Before the interview it is important to obtain as much information about the employer as possible. In certain instances it may be possible to obtain literature prepared by the employer if the position is in a hospital or university setting. If you are interested in being employed by a large organization, familiarize yourself with an employer's mission statement and strategic plan. Talk to anyone you know who is familiar with the potential employer. If you are not from the area, it may be possible to obtain information from the library, the Internet, nearby PA programs, or the state PA chapter. PA programs may know of the practice if they send students to the site for clinicals. State chapters may be able to connect you with current or past PAs who have worked for the practice.

The interview is your chance to prove that you are the best candidate for the position. Most employers are interested in employees with leadership qualities and problem-solving skills who are willing to work as part of a team. Interview questions should revolve around your abilities related to the position that you seek. Inappropriate questions include those related to race, age, religion, and child care.

It is important to meet with the supervising physician or physicians, staff (especially PAs), and administration separately. It is important to note if it is a family-run business with a spouse serving as office manager; this may make for a difficult working environment. Has the practice employed PAs in the past and has there been a high rate of turnover within the practice, especially mid-level practitioners? Is there a possibility that the practice will be sold or merged in the near future? Before making a decision, look at all aspects of the practice/position: What will your quality of life be, does your patient-care philosophy mesh with the practice's and that of your supervising physician(s), are you comfortable with the level of autonomy you will have, are there opportunities for professional growth within the practice, and, finally, the level of compensation and benefits.

INTERVIEW QUESTIONS

Typical interview questions you should be prepared to answer include:

- Why should I hire a PA?
- Why do you feel you are a good match for this position?
- How will the practice benefit from hiring you?
- What were your duties in your last position?
- How many patients are you used to seeing in a day?
- How independently are you used to functioning?
- Do you have a DEA number?
- What are your strengths and weaknesses?
- What duties can a PA legally perform?
- Why did you leave your last position?
- Where do you see yourself in 5 years or 2 years or 10 years?
- What do you hope to gain from this position?
- What type of duties do you enjoy most?
- How do you describe yourself?
- What are your professional interests?
- How do you feel about working evenings and weekends?

QUESTIONS A PA SHOULD ASK A POTENTIAL EMPLOYER

- Have you worked with PAs before?
- How familiar are you with the PA profession? (This creates an opportunity to educate the employer about the profession.)
- What type of duties would I be expected to perform?
- What type of patients would I see? (acute, chronic, well child)
- What hours would I be expected to work? Call?
- What practice settings will I be working in? Will there be support in the credentialing process?
- Who is in charge of scheduling? How will patients be assigned? Will I have my own panel of patients?
- Will I have support staff (i.e., medical assistant)?
- Will I have time set aside to perform administrative duties and paperwork?
- What is the procedure for telephone triage?
- Is the staff familiar with PAs? How is the staff structured? Are there other partners, mid-level practitioners, or employees? How will this affect my job duties?
- Is there a chance that the practice might be sold or merged within the next few years? (If the practice might be sold or merged, you should ask for protections in your employment contract.)

After your interview send a thank-you letter. Do not write a letter or e-mail that just restates your qualifications; instead, provide something unique that dramatically sets you apart from others. Focus on a topic discussed in your interview, and then provide your prospective employer with additional information on that topic. For example, if you discussed the epidemic of obesity in the United States, write a thank-you note that includes a sentence stating, "I enjoyed discussing the obesity epidemic with you during our interview. I have enclosed a patient education handout relating to obesity that you might find helpful in your practice." This may give you the edge in a situation where several qualified applicants have applied for the same position.

PA–PHYSICIAN TEAM

Whether you are a new graduate or an experienced PA seeking new employment opportunities it is important to educate a potential employer on the physician–PA relationship and the benefits that you as a PA will bring to the practice. It is especially important in situations where the physician or practice does not have previous experience working with PAs. In this instance you should familiarize the physician or practice with the regulatory requirements and the scope of practice of a PA.

A PA is an "agent" of the physician and can perform any and all duties and procedures customary to the practice of the supervising physician. PAs cannot perform duties and procedures not customary to the practice of their supervising physician, even if they are trained and competent in the area of practice. A PA's duties are delegated by the physician and cannot supersede the supervising physician's scope of practice and must be allowed by state law.

Hiring a PA benefits the physician, the practice, and the patients and allows for expansion of practice services.

Benefits to the Physician

- No addition to physician workload.
- Increased time to spend in operating room and hospital while the PA covers the office.
- Increased time for "more complex" patient management; the PA's patient load can consist of patients with "less complex" complaints.
- More openings for consultations.
- Increased time for procedures.
- Split night and weekend call.
- More efficient hospital rounds.
- Help with medical record completion.

Benefits to the Practice

- An additional provider will allow for quicker scheduling.
- An additional provider will increase net income.
- The practice size can be enlarged while saving the physician's time.

- Office hours can be expanded.
- The PA can triage phone calls and follow up on test results.
- The PA can fill an office or personnel management role.

Benefits to the Patient

- More time per patient encounter
- Extended office hours
- Same-day walk-in care
- Increased access in reaching a medical provider by phone

Expansion of Services

- Additional time for patient education
- Nursing home rounds
- Women's health
- Home visit program
- Rehab or sports medicine program
- Rural health clinic certification

LICENSURE

When you move to your planned state of residence, obtain a copy of the state statutes and practice rules and regulations for PAs. It is important to read the statutes as well as the state board of medicine's rules and regulations. Be sure to check if there are different rules and regulations for working under the supervision of a medical doctor or a doctor of osteopathy. Obtain an application for licensure and begin the application process as soon as possible. If the regulations allow application for licensure to be made prior to the designation of a supervising physician, begin the process. It will take at least 4 to 6 weeks to obtain a license. Most medical boards only meet once every 4 to 6 weeks. If the completed application and fees are not received prior to the determined deadline, usually 1 to 2 weeks prior to the meeting, the application will not be considered until the following meeting, which can mean up to a 3-month delay prior to a license being approved.

You may also want to contact your state PA society for a membership application. State societies are an important resource for practicing PAs. They will often be able to answer questions for you regarding PA practice within the state, give you salary information, and advance the profession within the state.

Some states require that you name a primary supervisor and secondary supervisor at the time of licensure application. The medical board will approve the supervisors along with the PA's application. The primary supervisor assumes full medical and legal responsibility for the PA. The alternate supervisor(s) assume(s) full medical and legal responsibility for the PA when the primary supervisor is away.

SHOULD I GET A WRITTEN CONTRACT?

At-Will Employment

Many physician assistants do not have a written contract with their employer. In most states this is termed "at-will" employment. You are "at will" if you do not have an employment contract or union contract that limits your employer's right to fire you or you are not a government employee with mandated job protection. Without the benefit of a written contract the employer or the employee may terminate the employment at any time. An "at-will" employee has no legal right to a job. The equal opportunity and disability laws, which prevent an employer from terminating an employee on the sole basis of age, gender, race, or disability or as retaliation, are an "at-will" employee's only protection. These protected reasons are often called "exceptions to the employment 'at will' rule." If an employer terminates an "at-will" employee unlawfully, the employee may be able to collect damages.

Without the benefit of a written contract an employer and the employee must negotiate issues that arise in the course of employment individually. An employer can change the pay, benefits, and job responsibilities, as the employer deems appropriate. The employee either must accept the new conditions of employment or seek another position.

Contracts

A contract is an agreement between two or more individuals, organizations, or agencies to do or refrain from doing a particular thing in return for compensation or something of value. Contracts are promises or agreements that the law will enforce. The law provides remedies if the contract is breached. Contracts can be oral; however, an oral contract is very difficult to enforce. Contract law is generally governed by state statutes, common law (judge-made law), and private law. Private law is considered the terms of the agreement between the two parties. Contracts do not guarantee that issues will be avoided but will enhance communications in labor disputes.

Written employment agreements are becoming more common. Employment agreements can be very complex. An employer has had its legal advisor prepare a document, which will offer the greatest protection to the employer. It is beneficial for the potential employee to take the contract to his or her own attorney for review prior to making any comments regarding the contract to the employer. You should retain a local lawyer who has knowledge and experience dealing with health care contracts (physician's or PA's). Avoid an attorney who needs to research what a PA is. Many attorneys will accept a flat fee for reviewing a contract. Be sure to come to an agreement on the fee arrangement with your attorney. The attorney should provide you with a written fee agreement. If you do not have an attorney, contact your local bar association to recommend local lawyers who have experience in medical contract negotiations.

Any changes to the contract will result in additional expense to the employer; it is in your best interest to make all requests for changes to the contract at one time. Prior to signing the agreement be sure that you understand the responsibilities, expectations, and benefits outlined in the contract. (See Contract Checklist in Appendix 5-B.)

Contract Negotiations

It is important to be prepared before entering into contract negotiations. When negotiating for a new position, gather as much information as possible. Most PAs who are employed over 32 hours per week are offered professional liability insurance, individual health insurance, a pension or retirement fund, and family health insurance. Most employers fully fund professional liability insurance, state license fees, NCCPA fees, DEA registration fees, AAPA dues and credentialing fees, and partially fund individual health insurance, family health insurance, dental insurance, disability insurance, and term life insurance.[3]

Eighty-eight percent of PAs received continuing medical education (CME) funding averaging $1559 from their primary employers in 2004. The majority of PAs receive 18 days of annual paid vacation, 10 days of annual paid sick leave, and 6 days of annual paid CME leave.[4] The average total income for PAs in 2004 was $74,264.[5]

It is important to consider the specialty and location of the position when negotiating salary. Specialties and surgical positions typically have higher salaries than primary care positions. Cost of living is an additional consideration in salary negotiations. Detailed salary information can be obtained through the AAPA for a nominal fee. If you are a member of the state PA organization, you may be able to obtain a state salary profile for free. Decide what terms are essential to you. Ask for everything, but be ready to give up nonessential items.

When it is time to renegotiate your contract, be prepared. Keep track of your contributions to the practice and gather supporting data to back up your claims. Be sure to have documentation showing the number of patient visits you were responsible for the previous year and the dollars billed and received as a result of the visits. You should also make a list of other contributions you make to the practice, including administrative work, and determine a dollar value for these contributions. Compare the revenues that you brought into the practice against your expenses, including salary, benefits, overhead (solo practice 40–50%, larger practice 20–30% of income), and the cost of physician supervision. Point out any benefits you bring to the practice that translate into "good will" for the practice. This may include positive patient surveys and quality assurance data.

Contractual Clauses

If your employer offers you a contract, there are four contractual clauses that an employer may include that are very important for you to understand. A termination clause spells out the terms on which either party may terminate employment. Restrictive clauses limit your ability to seek new employment. Prevailing party attorney fee provisions detail responsibility for attorney fees in the result of a contractual dispute, and bonus formulas determine additional pay that you may receive depending upon set factors.

Termination Clauses

Termination clauses are either "with cause" or "without cause." Termination with cause allows the employer to terminate employees who engage in illegal or illicit activities. Justifiable causes for termination should be clearly spelled out in the contract. Examples include loss of a professional license or a limitation placed upon a PA by any governmental authority that prevents the PA from rendering professional services. Termination without cause allows either party to end the contract without any reason. Typically a 90- to 120-day notice is required.

Restrictive Covenants

Restrictive covenants, noncompete agreements, and nonsolicitation and confidentiality agreements are agreements that are often freestanding contracts. Confidentiality agreements are very likely to be enforced. Agreements not to solicit customers and agreements not to solicit coworkers to change jobs are also likely to be enforced. An agreement not to work in competitive fields may be enforceable depending upon the circumstances.

Restrictive covenants or "noncompete clauses" prohibit you from practicing in a specific medical specialty in a certain geographical area for a specified amount of time after leaving a practice. The period of time is usually 6 months to 1 year. These agreements or clauses are enforceable in most states if they are considered reasonable. Reasonable restrictions may be a 10-mile radius in a rural area and a 5-mile radius in a metropolitan area. Unreasonable arrangements include restrictions from practicing in entire counties or states and prohibitions from practicing in certain hospitals. If you must sign a contract with a restrictive covenant try to negotiate a contract you can live with and sign it with the expectation that a court will enforce it. Attempt to negotiate the addition of a clause that voids the restriction if you are terminated "without cause." If the employer refuses to agree to add this clause, the employer may still be barred from enforcing the clause by state law if you are terminated without cause. Certain states have legal doctrine prohibiting the enforcement of a restrictive covenant by an employer who fires an employee without good cause.

The courts will look at a restrictive covenant to determine if the duration of the restriction is reasonable, if the geographical boundaries of the restriction are reasonable, and if the scope of the restriction is reasonable and does not preclude the employee from too many potential types of work. For example, a restrictive covenant that prohibits you from working as a PA within a 10-mile radius may be too restrictive in the case of a PA working in family practice who would like to accept a position as a surgical PA within that 10-mile radius. However, a restrictive covenant that prohibits you from accepting another position in the same specialty (i.e., family practice) as a PA within a 10-mile radius may be upheld—the narrower the restriction, the more likely that the clause will be upheld. The judge will try to balance the competing interests of the employer, protecting itself from unfair competition, and the public's interest in free enterprise and keeping people off public assistance. Your personal situation and the hardships you would encounter will also be considered. Other factors to be considered are the size of the town or city, the characteristics of the practice, the availability of health care in the region, and the employment climate for health care providers.

The decision to uphold or strike down a restrictive covenant will be made on the individual circumstances of each case. There are few rules. For example, there are no rules that declare a specific length of time is too restrictive; courts have upheld restrictive covenants with durations up to 5 years under the right circumstances. The employer knows that most employees cannot afford the lawyer fees and court costs related to obtaining a ruling on the enforceability of the agreement and may rely on this assumption when drafting a stringent noncompete clause.

If you have a restrictive noncompete clause and you cannot find employment as a result of the clause, you can go to court and ask for a "declaratory judgment." A judge will decide whether the clause is enforceable. This may be a less costly way to obtain a ruling on the enforceability of the noncompete clause.

If you are considering quitting your job and you have a restrictive covenant in your contract, it is in your best interest to obtain legal advice prior to giving notice to your employer. An employer may not be able to enforce a restrictive covenant if you are terminated without good cause, but if you quit your job, it makes it easier for your employer to sue you under the covenant. If you want to quit due to mistreatment by an employer, you may be able to claim "constructive discharge" and be treated as an employee who has been fired without good cause—if you obtain legal advice prior to leaving the position.

Once you have left an employer, it is in your best interest to tell a potential employer about your noncompete clause or restrictive covenant. If your former employer decides to sue you and your present employer for violation of the restrictive covenant and you have not disclosed this information to your current employer, he or she may choose to sue you for fraudulently inducing him or her to hire you. If you are sued over a noncompete clause, your personal assets are at risk. Damage awards will be paid out of your personal assets.

Prevailing Party Attorney Fee Provision

It is beneficial to include a prevailing party attorney fee provision in any employment-related contract. The provision allows the prevailing party to collect its attorney fees from the losing party. This will help prevent a weak case from being brought against either party because of the risk of having to pay the other party's attorney fees. If you have a strong case but have insufficient funds to pay an attorney, you may be able to persuade the attorney to take a smaller fee up front with additional payment if you prevail. The downside is that if you lose you will have to pay your previous employer's attorneys fees.

Bonus Formulas

Many PAs are paid a straight salary or an hourly rate. If you are offered a bonus in addition to your salary or hourly rate be sure that you and your employer understand the formula. Be sure that the formula clearly states how the bonus will be determined and when the bonus will be paid out. One of the major problems with bonus formulas is that they are often written in vague terms, which leads to different interpretations by different people.

One option offered to PAs is a guaranteed base salary plus a production bonus.

Sample:
Base $70,000
Benefits* .... $21,000 (roughly 30% of base)
Production .... 25% of gross charges over $200,000

A PA grossing $250,000 in charges would receive a bonus of $12,500.

Another bonus formula is advantageous for a PA who sees a significant amount of patients covered by managed care.

Sample:
Base salary $70,000
Benefits* .... $21,000 (roughly 30% of base)
Bonus .... 15% of fee for service and capitation
   (managed care payments made on a monthly basis) over $300,000

Calculation of bonus:
2000 capitated patients × $15 per member, per month $300,000/year
200 fee for service visits/month @ $50/visit .... +$120,000/year
Less base collections .... − $300,000/year
    Net $120,000
    Bonus ($120,000 x 10%) .... $ 12,000

*Benefits packages include health, life, disability, and malpractice
   insurance, pension, taxes, etc.

Summary:
Total salary .... $ 70,000
Benefits .... $ 21,000
Bonus .... $ 12,000
Total compensation $103,000

MALPRACTICE INSURANCE

There are two types of malpractice insurance: claims made and occurrence. A claims-made policy covers you for claims made during the time of coverage; in this case a tail policy would need to be purchased upon termination of employment. A tail policy is additional coverage that can be purchased after the expiration of a claims-made liability policy. The tail policy extends for a period of time, with or without limit, the right to report events that occurred before the policy was terminated. An occurrence policy covers claims that occurred during the time period the policy was in place. The best insurance for a PA to have is an occurrence policy for at least $1 million per claim and $3 million aggregate as an individual rather than as part of a group. If a PA needs to purchase his or her own insurance to meet this minimum, he or she should do so.

If your employer maintains your malpractice insurance, be sure to obtain a copy of your policy each year to be sure that the policy is still in place.

If you have a claims-made policy, be sure that your contract specifies that your employer will pay for continuation of your policy or purchase tail coverage at termination of your employment. When a PA is covered on the employer's policy rather than an individual policy in the PA's name and the PA leaves the practice, a tail policy may not need to be purchased. If the employer chooses to continue the policy and replaces the PA, both the PA leaving the practice and the new employee will be covered. Tail coverage would not need to be purchased as long as the policy is maintained. In order to be sure that the policy is maintained, the PA leaving the practice would need to obtain a copy of the policy on a yearly basis. When a PA's name is specified on the employer's policy, a specific "endorsement" or rider to the policy must be obtained that specifically grants the PA tail coverage. This rider would be titled "extended reporting period endorsement" or a similar title. The PA would need to obtain a copy of this rider as evidence of his or her coverage.[6]

A PA who has an individual claims-made policy can purchase a tail policy or a continuous successor policy. A continuous successor policy that maintained a retroactive date on a claims made basis or provided prior acts as part of an occurrence policy would relieve the need for the PA to purchase tail coverage. In some instances a successor policy can be 90% less expensive than a tail policy. Tail policies can run anywhere from $10,000 to $60,000.[7]

When negotiating a contract or written agreement regarding malpractice insurance:

1. Request that your employer reimburse you for your own individual insurance policy and agree to indemnify you for any liability related to your scope of employment. In some instances your individual policy may be less expensive than being added to the employer's policy.
2. Purchase an individual "occurrence" policy with a $1 million per occurrence/$3 million aggregate if possible. Fewer and fewer malpractice insur-

ance carriers are offering occurrence policies and the ones who still offer them have increased their rate by as much as 150%.

3. If a claims-made policy is the only coverage you can obtain, specify that the employer will continue your policy or purchase tail coverage on your behalf at termination of your employment. State that the employer will provide you with proof of coverage on an annual basis.

4. An employer who will not provide you with a $1,000,000/$3,000,000 policy should provide you with the same coverage as the supervising physician. The PA in this instance should consider purchasing additional coverage on his or her own as well.

5. Include a clause stating that the employer's failure to maintain adequate insurance coverage does not relieve the employer of the obligation to indemnify the PA for any liabilities incurred within the scope of his or her employment.

INDEPENDENT CONTRACTOR STATUS

According to the AAPA's 2004 census report, fewer than 1% of PAs are self-employed. If your employer wants to hire you as an independent contractor, it is in your best interest to seek legal advice from a tax attorney or an accountant to be sure that you meet the relevant state and federal requirements before choosing to work as an independent contractor. As an employee, your employer is responsible for withholding taxes. An independent contractor is responsible for his or her own taxes. In order to determine if you can be employed as an independent contractor, you need to evaluate several factors regarding your relationship with your employer. The IRS estimates that it loses over $2 billion dollars per year due to the incorrect classification of employees as independent contractors, and it is a frequently litigated issue. The IRS has been looking closely at physicians working as independent contractors and has issued technical memoranda on the topic. These memoranda could be applied to PAs and should be discussed with your tax advisor. In one instance, physicians were found to be employees of the hospital because they were deemed to be essential to the business operation and were subject to some control and direction by the hospital. Even though the physicians worked part time, provided their own liability insurance, received no benefits, and had outside practices that accounted for most of their income, the IRS found that they failed to meet the guidelines applicable to independent contractors. In general, the more control your employer exercises over you, the more likely it is that you are an employee.

Some of the questions you need to consider in order to determine if you can be classified an independent contractor are:

Does your employer control when and where you work? If you are required to comply with your supervisor's instructions about where, when, and how to work; you are more likely to be considered an employee. If the person who you are working for sets your hours, you are more likely to be considered an employee.

Are you employed on a full-time basis by the same person? Employment on a full-time basis precludes you from working for others and is found in an employee–employer relationship. Independent contractors work for whom they choose, when they choose.

Are you established separately from your employer on business cards, advertisements, and letters of incorporation? An independent contractor will be established separately from the employer.

Will you be trained by your supervising physician? Training implies that the supervisor wants the work done in a specific manners and you are more likely to be considered an employee.

Do you file a Schedule C tax form and receive IRS 1099 forms for all the income you receive? Independent contractors are required to submit these forms.

Do you use your own medical equipment and supplies and have your own base of operation? Independent contractors furnish their own equipment and supplies. Rendering services on the employer's premises indicates an employee–employer relationship.

Are you able to hire others to assist with the work without your supervisor's approval? Hiring other assistants pursuant to a contract where you are only reimbursed for materials and labor indicates independent contractor status.

Do you have the authority to purchase the supplies and services at a place of your own choosing? An independent contractor possesses this authority.

Do you determine what specific tasks are to be done? In an employee–employer relationship the employer determines the tasks to be done.

How much guidance do you receive from your employer about how to do your job? If a great deal of guidance is provided by the employer, it is likely that you are an employee.

Are you paid an hourly rate or do you do your own billing? Being paid hourly, weekly, or monthly indicates an employee–employer relationship.

Do you have to make oral or written reports to your supervisor? The requirement of submitting oral or written reports shows a degree of control exercised by the person you are working for.

Do you provide your own benefits such as health insurance and malpractice insurance? An independent contractor would provide his or her own health and malpractice insurance.

Do you have any paid time off? Independent contractors do not receive paid time off.

Are you reimbursed for expenses that are job related? Employees receive reimbursement for job-related expenses.

Do you perform the same services for others and have income from various sources? Independent contractors have various sources of income.

Did you invest in the facilities that are used to render services? Independent contractors invest in the facilities; employees do not.

Can you realize a profit or loss? Independent contractors realize profits and losses; employees do not.

Will you work for the employer indefinitely or just until a certain job is completed? Working on a continual basis for the same person indicates an employee–employer relationship.

Does your employer have a right to discharge you? Employers have a right to discharge employees. An independent contractor cannot be discharged as long as he or she continues to provide the services agreed upon.

Do you have a right to terminate your services without penalty? Employees have the right to terminate their services without penalty.

Are you an integral aspect of the business, or ancillary? If you are an integral aspect of the business you are more likely to be considered an employee.

Each of the above questions addresses the degree of control your employer has over you. There are no clear written guidelines to determine whether or not you can be employed as an independent contractor; each case is decided on an individual basis, which can lead to controversy over your status. Be sure to research your state's statutes and regulations referring to PA practice; certain states do not allow PAs to be self-employed.

FEDERAL REGULATION THAT MAY AFFECT PAs' OWNERSHIP IN MEDICAL ENTITIES

Stark Acts

The acts commonly referred to as the *Stark Acts* include Physicians' Referrals to Health Care Entities in Which They Have a Financial Relationship (63 Fed. Reg. 1659 91998) and the Ethics in Patient Referral Act of 1989 (42 U.S.C. sec. 1395nn), which was amended by the Omnibus Budget Reconciliation Act of 1993 and incorporated into the Social Security Act [Social Security Act, 42 U.S.C.A. sec. 1877 ad 1903(s)]. The federal Stark Acts, which limit physician self-referrals, are highly technical. It is difficult to apply these acts to many physician arrangements because the statutory language is unclear. The Health Care Financing Administration (HCFA) is in charge of the regulations under the Stark Acts and issues interpreting regulations and develops new regulatory exceptions.

Unless an exception applies, the Stark Acts prohibit physicians from referring Medicare or Medicaid patients to an entity to obtain "designated health services" if the physician (or a member of the physician's immediate family) has a direct or indirect financial relationship or ownership interest with the entity. There are also categories of designated health services that a physician cannot refer a patient to when the physician has a financial relationship with or interest in the facility, including laboratory services, radiology services, radiation therapy services, physical therapy services, occupational therapy services, home health, durable medical equipment and supplies, outpatient prescription drugs, parenteral and enteral nutrients, prosthetics, orthotics and prosthetic devices, and inpatient and outpatient hospital services. The Stark Acts have established several statutory exceptions, each of which contains specific, detailed requirements and limitations.

Referral is broadly defined by the Stark Acts and applies to both a physician's financial relationships with his medical practice to which he makes referrals, and to a physician's direct or indirect financial relationships with outside entities, such as hospitals, to which the physician refers. One of the exceptions allows a physician to make a referral to a physician within the same group practice without violating the self-referral law.[8]

The Stark Acts are not aimed at physician assistants. If your physician supervisor directed you to make a referral that violated the Stark Acts, the supervising physician and not the PA would be held accountable for the violation. The Stark Acts are aimed at physicians who own an interest in medical equipment companies, laboratories, pharmacies, and so on and will profit when patient referrals are made for these services. If you are a part owner in the practice where you are employed or a part owner in any entity to which the practice you are employed at makes referrals to, it is in your best interest to seek legal counsel to be sure that there is not a violation of the Stark Acts, which you may be held accountable for.

Antikickback Statutes

In 1997 Congress enacted antikickback statutes that prohibit paying a fee for a referral, receiving a fee for referring a patient, and waiving deductibles or co-payments for Medicare patients. Congress feels that these practices lead to inappropriate referrals, which lead to overutilization of services and goods, increase the cost of health care and health care programs, and lead to unfair business practices and competition.

Federal law establishes both civil and criminal penalties for violation of the antikickback statutes. A violation occurs when an individual or entity pays for, asks for, or receives anything of value for referrals reimbursable by a federal health care program.

HOSPITAL PRACTICE

If you will be employed by a hospital or managing patients from your supervisor's practice at a hospital, obtain a copy of the hospital bylaws in order to understand your status relative to the medical staff. Determine the procedure for applying for privileges at the hospital. Privileges are granted by the governing body of the institution and will allow the PA to provide specific health care services at the institution. As of January 2004, the standards of the Joint Commission on Accreditation of Healthcare Organizations (JCAHO) require hospitals to credential and privilege PAs and APNs through the medical staff "or an equivalent process." (See Appendix 5-C for sample privilege request guidelines.) Institutions require medical staff to obtain privileges prior to allowing the medical staff member to practice within the facility in order to protect patients from unqualified medical personnel and the liability that may result.

The hospital may have specific restrictions on what a PA's scope of practice is within its facility. The facility can be more restrictive in regard to PA practice than state law, but cannot be less restrictive. Generally, your scope of practice will be consistent with the scope of your supervising physician.

Prior to granting privileges an institution will credential the PA. Credentialing consists of validating the background and assessing the qualifications of the PA. (See Appendix 5-D for information that may be gathered during the credentialing process.) An objective evaluation of the PA's current license, training, experience, competence, and ability to perform the requested services and procedures will be performed.

The hospital may require as part of privileging and credentialing that you show proof that you have been trained in the specific health care services that you are requesting them to grant. You may be requested to prove that you have performed each task up to 80 times in training or in experience. This information can be obtained through official logs generated during clinical training or information generated during practice. This type of documentation should be maintained in order to aid you when making applications for privileging and credentialing.

In order to maintain hospital privileges a PA may be required to:

- Have a physical every 2 years.
- Reapply for privileges every 2 years and update the information on the original application.
- Provide the facility with credentials, certifications, and so on.
- Report having privileges revoked, suspended, or restricted by other facilities.
- Report malpractice payments listed in the National Provider Data Bank.
- Provide evidence of continuous education.
- Document training for any additional privileges requested.
- Quality and risk management information may be reviewed including complaints against the PA, adverse outcomes or questionable medical practices, morbidity, mortality, and length of stay.
- Review of productivity and quality data if available.[9]

REQUIRED IDENTIFICATION

Be sure to review your state's statutes and regulations pertaining to required identification for PAs. Most states require PAs to wear name tags that clearly identify the PA to the public. In certain states *Physician Assistant* must be spelled out and not abbreviated on the name tag and may be required to be a certain font. PAs are required to clearly identify themselves to each of their patients as being a physician assistant and correct any patient who incorrectly refers to them as "doctor." There may be a requirement that a public notice be posted in the waiting area identifying that a PA works at the practice, that the patient may be seen by a PA, and that the patient has a right to refuse to be seen by the PA if he or she prefers to be seen by a physician. Additionally, many states require that state-approved credentials for the PA and the supervising physician be displayed.

CREDENTIALING SERVICE

The AAPA and the American Medical Association (AMA) have developed a credentialing service for PAs. The credentialing service makes it more convenient for hospital credentialing staffs and managed care organizations (MCOs) to verify PAs' credentials. The AAPA feels that the credentialing service reinforces the alignment between physicians and PAs and physician-type practice in hospitals, reflects the AMA's understanding of PA credentials, and reflects a level of professional recognition by organized medicine and the JCAHO. The PA credentialing service expands the AMA's Physician Profile Service. Because many of the nation's hospitals and several MCOs verify physician credentials through the AMA program, they are familiar with the process and will adapt easily to verifying PAs credentials through the same service.

Hospitals and MCOs that are attempting to verify credentials applications can contact the AMA and verify the PA's educational program attended and graduation date, NCCPA number and current status, current and historical state licensure information, and AAPA membership status. The information is delivered within one hour.

The AAPA provides the PA data to the AMA to be used in the profiling service. Credentialing professionals will be able to obtain all the information from the AMA at one time instead of having to contact individual PA programs and the NCCPA to verify an individual PA's credentials application. Using the AMA's PA profiling service will be more efficient and less expensive for hospitals and MCOs because it will save time for the credentialing staff.

Hospitals are required to perform primary source verification on the data submitted by PAs prior to credentialing or recredentialing, which would require the hospital or MCOs to contact the PA program and the NCCPA directly to verify program completion and NCCPA certification. JCAHO has stated that the information AAPA provides on PA education and NCCPA certification can be considered "equivalent primary source" information for credentialing purposes. Equivalent status means that the information provided from the AMA's PA profiling service can be used by hospitals and MCOs in their credentialing process and that PA programs and the NCCPA do not have to be contacted individually. This process should speed up the credentialing process, allowing PAs to begin hospital practice quicker.

The AMA's PA profile service can be used for initial credentialing and the biannual recredentialing. The AMA will not provide verification of nurse practitioner or other advanced-practice nurse (APN) credentials.

Physician assistants do not have to request to be included in the service or provide any information to the AMA or AAPA. The AAPA suggests that all PAs verify the accuracy of information about them in the AAPA's online member directory (*https://members. aapa.org/*) and fill out the annual census form each year. Information can be updated online or by calling AAPA CME and Member Services, (703) 836-2272, ext. 3350.[10]

REFERENCES

1. American Academy of Physician Assistants Web site. AAPA Physician Assistant Census 2004 results. Available at http://www.aapa.org. Accessed October 2004.

2. United States Department of Labor, Bureau of Labor Statistics. Occupational outlook handbook, 2003–2004 Edition. Available at http://www.bls.gov. Accessed March 2005.

3. American Academy of Physician Assistants. (1997). *Contracts and contracts: An employment guide for physician assistants* (2nd ed.). Alexandria, VA: AAPA.

4. American Academy of Physician Assistants Web site. AAPA Physician Assistant Census 2004 results. Available at http://www.aapa.org. Accessed October 2004.

5. American Academy of Physician Assistants Web site. AAPA Physician Assistant Census 2004 results. Available at http://www.aapa.org. Accessed October 2004.

6. McCammon, G. (April 15, 2004). A good question deserves a good answer. *AAPA News.*

7. McCammon, G. (April 15, 2004). You're changing jobs: Will your insurance disappear? *AAPA News.*

8. Social Security Act, 42 U.S.C.A. sec. 1877(b)(1).

9. American Academy of Physician Assistants. (2003). *Physician assistant credentialing* (issue brief).

10. American Academy of Physician Assistants Web site. Available at http://www.aapa.org. Accessed July 2004.

Sample Cover Letters, Curricula Vitae and Resumes, and Thank-You Letters

COVER LETTERS

New Graduate

(Date)

John Franco, Human Resources
University Hospital
721 South Way
West City, State 19876

Dear Mr. Franco,

I am a recent graduate of Some Physician Assistant Program. I am interested in applying for the physician assistant opening in the outpatient clinic at your facility.

I have completed 13 months of clinical rotations with six months of ambulatory care experience. Prior to my physician assistant training I was a medical assistant for five years at a private physician's office.

My resume is enclosed for your consideration. I look forward to the opportunity to discuss my qualifications and career opportunities with you. I am willing to meet with you at your convenience. I will contact you next week to inquire about arranging a meeting. In the meantime I can be reached at 222/789-4565.

Thank you for your consideration. I look forward to speaking with you.

Sincerely,

(signature)

Maggie May, PA-C
1212 Lexington Ave.
East City, State 87654

Encl.

General

(Date)

Jan Jones, Business Manager
CV Practice
100 State St., Suite 101
City, State 12345

Dear Ms. Jones,

I am writing to inquire about physician assistant employment opportunities with CV Practice. I recently spoke with Dr. Smith, who suggested that I contact your office. I will be relocating to your area in the near future.

My experience in general surgery, cardiothoracic surgery, and the cardiovascular intensive care unit is a good match for your practice. For the past seven years I have been employed by General Hospital as a surgical physician assistant. The first three years were spent in general surgery and the last four in cardiovascular surgery. My responsibilities included pre- and postoperative coverage of patients in the intensive care unit as well as first assisting during cardiothoracic and vascular surgery.

I have enclosed my resume for your review. I welcome the opportunity to meet with you to discuss the possibility of employment with your practice. I will call you next week to see if a meeting can be arranged at a mutually convenient time. In the interim I can be reached at 321/345-7777.

Thank you for your consideration. I look forward to speaking with you.

Sincerely,

(signature)

Sam Smith, MPAS, PA-C
140 Canter Lane
North Town, State 16601

Encl.

CURRICULA VITAE

Sample 1

Jane Smith, JD, MPAS, PA-C
140 Canterbury Lane
Fairview, CA 16418
(814) 424-4617

Professional Experience

Cannon University
100 University Square
Erie, CA 16548
(814) 881-5243

> Associate Dean, College of Sciences Engineering and Health Sciences, July 2004–Present
> Chair, Physician Assistant Department, July 2003–Present
> Director Physician Assistant Program, June 1997–July 2003
> Tenured Faculty, July 2004–Present
> Associate Professor, July 2002–Present
> Assistant Professor, June 1997–June 2002

> Supervisory responsibility for seven full-time faculty, two full-time administrative staff members, and six adjuncts. Budget management $560,000

Legal Aid Volunteer Attorney, 1998–Present
A Joint Program of the Erie County Bar Association and Northwest Legal Services
100 Market Street, Suite1200
Erie, CA 16501
(814) 452-6957

Saint Rita Hospital
42200 45th Street
Pittsburgh, PA 15201
(412) 648-4200

> Certified Physician Assistant
> August 1990 to June 1997

> Complete first assistant surgical experience including cardiovascular, cardiothoracic, obstetrical, gynecological, ENT, orthopedics, neurological, and general surgery. Preceptor for PA students.

Education

Saint Ann College, Loratto, CA 19940 (814) 422-6000
Graduation: August 1990   Degree awarded: BS—Summa Cum Laude
Major: Physician Assistant
G.P.A. 3.98, Scale A = 4.0

Graduate Studies

Hometown University, School of Law, Pittstown, CA 95482 (412) 996-6200
Graduation: June 1996   Degree awarded: Juris Doctor
G.P.A. 3.47, Scale A+ = 4.0
1994 American Academy of Matrimonial Lawyers Award

University of Savannas Medical Center, Oman, ND 67298-4300 (402) 555-7250
Graduation: August 2002   Degree awarded: Master of Physician Assistant
Studies

Certification/Licensure

California State Board of Medicine
National Commission on Certification of Physician Assistants
Licensed to practice law in the State of California
Licensed to practice law in the State of Ohio (inactive status)

Memberships/Associations

American Academy of Physician Assistants
California Society of Physician Assistants
Society for the Preservation of Physician Assistant History
California Bar Association
Erie County Bar Association
Member California Supreme Court
Member Ohio Supreme Court
Loyal Christian Benefit Association

Committees

Chair Committee on Student Conduct—*Cannon University* 1997–present
Co-Chair Student Affairs Committee—*Peninsula Society of Physician Assistants*
   2001–present
Speakers Bureau—*Cannon University* 2002–present
Health Science Administration Council—*Cannon University* 1997–present
Scholarship Committee—*Erie County Bar Association* 1999–present
Advisory Committee—*Physician Assistant Program, Cannon University* 1999–present
Conference Committee—*Peninsula Society of Physician Assistants* 2002–present
Board of the Consortium Program in Dietetics—*Cannon University* 2003–present
Institutional Policy Manual Revision Task Force—*Cannon University* 2003–present
Mission and Identity Council—*Cannon University* 2003–present
TLTR Course Management Software Project Committee—*Cannon University*
   2004–present
Online Evaluation and Assessment Committee—*Cannon University* 2004–present
Jack Kent Cooke Scholarship Committee—*Cannon University* 2003–2004
University Review Council—*Cannon University* 2000–2003
Search Committee Dean of Sciences, Engineering and Health Sciences—*Cannon
   University* 2002–2003

Chair Hearing Committee University Review Council—*Cannon University* 2002–2003

Chair Thesis Committee—*Physician Assistant Program, Cannon University* 2002–2003

CSEHS Research Committee—*Cannon University* 1999–2001

Middle States Working Group (Finance)—*Cannon University* 2001

Search Committee School Director/Chair Nursing Department—*Cannon University* 2000

Medical/Legal Committee—*Erie County Bar Association* 1998–2001

Legal Journal Committee—*Erie County Bar Association* 2000

Curriculum Development

Postbaccalaureate, Master of Physician Assistant Science (2 year), Cannon University, 2001

Master of Physician Assistant Science (5 year), Cannon University, accepted by the Department of Education, 1999

Grants

Orris C. Hertel and Beatrice Dewey Hertel Memorial Foundation—$202,373, pending

Study of Bioengineered Skin—$10,000 *Novatec Pharmaceutical* 2002

Equipment Grant—$1,700 *Welch and Allen* 2001

Faculty Development Grant—*Cannon University* 1999–2002

Faculty Research Grant—*Cannon University* 2000

Nonfunded

Topical Hyperbaric Oxygen Protocol—$30,000 *Advanced Hyperbaric Industries* 2003

Community Grants Program—$2,500 *Physician Assistant Foundation* 2002

Implementation of Sani CLIE-PDA into the Cannon University Physician Assistant Curriculum—$1,500 *Sani Corporation* 2002

Analyzing and Reporting Events That Compromise Health—$7M *Department of Health-Tobacco Settlement* 2002

Publications and Scholarly Activity

Smith MM, Sparer S. Recognizing Calciphylaxis, currently in the peer review process. *Advance for Physician Assistants,* 2004.

Smith MM, Wilker C. Leech Therapy Returning to Medicine, currently in the peer review process. *Advance for Physician Assistants,* 2004.

Smith MM, Reichter H. Early Sports Specialization, currently in the peer review process. *Advance for Physician Assistants,* 2004.

Smith MM, Sanner C. Exercise Induced Bronchoconstriction. *Advance for Physician Assistants,* 2004 March: 12(3): 24–29.

Rath AM, Smith MM, Kaufmann MK. Adolescent Depression. *Advance for Physician Assistant,* 2003 Sept: 11(9): 48–51.

Smith MM, Hayes K. Bell's Palsy. *Advance for Physician Assistant,* 2003 May/June: 11(5–6): 52–58.

Smith MK, Kaufmann MM. Jaundice in the Newborn: A Family Practice Approach. *Advance for Physician Assistant,* 2002 Sept: 10(9): 56–62.

Sereny TE, Kasten S, Smith M, Corral C, Zing C, Sereny C. Incorporation of Bioengineered Skin (Apligraf) into a Diabetic Foot Ulcer Treatment Protocol *Wound Repair and Regeneration,* 2002 March–April: 10(2): A52. (Abstract)

Micheli N, Smith MM. Intervention: Identifying Patients with Alcoholism. *Advance for Physician Assistants,* 2002 Jan/Feb: 10(1–2): 49–52.

Smith MM, Kaufmann MK. Melanoma or Mimic? The Need for Early Diagnosis. *Advance for Physician Assistants,* 2001 Nov/Dec: 9 (11–12): 32–36.

Smith MM, Kaufmann MK. Chest Pain with no Clear Cause. *Advance for Physician Assistants,* 2001 Jan/Feb: 9 (1–2): 44–46, 49.

2003 Undergraduate Faculty Scholarship Award, *Faculty Senate Cannon University*

Corresponding Item Writer, *National Commission on Certification of Physician Assistants* 2001–present

Site Visitor, *Accreditation Review Commission on Education for the Physician Assistant, Inc.* 2002–present

Peer Reviewer, *Journal of the American Academy of Physician Assistants (JAAPA)* 2003–present

Peer Reviewer, *Advance for Physician Assistants* 2002–present

History and Physical Examiner, *Lake Erie College of Medicine* 2002–present

Presentations

Workshop/Dossier Presentation, "Strategies for Successful Professional Advancement," Cannon University, Erie, PA. June 2, 2004

"Malpractice Issues for PAs," Society of Physician Assistants 28th Annual CME Conference, Philadelphia, PA. October 15–18, 2003

"The Physician Assistant Profession and Education," Academic Affairs Committee of the Board of Trustees, Cannon University, Erie, PA. September 25, 2003

Workshop Presentation, "Advancing from Assistant to Associate Professor," *Demystifying the Process...Strategies for Successful Professional Advancement,* Cannon University, Erie, PA. June 4, 2003

"The Physician Assistant," Lake Erie College of Medicine, Erie, PA. December 17, 2002

"Insurance Issues—Medicare/HIPPA," Society of Physician Assistants 27th Annual Conference, Pittsburgh, PA. September 27, 2002

"Malpractice Pitfalls," Society of Physician Assistants 27th Annual Conference, Pittsburgh, PA. September 27, 2002

Podium Presentation, "The Choice of Apligraf over Autograph in the Reconstruction of a Fasciotomy Site," Nice-Port St. Laurent, France. September 14, 2002

Workshop Presentation, "Tips for Successful Professional Advancement," Cannon University, Erie, PA. June 12, 2002

Podium Presentation, "The Use of Bioengineered Skin (Apligraf) to Treat a Complex Wound Created by Ecthyma Gangrenosum and the Persistence of Bioengineered Skin 10 Months After Application" (coauthor), The Wound Healing Society Meeting, Baltimore, MD. May 29–June 1, 2002

Poster Presentation, "Incorporation of Bioengineered Skin (Apligraf) into a Diabetic Foot Ulcer Treatment Protocol" (coauthor), The Wound Healing Society Meeting, Baltimore, MD. May 29–June 1, 2002; also presented at The Society of Physician Assistants 27th Annual Conference, Pittsburgh, PA. September 25–28, 2002

Poster Presentation, "What Do Physician Assistant Students Know About the Educational Requirements for Other Allied Health Care Personnel?" (coauthor), American Academy of Physician Assistants 30th Annual Conference, May 25–30, 2002; also presented at The Society of Physician Assistants 27th Annual Conference, Pittsburgh, PA. September 25–28, 2002

"A Career as a Physician Assistant," Career Day, Northwestern School, Girard, CA. April 4, 2001

"Risk Management," Society of Physician Assistants 26th Annual CME Conference, Philadelphia, PA. October 17–19, 2001

Poster Presentation, "A Look at Scholarship in the Physician Assistant Profession," Society of Physician Assistants 26th Annual CME Conference, October 17–20, 2001

Poster Presentation, "*Yersinia enterocolitica* Presenting as Acute Appendicitis in a Three-Year-Old Amish Boy in Rural Northwest Pennsylvania: A Diagnostic Dilemma," Society of Physician Assistants 26th Annual CME Conference, October 17–20, 2001

"The Society of Physician Assistants," Cannon University, Erie, PA. August 30, 2001

"The Physician-PA Team," Cannon University, Erie, PA. August 29, 2001

Sample 2

Mark Jones PA-C
2402 Willow Lane
Fairview, PA 16415
414-466-4677
pamark@juno.com

Professional Goals

To provide unprejudiced, quality health care with an exclusively procedural medicine practice, focusing on the family and treating the patient as a whole, emphasizing preventative care by maintaining healthy habits of appropriate nutrition and exercise while treating the body, mind, and soul when illness arises, with God as my guide.

Board Certification

National Commission on the Certification of Physician Assistants 1990–present

Current Professional Experience

6/30/03–present   Primary Care Physician Assistant
Veteran's Administration
125 East Street
Erie, PA 16522
814-822-6112
Duties: Providing outpatient continuity of care and inpatient
hospitalizations, assisting with colonoscopies and dermatologic
procedures, member of the Ethics Committee.

6/2003–present   Assistant Professor and Director of Problem-Based Learning
History and Physical Examination
Lake College of Medicine
1877 Grandview Rd.
Warren, PA 16509
824-844-8841
Developed, implemented, and instructed complete curriculum
and clinical activities.

Education

1987–1990   B.S. Physician Assistant
Saint John College
Medina, PA 15333
Graduated cum laude—3.62 GPA

Procedural Education

April 2003   Dermatologic Skills for Family Physicians
American College of Osteopathic Family Physicians
John L. Pfenniger, M.D.
National Procedures Institute
4909 Hedgewood Drive
Midland, MI 48640
1-800-462-2492

Feb. 2001   Dermatologic Procedure
Course included cryosurgery, radiofrequency excision, biopsy
techniques, and suturing principles with treatment for lipomas,
cysts, actinics, seborrheics, basal cell and squamous cell car-
cinomas, melanomas, ingrown nails, warts, tags, chalazion,
abscesses, and many more.

August 2001   Sclerotherapy
Included patient evaluation, treatment techniques, and postoperative care.

Sept. 2001	IUD Insertion
	Skin biopsy
	Vasectomy—including no scalpel technique
	Abnormal uterine bleeding/endometrial biopsy
	Hemorrhoids
	Radiofrequency Surgery
	Joint Injection
	Needle Breast Biopsy
	Flexible Nasopharyngoscopy
	Flexible Sigmoidoscopy
Nov. 2001	Coloscopy
Sept. 2002	Anesthetics

Memberships

2002–Present	Faculty advisor and member Sigma Sigma Phi
2000–Present	PSPA
1996–Present	AAPA
1996–Present	EMPA

Committees

2004	Chair, Operative and Other Procedures, VAMC
2004	Ethics Committee, VAMC
2001–2003	ACOFP Strongest Link Representative
2000–2003	LECOMT Representative
1999–2000	Self-Study Report Curriculum Committee
1997–1998	Self-Study Report Students Committee
1997–1998	Chair ACOFP Clinical Education

Publications/Presentations

"Chronic Pain Management: Climbing the Ladder." *Journal of the Pennsylvania Osteopathic Medical Association.* March 2003: 21–24.

"Jaundice in the Newborn." Presented at the Central States Winter Get-away Conference. January 19, 2001.

A Call to Healing. Video publication depicting the day in the life of a physician assistant, produced in promotion of physician assistant awareness and community service. June 1999.

"Randomized Comparison of Ganciclovir and Oral Acyclovir for the Prevention of Cytomegalovirus and Ebstein-Barr Virus Disease in Pediatric Liver Transplant Recipients" (coauthor). *Clinical Infectious Disease.* 1997 Dec; 25:1344–1349.

"Affect of OKT3 on the Incidence of Posttransplant Lymphoproliferative Disease (PTLD) in Pediatric Intestinal Transplantation" (lead author). Oral presentation at the XV World Congress of Transplantation, Kyoto, Japan, August 1994.

"Posttransplant Lymphoproliferative Disease After Whole Organ Transplantation Under FK506 Immunosuppression in Children" (coauthor). Accepted for poster presentation at the XV World Congress of Transplantation, Kyoto, Japan, August 1994.

"Randomized Trial of Ganciclovir Followed by High Dose Oral Acyclovir vs.
Ganciclovir Alone in the Prevention of Cytomegalovirus in Pediatric Liver
Transplant Recipients: Preliminary Analysis" (coauthor). *Transplantation
Proceedings*. Presented at 1st International Congress on Pediatric
Transplantation, Minneapolis, MN, August 1993.

Peer Review

2003	Advance for Physician Assistants

Awards

2003	Certificate Customer Service Star, Veteran's Administration, Patient Nomination
2003	Certificate of Merit, City of Erie, Office of Mayor
2003	Certificate of Recognition, Community Hospital
2001–2003	American College of Osteopathic Family Physician's Preceptorship Program Award Recipient
2002	Letter of Appreciation, Great Lakes Tae Kwon Do Open
2002	Letter of Commendation, Certificate of Appreciation, ALLHAT
2002	Nominated for Pfizer Outstanding PA Resident Award
2001	Certificate of Merit, City of Erie, Office of Mayor
2001	Certificate of Appreciation, LECOM Junior Faculty Member
1990	Dean's Award
1989	Psi Sigma Alpha: National Scholastic Honor Society
1989	Academic Scholarship
1989	APOMA Scholarship Award

Prior Work Experience

1994–2003	Owner/operator Discount Medical Supply
7/2003	Physician Assistant Consultant, Miller Attorneys at Law
6/00–5/03	Junior Faculty Lake College of Medicine History and Physical Examination Problem-Based Learning Pathway
1998–2003	Study Coordinator ALLPHAT Antihypertension Lipid Lowering to Prevent Heart Attacks Trial
1990–1996	Physician Assistant—Pediatric Transplant Surgery Children's Hospital of Pittsburgh 3705 5th Avenue Pittsburgh, PA 15213-2583 412-692-6110 Responsible Physician—Gorge Chaffers M.D. Duties included clinical workup for transplant candidates, history and physical examinations, ICU and floor rounds, ordering and interpretation of diagnostic tests including lab values and imaging, admissions and discharges with dictations, floor procedures including IV, chest tube and central line placements, liver biopsies, assisting in surgery, and training of fellows.

Lectures

3/2003	Basic Suturing Workshop
	Lake Erie College of Medicine
2000–present	Moderator
	LECOM Peak and Peak Primary Care Conference
5/98–present	Southern University:
	Guest Lecturer
	Evaluator—Clinical Skills Testing
	Written History and Physical Exams
12/17/03	Testing day topics
	Multiple medications
	Cost and insurance company effects on patient care
	Drug seeking patients
	Diabetes mellitus
	Pain relief and oncology
	Noncompliant patients
	Obese patient physical examination
12/5/2003	Physical Exam Techniques
	Prior topics:
	Pre- and postoperative orders
	Pediatric drug dosing
	Arterial blood gases
	Labor and delivery
	Normal pediatric exam
	Immunizations
	Common pediatric problems

Personal Achievements

Proud husband and father of twin boys, who have made life's journey just a little bit steeper, but immeasurably sweeter.

Brown Belt Tae Kwon Do

SAMPLE RESUMES

Sample 1

RESUME FOR **JOSEPH SMALL, P.A.**

DATE	01-02-05
HOME OF RECORD	63223 Meadow Lane, Eviron, PA 12205-1026
TELEPHONE	724-565-6128
E-MAIL ADDRESS	jjosephsmall@earthlink.net
CITIZENSHIP	USA
PLACE OF BIRTH	Philadelphia, PA
EDUCATION	A.B., Syracuse University, Syracuse, NY
	P.A., Teem University, Philadelphia, PA
MILITARY SERVICE	General Medical Officer, U.S. Army Medical Corps, United Nations Command Far East
	Chief, Outpatient Medical Services, Dewitt Army Hospital, Honorable Discharge with Army Commendation Medal
EMPLOYMENT	Medical Director, Lowmark's Health Promotion and Disease Prevention Division, 2001–2004
	Medical Director, Healthcare Management Services, Lowmark's utilization review organization for all books of business, 2000–2001
	Director, medical lead and liaison with N.I.A., Lowmark's vendor for imaging utilization, 1998–2000
	Medical Editor, *Clinical Thoughts*, Lowmark's internationally awarded quarterly journal to providers offering only clinical information, 1998–2004
	Director, northwest region, Lowmark, 1997–2000
	Director, Lowmark Representative at Medical Affairs Committee, policy determining body, 1997–2004
	Physician Assistant, Employee Health Services, Hanot Medical Center, Eviron, PA, 1992–1997
	Acting Medical Director, Assistant Medical Director, Hanot Occupational Health Center, Eviron, PA, 1992–1997
PUBLICATIONS	Upon request
REFERENCES	Upon request
INTERESTS	Current events and history, reading, writing, public speaking, teaching, sailing, travel, counterterrorism, and pecuniary rewards
STRENGTHS	Adaptable, affable, analytic, articulate, both verbal and written, detail and goal oriented, personable, energetic, people-skilled, organizer

Sample 2

Elizabeth Thomas MS, PA-C
3605 W. 24th St.
Cleveland, OH 44111
216-942-1421

Employment

1997–present   Prequel Family Medicine   Eviron, PA
Physician Assistant
- Evaluating, diagnosing, and treating patients in a family medicine office, including physicals, well-child checks, pelvic exams, minor acute problems, and patient education.

May 1991–Dec 1991 Valley Health Center Connaught, PA
Physician Assistant
- Seeing patients in family practice clinic setting, physicals, well-child checks, immunizations, pelvic exams, minor acute problems, and recommending or instituting treatment regimens.

July 1985–Dec 1989 Reconstructive Surgery   Eviron, PA
Physician Assistant
- Assisting in surgery, performing preoperative histories and physicals, scheduling surgeries, and patient education.

Aug 1985–May 1988 Guardian Life Assurance   Jerkin, PA
Medical Examiner
- Performing in-home histories, physicals, EKGs, and venipunctures.

Education

Aug 1996   Cannon University   Eviron, PA
M.S., Counseling/Psychology

May 1980   Cannon University   Eviron, PA
B.S., Physician Assistant

Certification

National Commission on Certification of Physician Assistants
- Certificate #82018
- Recertification Exam—Passed with Recognition, August 1990, July 1997, March 2002
- Certification Exam—Passed with Recognition, October 1984

Memberships
American Academy of Physician Assistants # 999786
Pennsylvania Society of Physician Assistants #981217

Community Involvement
Fairview PTA 1995–present
Volunteer Swim Instructor, YMCA 1998–present

References are available on request.

THANK-YOU LETTERS

Sample 1

(Date)

William Smith D.O.
SOLO Family Practice
1219 Pear Street, Suite 200
Olmsted Township, State 12121

Dear Dr. Smith,

Thank you for taking the time to speak with me on Friday, (date of interview). I enjoyed meeting you and would like to reaffirm my interest in joining your practice. I believe the interview highlighted the fact that I am a good match for SOLO Family Practice. My previous employment experience in family practice has prepared me for the position that you seek to fill. Your practice style parallels my previous working environment, and I feel I would be able to make a smooth transition into your practice and quickly become an asset to your office.

As a follow-up to our discussion regarding asthma treatment, I have included the latest literature review on the development of tolerance when using long acting beta-agonists. Please feel free to contact me at 888/721-5656 if I can provide any additional information.

Thank you for your time and consideration.

Sincerely,

(signature)

Jane Johns PA-C
3434 West Street
City, State 17878

Contract Checklist

The term of the contract must be stated including your starting date and the length of the contract.

Every aspect of your employment should be clearly spelled out and include the following:

Responsibilities

- ❑ Patient load
- ❑ Working times
- ❑ Sites where you will practice
- ❑ Practice duties
- ❑ Rounds and on-call duties
- ❑ Any restrictions regarding moonlighting or volunteering
- ❑ Hospital privileges and credentials that must be maintained

Salary

- ❑ Will there be a base salary as an employee or hourly rate? If you will be paid an hourly rate, specify the minimum hours per week you are guaranteed to work to assure an adequate income.
- ❑ If you will have a production-based salary, the contract will need to specify how such a salary will be calculated, what will be included, and how often this calculation will occur.
- ❑ On-call pay and schedule.
- ❑ Bonus pay.
- ❑ Incentives.
- ❑ When will review periods and process job performance reviews occur? Typically reviews occur at 1-month, 3-month, and 6-month intervals.
- ❑ Periodic increases.
- ❑ Profit sharing.
- ❑ Partnership, conditions for buy-in, and basic terms should be outlined; this may be included in a separate letter of intent, which should also

include the amount of time you have to wait, how the practice will be valued, and how you will participate in business decisions.

❑ Pension and retirement program and employer's contributions.
❑ Sign-on bonus.

Benefits

❑ Vary by employer, can range from almost none to a complete package.
❑ Some employers use a cafeteria plan—you pick what you want based on self-perceived needs.
❑ Can you periodically change your benefit plan?

Liability Insurance

❑ Occurrence and tail coverage.
❑ What legal services will be provided in the event you are involved in a malpractice suit?
❑ Who will be responsible for the cost of the liability coverage?
❑ Will the policy you are covered under be a rider on a supervisor's policy or a policy in your own name?

Health and Dental Insurance

❑ Employee only or family coverage
❑ Employee contribution
❑ Are their any deductibles?
❑ Pharmacy coverage
❑ Catastrophic coverage

Disability Insurance

❑ Worker's compensation
❑ Life insurance
❑ Employee
❑ Low-cost family insurance
❑ Death or disability while on job
❑ Key provider insurance
❑ In case of death of physician or PA, the practice survives

Paid Time Off

❑ Vacation days
❑ Holidays
❑ Sick leave
❑ CME days
❑ Jury duty

❏ Condolence days
❏ Humanitarian mission (i.e., Doctors without Borders)—paid, unpaid, shared?

Fringe Benefits

❏ CME allowance
❏ Tuition assistance and forgiveness
❏ Professional dues/fees (AAPA, state organization)
❏ Licensure, certification, credentialing fees (DEA)
❏ Relocation and settlement allowance
❏ Technology (PDA, pager, cell phone, computer, ISP)
❏ Hospital medical staff fees
❏ Professional journals

Personnel Policies

❏ Dispute resolution and grievance procedures, mandatory arbitration, who will pay attorneys fees
❏ Access to patient records in the event that you are involved in a malpractice suit
❏ Noncompetition clauses or restrictive covenants
❏ Termination procedures
❏ Termination clause
❏ Resignation procedures
❏ Safe harbor provisions (Stark Acts)
❏ Noncompete provisions
❏ Provisions for providing you with adequate staffing and materials
❏ Administrative release time to allow you to keep up with paperwork, charting, lab reports, billing, correspondence, etc.

Contract Renewal

❏ Option to renew provisions
❏ Renegotiation based on performance evaluation
❏ Performance criteria should be attached or included in the contract

Sample Practice Privilege Checklist and Guidelines

PHYSICIAN ASSISTANTS

Baseline Privileges

Prior to being granted practice privileges, each physician assistant who is certified by the State Board of Medicine must provide to the Medical Center a complete copy of the executed written agreement (the 'Written Agreement') between the physician assistant and the physicians who the physician assistant will be assisting. The physician assistant's primary supervising physician must be a medical doctor with medical staff privileges at the Medical Center, licensed by the State Board of Medicine, and registered with that Board as the physician assistant's primary supervising physician. To the extent that the following practice privileges are within the scope of a physician assistant's Written Agreement and the regulations issued by the State Board of Medicine, such practice privileges may be exercised by a physician assistant who is certified by the State Board of Medicine and board certified by the NCCPA and who is granted permission to practice at the Medical Center (physician assistants certified by the State Board of Medicine who are not board certified by the NCCPA will be granted more limited practice privileges as permitted by the State Board of Medicine):

1. Screen patients to determine need for medical attention.
2. Review patient records to determine health status.
3. Take patient histories and perform physical examinations, subject to the dictates of the Organization and Functions Manual; provided, however, that all findings not within normal limits shall be reported to the supervising or substitute supervising physician as soon as possible, but no later than 12 hours.
4. Write progress notes in patients' charts, subject to the dictates of the Organization and Functions Manual, which progress notes must be reviewed and countersigned by the supervising or substitute supervising physician prior to major diagnostic or therapeutic intervention outside the normal scope of practice of physician assistants or within 24 hours, whichever occurs first.

5. Execute medical regimens ordered by the supervising or substitute supervising physician, including medical regimens issued pursuant to oral and standing orders, and relay such medical regimens for execution by other health care practitioners; provided, however, that all such medical regimens executed or relayed by the physician assistant must be entered in the patient's chart at the time they are executed or relayed, and must be reviewed and countersigned by the supervising or substitute supervising physician prior to major diagnostic or therapeutic intervention outside the normal scope of practice of physician assistants or within 24 hours, whichever occurs first.
6. Initiate requests/orders for routine labs, X-rays, and other diagnostic studies, subject to the dictates of the Organization and Functions Manual.
7. Make decisions regarding data gathering and appropriate management and treatment of patients being seen for the initial evaluation of a problem or for the follow-up evaluation of a previously diagnosed and stabilized condition.
8. Provide counseling and instruction regarding common patient problems.

Specific Privileges

The following practice privileges must be specifically requested by each physician assistant seeking permission to practice such privileges at the Medical Center, and such practice privileges must be expressly within the scope of the physician assistant's Written Agreement. Please check each practice privilege that is being requested and provide documentation of training and competency:

- Initiate evaluation and emergency management for emergency situations
- Cardiopulmonary resuscitation
- Control of external hemorrhage
- Apply dressings and bandages and attend to postoperative wound care including suture and staple removal
- Carry out aseptic techniques and isolation techniques
- Perform developmental screening exams on children
- Accept/transcribe verbal and standing orders from supervising or substitute supervising physicians, subject to the dictates of the Organization and Functions Manual of the Medical Staff Handbook
- Dictate reports such as histories and physicals, discharge summaries, and consults, subject to the dictates of the Organization and Functions Manual, all of which shall be countersigned by the supervising or substitute supervising physician prior to major diagnostic or therapeutic intervention outside the normal practice of allopathic physician assistants or within 24 hours, whichever occurs first
- Dictate procedure notes and operative notes (only if the procedure is performed by the physician assistant, or if the physician assistant is the surgical first assistant), subject to the dictates of the Organization and Functions Manual of the Medical Staff Handbook

Other Specific Privileges

Physician assistants seeking permission to (a) administer, prescribe, or dispense medications; or (b) relay the standing or verbal orders of the supervising or substitute supervising physician for the administration of medications; or (C) practice other privileges not specifically covered by the above categories of this checklist must specifically request permission to practice such privileges at the Medical Center. Please provide documentation of training and competency for each privilege requested:

1. Attach to this checklist the list of medications that the physician assistant will be administering, prescribing, dispensing or that may be relayed pursuant to standing orders of the supervising or substitute supervising physician. (Must be expressly within scope of Written Agreement.)
2. Attach to this checklist any additional specialized regimens, procedures, or privileges that are not already covered by this checklist. (Must be expressly within scope of Written Agreement.)

SCOPE OF PRACTICE DELINEATION FORM

Type of Request: ❏ Initial ❏ Renewal

Name_____ Category: Physician Assistant in Medicine
Inpatient/Outpatient Setting

Please check the procedures for which you are making application and submit with PA protocols or physician agreement.

Requested	Granted	Denied	Class 1 Practice Privileges	Number Performed in Training or Experience	Number to Be Proctored
1. Evaluation Functions					
Pediatric			Perform and record patient evaluations	20	5
Adult			Perform and record patient evaluations	60	5
2. Monitoring Functions					
Pediatric			Develop and implement patient management plans	20	5
Adult			Develop and implement patient management plans	60	5

Requested	Granted	Denied	Class 1 Practice Privileges	Number Performed in Training or Experience	Number to Be Proctored
3. Diagnostic Functions					
Pediatric			Order routine or specific diagnostic procedures *1	20	5
			Order routine or specific diagnostic procedures *1,2	10	3
Adult			Order routine or specific diagnostic procedures *1	60	5
			Order routine or specific diagnostic procedures *1,2	40	7
4. Therapeutic Functions					
Pediatric			Orders therapies or treatments *1	10	3
			Order medications permitted by PA law for physician assistants.	10	3
			Assist physician in the management of complex illness or injuries	5	2
			Perform procedures:		
			Injections and immunizations	10	3
			Suturing and wound care	5	2
			Application and removal of splints	5	2
			Removal/destruction of superficial skin lesions	5	5
			Minor surgical procedures, with or without local anesthesia (e.g., drainage of subungual hematoma, removal of partial nail avulsion, I&D of superficial abscesses)	5	5
Adult			Orders therapies or treatments *1	40	7
			Order medications permitted by PA law for physician assistants	40	7
			Assist physician in the management of complex illness or injuries	5	2
			Perform procedures:		
			Injections and immunizations	10	3
			Suturing and wound care	5	2
			Application and removal of splints	5	2
			Removal/destruction of superficial skin lesions	5	5

Requested	Granted	Denied	Class 1 Practice Privileges	Number Performed in Training or Experience	Number to Be Proctored
			Minor surgical procedures, with or without local anesthesia (e.g., drainage of subungual hematoma, removal of partial nail avulsion, I&D of superficial abscesses)	5	5
5. Counseling Functions					
			Instruct and counsel patients regarding compliance with prescribed therapeutic regimes; pediatric growth and development; family planning; and health maintenance	80	5

*1 As specified in PA protocols or physician agreement.
*2 Such as venipuncture, throat culture, EKG, pap smear, blood gas, anoscopy.

_____   _____
Applicant's Signature   Date

_____   _____
Chief, Division of Medical Specialties   Date

Credentialing Information

A credentialing application may ask for the following information:

- The PA's name, and other names used in past licensure and certification
- States of licensure and license, registration or certification number
- NCCPA certification
- State prescribing number
- DEA number
- Medicare provider identification number
- Social Security number
- Birth date
- Citizenship
- Place of birth
- Home address and telephone number
- Primary practice name, address, telephone, tax identification number, and office manager name
- Practice status (individual, partnership, or group)
- Practice specialty
- Dates at this practice
- Other practice locations
- Undergraduate and graduate education institution address, dates attended, degrees conferred for PA education
- PA postgraduate training: institution, address, dates attended, type of training, name of program director, specialty
- Additional training (e.g., advanced cardiac life support, pediatric advanced life support, advanced trauma life support)
- Chronologic professional employment history/professional affiliations: institution, address, phone numbers, dates of privileges, position title, leadership positions held, name of department chair, type of facility, reason for leaving
- Current privileges: hospital, address, date received privileges, staff category, leadership positions held, name of department chair

- Military service: branch, period of service, discharge status, rank
- Professional liability coverage:
  - Proof of current coverage, name of previous carrier, period of coverage, limits of coverage, type of coverage, reason for discontinuance
  - Whether you have maintained continuous professional liability coverage since first obtaining coverage
  - Whether you have been subject to a professional liability suit, including but not limited to malpractice claims, in the past 5 years
  - Whether there are any restrictions, limitations, or exclusions in your current professional liability coverage
  - Whether your professional liability insurance coverage has ever been denied, limited, reduced, interrupted, terminated, or not renewed

- Personal information:
  - Date of last physical examination
  - Whether you are currently suffering from, or receiving treatment for, any physical or mental disability or illness, including drug or alcohol abuse, that would impair the proper performance of your essential functions and responsibilities as a health care provider
  - Whether you have ever been convicted of, or pleaded guilty to or nolo contendere, to any crime other than traffic violations

- Professional sanctions.
  - Whether your license to practice any health occupation in any jurisdiction has ever been limited, suspended, denied, subjected to any conditions, terms of probation, or formal reprimand, not renewed, or revoked
  - Whether you have surrendered your license to practice any health occupation in any jurisdiction
  - Whether your request for any specific clinical privilege has ever been denied or granted with stated limitations
  - Whether you have ever been denied membership on a hospital medical staff
  - Whether your staff privileges, appointment, and/or delineation of privileges at any hospital or other health care institution has ever been suspended, revoked, limited, reduced, denied, or subject to any conditions or not renewed
  - Whether your DEA or other controlled substance authorization has ever been limited, suspended, denied, reduced, subject to any conditions, terms of probation, not renewed, or revoked
  - Whether proceedings toward any of these ends has ever been initiated
  - Whether your controlled substance authorization has ever been voluntarily relinquished
  - Whether you have ever been subject to disciplinary action in any medical organization or professional society

- Whether there are any disciplinary actions pending against you
- Whether you have resigned from any hospital or health care institution or professional academic appointment
- Whether you have ever been placed on probation, suspended, asked to resign, or been terminated while in a training program
- Whether you have ever been placed on probation, suspended, or asked to resign or been terminated while in a hospital program
- Whether you have ever withdrawn your application for appointment, reappointment, or clinical privileges or resigned before a decision was made by a hospital's or health care facility's governing board
- Whether you have ever been denied certification or recertification by a specialty board or received a letter of admonition from such a board or committee
- Whether you have ever been investigated by any private, federal, or state agency concerning your participation in a private, federal, or state health insurance program
- Whether you have ever been subject to probation proceedings or suspended sanctioned, or otherwise restricted from participating in any private federal or state health insurance program
- Whether you have received a determination from any professional review organization indicating a "final severity level 3" or a "gross and flagrant" quality concern

- Professional references: list names and addresses of four persons who have worked extensively with you or have been responsible for professionally observing you. Do not list more than two current partners or associates in practice. Do not list any relatives by blood or marriage, the chief of service to whom you are applying, any person in current or past training programs with you (unless he or she is now a colleague), or persons who cannot attest to your current level of clinical competence, technical skill, and medical knowledge.

CHAPTER 6

Negligence and Medical Malpractice

Malpractice Overview •Standard of Care • Civil and Criminal Proceedings • Burden of Proof • Legal Theories • Breach of Confidentiality • Negligence Per Se • Vicarious Liability/Respondent Superior/Captain of the Ship • Statute of Limitations • Adverse Events • Choosing a Malpractice Case • Being Deposed • National Practitioner's Data Bank (NPDB) • Healthcare Integrity and Protection Data Bank (HIPDB)

We live in a highly litigious society, and practicing medicine puts you at risk of being named in a malpractice suit. The litigious environment has increased the number of claims being filed and there is a trend toward increasing awards. The majority of malpractice actions never make it to court. In fact, over 90% of all malpractice claims are settled.[1] The number of claims originating from care provided in the ambulatory setting is increasing. Practitioners in obstetrics, outpatient surgery, and emergency departments are at increased risk of being named in a malpractice action. On average, one in four practitioners will be sued during his or her career. According to the 2002 National Practitioner Data Bank Annual Report, physicians are responsible for 8 out of 10 malpractice payments, dentists are responsible for 1 out of 10, and physician assistants are responsible for less than 1% of all malpractice payments. Involvement in a malpractice action is a lengthy process and can take 3 to 5 years before the action is resolved. (See Table 6-1.)

MALPRACTICE OVERVIEW

It is estimated that medical errors result in 44,000–98,000 deaths annually in the United States, occur in 2% of all hospital admissions, and cost the nation $2 billion per year.[2,3] Medical errors kill more people each year than breast cancer, AIDS, or motor vehicle accidents. Fewer than 50% of patients with diabetes, hypertension, tobacco addiction, hyperlipidemia, congestive heart failure, asthma, depression, and chronic atrial fibrillation are adequately managed.[4]

Table 6-1 Common Types of Medical Malpractice

Failure to diagnose a medical condition
Prescription errors
Failure to perform surgery or other medical procedure properly
Delay in treatment
Failure to properly explain a medical procedure or potential side effects
Improper treatment

In a study that looked at one million hospital admissions, it was determined that 37,000 patients suffered injuries as a result of medical management. Of the 37,000 injuries, 10,212 were a result of negligence. Of these 10,212 patients, 204 filed malpractice claims and 102 received some form of compensation. One percent (102 out of 10,212) of patients suffering a medical injury due to negligence received compensation for their injury (99% of the patients suffering medical injuries due to negligence received no compensation). In a similar study, it was found that of 100 malpractice claims filed, only 17 involved medical negligence; 83% of the physicians who were sued for malpractice were found to be not negligent.[5] These two studies point out the fact that the current malpractice system does not seem to work for either patients or providers.

Malpractice premiums for physicians have risen dramatically, and PAs can expect to see increases in their malpractice premiums as well. The AAPA-endorsed insurance program will no longer offer occurrence policies to new policyholders.[6] PAs who currently have an occurrence policy through the AAPA's insurance program will continue to be able to purchase the occurrence policy, but the rate for the same policy purchased in 2004 may be three times as expensive in 2005.[7]

The average cost of defending a medical malpractice lawsuit is greater than $30,000. This cost does not include the loss of income from practice during the three-plus weeks that a practitioner is required to be in court defending himself or herself or any judgment awarded to the patient who filed the case.

STANDARD OF CARE

The *standard of care* is defined as the care a reasonably prudent clinician of like credentials and training in the same locale would provide to a patient. A physician assistant must meet the same standard of care that another physician assistant in the same locale would have provided. All malpractice actions for negligence revolve around the standard of care. If the care a practitioner provided to a patient met the standard of care, malpractice did not occur. Malpractice occurs when a practitioner fails to provide care to a patient that meets the standard of care. In a malpractice action that goes to court, whether a PA has met the standard of care will be determined through expert testimony. After hearing expert testimony for the plaintiff and the defense, the jury will decide if the PA met the standard of care. The expert witness used in a malpractice action against a physician assistant will be another physician assistant who is practicing in the same or a similar location. *Location* refers to rural areas, metropolitan areas, large medical centers, and teaching hospitals. In different locations there may be a variation in the approach to a patient due to the availability of technology at the practice site and the local area.

To meet the standard of care a practitioner must remain current in his or her medical knowledge by attending conferences, reading medical journals, using the latest medical textbooks, and referring to appropriate medical Internet sites. Practitioners must follow recommended protocols and screening recommendations accepted and published by the medical community or facility where the practitioner is employed. Failure to follow a published protocol or screening recommendations by a practitioner may be deemed to be a failure to have met the standard of care in that instance.

CIVIL AND CRIMINAL PROCEEDINGS

The majority of malpractice suits are filed in a civil court. The Healthcare Integrity and Protection Data Bank (HIPDB) recorded 967 adverse action reports (civil) and seven judgment or conviction reports (criminal) from state and federal agencies for PAs between August 1996 and August 2004.[8] Criminal charges can arise if a practitioner is guilty of *criminal negligence*, which is defined as a gross lack of competence or indifference to a patient's safety. Violations of the narcotics laws, medical fraud, and violations of federal confidentiality laws can also result in criminal charges being filed against a practitioner. Criminal acts such as intentional torts, where a practitioner intentionally causes injury to a patient, and *gross negligence*, which is defined as willful, wanton, or malicious acts, can also lead to criminal charges being filed against a practitioner. Sexual misconduct or sexual involvements with a patient by a practitioner or practicing medicine or performing a procedure under the influence of alcohol or illicit drugs are additional instances that may lead to criminal charges. Fines or awards that result from criminal charges against a practitioner are not covered by most professional liability coverage.

BURDEN OF PROOF

In all malpractice actions the burden of proof falls on the plaintiff (the patient who filed the malpractice action). The plaintiff must prove the elements of the case by a preponderance of the evidence, which is slightly greater than a 50% likelihood (more likely than not) that the defendant (practitioner) did what the plaintiff alleges (i.e., did not meet the standard of care). The burden of proof in a malpractice action, which is a civil action, is less than the burden of proof in a criminal case, which is beyond a reasonable doubt.

LEGAL THEORIES

A practitioner may become the defendant in civil litigation under the legal theory of negligence, informed consent, or abandonment.

Negligence

Activities that primary care practitioners carry out during ordinary office visits account for an average of 20% of all malpractice claims. The majority of malpractice actions are attributed to diagnostic errors or failure to treat. The legal theory used to bring this type of action is negligence. *Negligence* is defined as a failure to exercise the care toward others that a reasonable or prudent person would provide under similar circumstances, or taking action that such a reasonable person would not. Negligence is accidental as distinguished from *intentional torts* (assault or trespass, for example) or from crimes, but a crime can also constitute negligence, such as reckless disregard for a patient's welfare. Negligence can result in all types of accidents causing physical and/or property damage, but can also include business errors and miscalculations, such as a sloppy land survey. In making a claim for damages based on an allegation of another's negligence, the injured party (plaintiff) must prove (a) that the party alleged to be negligent had a duty to the injured party—specifically to the one injured or to the general public, (b) that the defendant's action (or failure to act) was negligent—not what a reasonably prudent person would have done, (c) that the damages were caused ("proximately caused") by the negligence. An added factor in the formula for determining negligence is whether the damages were "reasonably foreseeable" at the time of the alleged carelessness. If the injury is caused by something owned or controlled by the supposedly negligent party, but how the accident actually occurred is not known (like a ton of bricks falls from a construction job), negligence can be found based on the doctrine of *res ipsa loquitur* (Latin for "the thing speaks for itself"). Furthermore, in six states (Alabama, North Carolina, South Carolina, Tennessee, Virginia, Maryland) and the District of Columbia, an injured party will be denied any judgment (payment) if found to have been guilty of even slight "contributory negligence" in the accident. This unfair rule has been replaced by "comparative negligence" in the other 44 states, in which the negligence of the claimant is balanced with the percentage of blame placed on the other party or parties ("joint tortfeasors") causing the accident. Negligence is one of the greatest sources of litigation (along with contract and business disputes) in the United States.

The elements of a negligence action include a duty, a breach of the duty, causation, and that damages occurred as a result of the breach of duty. The plaintiff must prove each of these elements by a preponderance of the evidence. In order to prove that the practitioner had a duty to the plaintiff (patient), the plaintiff must show that a patient–clinician relationship had been established between the practitioner and the plaintiff. This element is relatively easy to prove. Speaking with a patient on the phone, treating a walk-in patient to the office or clinic, an HMO contract, and informal (curbside) consults will establish that the practitioner had a duty to the plaintiff. A duty between the practitioner and the patient is established if the patient can reasonably depend on the medical advice given by the practitioner. The plaintiff must prove that the practitioner breached the duty by not providing care consistent with the standard of care. This will require the plaintiff to obtain an expert witness in the practitioner's field who will provide testimony that the care the practitioner provided to the patient fell below the accepted standard of care. The plaintiff must prove that the breach of duty was the proximate cause of the patient's injuries. In order to prove proximate cause the plaintiff must show that but for the act or omission of the wrongdoer the personal injury would not have occurred when it did as it did. Finally, the plaintiff must prove that damages were sustained as a result of the breach of duty. Most commonly damages are in the form of pain and suffering, additional medical costs, or lost wages.

Informed Consent

An action brought against a practitioner alleging a lack of informed consent is brought under the theory of battery. A battery is any physical contact with another person to which that other person has not consented. Patients have a number of rights that protect them from receiving inferior health care. In order to obtain an informed consent a practitioner must provide a patient with:

- Complete and current information about the patient's condition—A health care provider is obligated to fully explain medical conditions to his or her patients.
- Complete and current information about treatment—A practitioner is obligated to fully explain what treatments are available for a patient's medical condition. Although a practitioner may recommend one treatment over another, he or she must present all reasonable treatment options to a patient. The practitioner should carefully document the risks, consequences, and complications of each of the treatment options offered to the patient.
- The opportunity to fully participate in decisions affecting health—The patient alone has the right to choose what treatment is acceptable. A practitioner can recommend a particular treatment, but the decision is ultimately the patient's. This includes nontraditional medical treatments such as acupuncture, holistic remedies, chiropractic care, and any other treatment available to the patient. If a patient decides against the treatment option that was recommended, the practitioner should carefully document the risks, consequences, and complications of not following the recommended treatment plan.

The Right to Informed Consent

The patient has the right to consent to or reject medical treatment. *Informed consent* means that the patient has consented to a treatment after having had an opportunity to learn about available treatment options, potential side effects, potential risks, and the nature of the condition. A patient also has the right to know whether or not the proposed treatment is experimental.

The standards for informed consent require a practitioner to provide all the information to a patient that a reasonably prudent clinician would provide and that a reasonably prudent patient or guardian would wish to know.

Documenting Informed Consent

It is the duty of physicians to document informed consent. Informed consent should be documented prior to:

- Performing a surgical procedure or administering anesthesia
- Administering radiation or chemotherapy
- Administering a blood transfusion
- Inserting a surgical device or appliance
- Administering an experimental medication, using an experimental device, or using an approved medical device for an experimental reason

Informed consent does not have to be obtained in an emergency situation where the patient is unconscious or incompetent to provide consent as a result of trauma or an urgent medical condition.

Liability

A physician will be held responsible for failure to obtain informed consent if the patient proves that he or she did not receive information that would have been a substantial factor in the patient's decision to undergo a procedure.

In some states a physician may also be held liable for failure to seek a patient's informed consent if the physician knowingly misrepresents his professional credentials, training, or experience to the patient.

Delegating

If a physician assistant is responsible for obtaining informed consent, that PA should be sure that it is legal in his or her state for physicians to delegate the task of obtaining informed consent. As a PA, if you are obtaining informed consent, be sure that you are acting within your scope of practice as defined by statute, rules, or your written agreement. In most instances the physician is still liable for failure to obtain informed consent even if the duty is delegated.

A physician assistant who performs procedures should obtain informed consent for the procedure to be performed rather than delegating the duty to another member of the health care team.

Consent Form

A patient can challenge the actual consent form. To decrease the chance that your consent forms will be challenged, do the following:

- Be sure that the forms are readable. The majority of consent forms are written at the college level, making them too difficult to understand for the majority of the population. It is recommended that consent forms be written at an eighth-grade-education level so that all patients can easily interpret the form they are required to sign. If you feel that the consent forms being used in your practice are too difficult to understand, rewrite the forms or request your legal counsel to rewrite the forms at a more basic level. Be sure that legal counsel approves the forms prior to adoption.
- The consent form should be detailed and procedure specific rather than generic. It is recommended that each procedure have a specific consent form with risks and complications specific to the procedure listed on the form.
- The consent should be witnessed by one or two individuals other than the person obtaining the consent.
- If possible, obtain informed consent on two separate occasions, once in the office and again the day of the procedure.
- It is important to emphasize to patients the significance of the consent form. In order to make it clear to the patient the importance of an informed consent, include language on the forms that states, "Do not sign this form until you fully understand the procedure and all of your questions have been answered." Have the patient initial the sentence, then sign the form.
- Patients often say that they did not read the form or that they did not understand the form. Include these three questions on all your consent forms:
  - Did you read the form?
  - Did you understand the form?
  - Were all your questions answered?

Have the patient check yes to all three questions and have a third party witness the form and that the patient answered the above three questions affirmatively.

Abandonment

A practitioner does not have a duty to treat any person who is not a patient. Once a practitioner–patient relationship has been established, a practitioner has a duty to continue to treat the patient until the patient no longer has a need for medical services. In some instances it is necessary for a practitioner to terminate a relationship with a patient. It is considered abandonment if a practitioner does not conform to the applicable standard of care when discontinuing the practitioner–patient relationship. A practitioner must provide the patient with an acceptable alternative practitioner or give the patient enough time to establish a new relationship with an alternate practitioner. A letter should be sent to the patient stating that the practitioner will continue to provide health care services for a specified amount of time, usually 30 to 90 days, depending on the difficulty the patient will have in finding another provider.

BREACH OF CONFIDENTIALITY

A practitioner can be sued and face both civil and criminal penalties if a patient's protected personal health information is released improperly. (See Chapter 8 for detailed coverage of this topic.)

NEGLIGENCE PER SE

Per se is Latin for "by itself," meaning *inherently*. If a PA performs an act that is beyond the scope of the PA's practice, that PA is "negligent per se" without further explanation of the meaning of the statement, even if the act met the accepted standard of care. For example, a PA works for a hospital and has a supervising physician who is a cardiologist. The PA also performs deliveries on the obstetrics floor in emergency situations at the hospital's request. Even if the PA performs a delivery and meets the applicable standard of care, the PA is "negligent per se" because the PA has performed a medical procedure outside his or her scope of practice. A PA's scope of practice is limited by the supervisor's scope of practice; since the supervisor in this example is a cardiologist the PA's scope of practice is limited to cardiology.

VICARIOUS LIABILITY/RESPONDENT SUPERIOR/CAPTAIN OF THE SHIP

The doctrines of vicarious liability, respondent superior, and captain of the ship allow patients to commence a malpractice action against a physician assistant's supervising physician for negligent acts performed by the physician assistant. Vicarious liability is sometimes called *imputed liability* and is defined as an attachment of responsibility to a person for harm or damages caused by another person in either a negligence lawsuit or criminal prosecution. Thus, an employer of an employee who injures someone through negligence while in the scope of employment (doing work for the employer) is vicariously liable for damages to the injured person. The doctrine of respondent superior also allows an employer to be held negligent for acts of an employee. The captain of the ship doctrine allows a person who is supervising nonemployees to be held liable for negligent acts of those being supervised. This doctrine is often used in the case of a surgeon who is supervising hospital employees during surgery. Under the captain of the ship doctrine a surgeon can be named in a malpractice action if a circulating nurse makes an error in the sponge count and a sponge is left in the patient, resulting in additional intervention to remove the sponge even though the nurse is employed by the hospital and not the physician.

STATUTE OF LIMITATIONS

The statute of limitations is the time limit in which an injured patient must file a claim. Once the statute of limitations has passed a patient is barred from filing a malpractice action. The time limit for filing medical malpractice claims varies from 1 to 7 years, depending on your state.

Injuries to Minors

A *minor* is anyone who has not attained the age of 18 years. It is important to keep all records, including obstetric, pediatric, and family practice, on minor patients until they reach the age of 25 years. Many states allow minors to file medical malpractice actions 7 years from the alleged tort or until the minor reaches the age of 20, whichever is later.

Death and Survival Actions

A patient's family member who feels that negligence contributed to the patient's death may bring death and survival action. The statute of limitations on death and survival actions will be tolled if the plaintiff can prove that there was affirmative misrepresentation or fraudulent concealment of the cause of death.

ADVERSE EVENTS

PAs who work in or for organizations accredited by the Joint Committee on Accreditation of Healthcare Organizations (JCAHO) are required to report adverse or serious patient events. *Adverse events* are defined as occurrences or situations involving the clinical care of a patient in a medical facility that results in death or compromises patient safety and results in an unanticipated injury requiring the delivery of additional health care services to the patient. An *incident* is defined as a near miss, which does not result in serious consequences to the patient. There is no requirement to report an incident. If a patient is prescribed the wrong medication dose but the error is caught prior to the patient being given the medication, the event would be considered an incident and nonreportable. If the patient was actually given an incorrect medication dose and had to be resuscitated as a result of the medication, the event would be considered an adverse event and would have to be reported.

To meet the reporting requirement a health care provider must notify the patient or patient's representative in writing within 7 days of the occurrence or discovery of the adverse event. Employees who report a serious event are immune from retaliatory action. A family or patient can report an event and trigger JCAHO analysis. The hospital's patient safety committee has 45 days to analyze and develop an action plan in response to the adverse event report. If the hospital requirement to develop an action plan is not met by the institution, JCAHO will place the institution on accreditation watch. Once a report is filed the statute of limitations for filing a malpractice action will begin to run.

CHOOSING A MALPRACTICE CASE

The choice to file a malpractice complaint is a business decision for the plaintiff's attorney. Plaintiffs' attorneys are paid on a contingency basis. The majority of plaintiffs do not have the resources to pay malpractice attorneys on an hourly basis. A malpractice attorney will enter into a contract with a plaintiff, requiring the attorney to pay all of the costs of litigation including expert fees and court costs in exchange for a percentage of the plaintiff's award or settlement. Once the award or settlement is made the attorney recoups the litigation costs and then an additional 30% to 40% of the remaining funds. If the defendant (practitioner) prevails, the plaintiff's attorney has lost the time and money the firm has invested in the case. A loss in court will result in a $20,000 to $30,000 average loss for the attorney's firm. Plaintiff's attorneys will only take strong cases because they are more likely to settle before ever reaching court. If an insurance company feels that the plaintiff's case is weak, the company will not agree to a settlement, resulting in the risk of loss increasing for the plaintiff's attorney.

Due to the risk plaintiffs' attorneys face, they carefully screen potential claims. Only one third of all medical claims lead to a 2-hour client interview. Attorneys are less likely to accept cases involving older individuals because older individuals are more likely to have multiple medical problems, which increase the cost of the preparation of the case. Older individuals are also less likely to have lost wages and have a shorter life expectancy, decreasing the damages which can be sued for.

Prior to the interview the firm will assess the possible damages. If there are no damages, there is no case. The damages in the case must be valued at a minimum of $100,000 before a large firm will consider taking the case. A small case takes as much time to prepare as a large case. Taking on a case with a small return is considered a poor business decision.

After the interview, if the plaintiff's attorney feels that the case may be worth pursuing, the attorney will request the most pertinent medical records. At this point the case requires the firm to begin spending money. To obtain the most pertinent medical records the firm will have to spend an average of $1000. The next step for the firm is to hire a medical expert to review the records, which will cost the firm approximately $1500 to $2000.

An expert is asked the following four questions:

- Was the diagnosis correct?
- Was the treatment appropriate?

- Was the plaintiff damaged?
- Did the provider's negligence cause the damage?

If the expert does not answer yes to all four of the questions, the plaintiff's attorney will not be able to prove negligence occurred and there is no case.

Consider this example: A patient is seen by a surgeon for a breast mass. The surgeon does not remove the mass. The patient is later diagnosed with cancer and passes away as a result of the cancer. The patient's family seeks legal advice from a malpractice attorney. It appears to the attorney that negligence has occurred. The attorney requests the patient's medical records and has them evaluated by an expert surgeon. The surgeon concludes that the defendant surgeon failed to meet the standard of care by not removing the mass. Next an expert oncologist reviews the records. The oncologist finds that the patient was seen by the defendant surgeon in January with the complaint of a breast mass. The patient was diagnosed with cancer in May of the same year and passed away as a result of the cancer six months later, in November. In the oncologist's expert opinion he states that the patient most likely had stage four cancer when the defendant surgeon saw her. A patient with stage four cancer has little or no hope for long-term survival. The plaintiff's attorney cannot prove causation because there is no proof that the delay in diagnosis caused the damages. Since the attorney cannot prove causation, a malpractice action brought under the theory of negligence would be unsuccessful. The plaintiff's attorney would not proceed with the case. In this instance the attorney's firm would have lost approximately $5000 to $7000 pursuing the case to this point.

The decision to move forward and file a complaint in a malpractice action is based solely on the expert's review of the patient's medical records.

BEING DEPOSED

If you are named in a malpractice action, you will be deposed prior to trial. Table 6-2 shows the sequence of events of a malpractice lawsuit, including when depositions are given.

Table 6-2 Malpractice Lawsuit Timeline

Act or omission
Summons and complaint issued (insurer and employer informed)
Review records (begin meeting with attorney)
Pretrial alternatives/motions (interrogatories and depositions)
Settlement
Trial (usually 5 years from issue of complaint)
Verdict
Payment or judgment

At a deposition you will be asked a series of questions, which a court reporter will transcribe. The answers that you provide at the deposition will become part of the court record if the case does not settle. The deposition is the most important event in the lawsuit short of the trial. The plaintiff's attorney is trying to determine what effect you will have on the jury. The effect your testimony will have on the jury helps decide whether or not the plaintiff's attorney will try to settle the case and affects the amount the plaintiff's attorney will seek in settlement.

The plaintiff's attorney will attempt to establish through the mouth of the defendant the standard of care and that the defendant knows that it has been breached, the defendant's knowledge of what should have occurred, and if the defendant failed to consider a diagnosis. The deposition is more about psychology, appearance, and cosmetics than about finding the truth.

The plaintiff's attorney is asking the jury to take money from one person and give it to another. Juries do not like to find practitioners guilty. They rely on their own practitioners. It is easier for the jury to award the plaintiff money if the practitioner appears angry or arrogant, because the jury will not like the practitioner and this will make the decision to give money to the plaintiff easier.

Preparation for a deposition is very important. Prior to being deposed, review all depositions pertinent to the case and the answers to interrogatories (questions answered in written form, which are usually done prior to the deposition). Review all the medical records pertinent to the case, not just your own. Review the timelines pertinent to the case to have a sense of the care provided by other practitioners who were involved in the patient's case. Review samples of depositions from other similar cases taken by the plaintiff's attorney in order to give you an idea of the types of questions that you may be asked. Attend the depositions of the expert witnesses involved in the case. Ask your attorney to hold a mock deposition with you prior to your deposition.

NATIONAL PRACTITIONER'S DATA BANK (NPDB)

The National Practitioner's Data Bank was established through Title IV of Public Law 99-660, the Health Care Quality Improvement Act of 1986, as amended. The final regulations governing the NPDB are codified at 45 CFR Part 60. Responsibility for and maintenance of the NPDB reside in the Bureau of Health Professions, Health Resources and Services Administration (HRSA), U.S. Department of Health and Human Services (HHS). The NPDB is a repository for data on medical malpractice claims paid, adverse licensure and credentialing actions, and maintains the permanent records of health care professionals.

The NPDB was developed to improve the quality of health care by encouraging state licensing boards, hospitals, health care entities, and professional societies to identify and discipline those who engage in unprofessional behavior and to restrict the ability of incompetent health care practitioners from freely moving from state to state without disclosing previous medical malpractice histories, limitations on clinical privileges, licensure actions, denial of professional society membership, and exclusions from Medicare and Medicaid.[9]

The NPDB collects information on malpractice payments, adverse licensure, clinical privileges and professional society membership actions, and ineligibility to participate in Medicare and Medicaid. The information maintained by the NPDB is meant to alert credentialing bodies of past adverse actions and prompt a more thorough review of a practitioner's credentials prior to granting clinical privileges, employment, affiliation, or licensure. The NPDB is meant to augment and not replace the traditional credentialing practices of an institution.

The settlement of a malpractice action may occur for any number of reasons and should not be automatically construed as reflecting negatively on a practitioner's competence. A high settlement award or a high jury award does not mean that a practitioner acted incompetently. The record may not have been documented well enough to form a defense in the malpractice action. There may have been numerous defendants in the case and their involvement may have altered the outcome of the case. Your supervising physician, nurses, the hospital, or other employees may have been named. If a single insurer is involved, such as the hospital policy, which defends all the defendants a settlement may be made on behalf of all parties involved. In this instance the hospital, which holds the insurance policy, or the insurer would determine how the settlement payment should be allocated among those involved. If you are insured by your employer and do not have a consent-to-settle clause, you may not even know that an allocation has been made. If you have a consent-to-settle clause in your policy, you will be informed of the amount of settlement and be able to follow up with the NPDB to be sure that the allocation was properly made. A credentialing body should take into account the evidence of current competence by evaluating continuous quality improvement studies, peer recommendations, current health status, verification of training, experience and continuing education, and relationships with patients and colleagues.

The information obtained from the NPDB must be kept confidential. Any unauthorized release of information is subject to civil penalties of $11,000 per occurrence. The NPDB can be accessed by state licensing boards, hospitals, other health care entities, professional societies, federal agencies, and others as specified in the law.

Hospitals are mandated to query the NPDB when a practitioner applies for privileges and every two years as long as the practitioner remains on the medical staff or maintains his or her privileges. The hospital must also query the NPDB if a practitioner wished to add additional privileges or request temporary privileges. A hospital may query the bank at any other time as it sees fit.

Other health care entities that provide health care services may query the NPDB at any time before offering employment to or affiliating with a practitioner. Professional societies may query the bank prior to granting membership. State licensing boards may query the NPDB at any time. A plaintiff's attorney or a plaintiff without counsel may query the NBDB under very limited circumstances.

A practitioner may self-query the NPDB at any time by visiting the NPDB-HIPDB Web site at www.npdb-hipdb.com or by calling (800) 767-6732. For a small fee you can obtain your report. All self-query fees must be paid by credit card. If you find an error, you can contact NPDB to dispute it. If what has been reported is correct, the NPDB will not change the report. For example, you and your supervising physician are named in a malpractice action, which settles for $1 million. The supervising physician holds the insurance policy and he instructs the insurer to allocate the entire $1 million to you. Your data bank will show a $1 million malpractice payment whereas the supervising physician's data bank will show nothing. In this instance the report is correct. You would have to dispute the allocation with the insurer. If you are unable to have the allocation changed, you can submit a statement up to 2000 characters, which will become part of your NPDB permanent record.

An entity that makes a malpractice payment on behalf of a health care practitioner, in settlement of, or in satisfaction in whole or in part of a settlement or judgment against that practitioner, must report payment information to the NPDB. If an individual practitioner is not named as part of the settlement or judgment, the payment made is nonreportable. Medical malpractice payors must report medical malpractice payment within 30 days of the payment being made. A copy of the report must be immediately sent to the appropriate state licensing board in the state in which the malpractice claim occurred. According to the NPDB's 2002 Annual Report, physician assistants are responsible for fewer than 1% of all medical malpractice payment reports, the majority of which are for diagnosis-related problems.[10] (See Tables 6-3 through 6-6.)

Table 6-3 Practitioners with Reports (September 1, 1990–December 31, 2002)

Practitioner Type	Number of Practitioners with Reports	Number of Reports*	Reports per Practitioner
Chiropractors	5647	7304	1.29
Dentists	26,375	42,626	1.62
Emergency medical practitioners	118	147	1.25
Nurses and nursing-related practitioners	14,390	16,063	1.12
Physician assistants	766	880	1.15
Physicians	132,895	235,209	1.77
Podiatrists and podiatric-related practitioners	3635	6242	1.72
Respiratory therapists and related practitioners	30	31	1.03

*"Number of reports" includes medical malpractice payment reports, adverse licensure action reports, clinical privilege reports, professional society membership reports, Drug Enforcement Administration reports, and Medicare/Medicaid exclusion reports. Only physicians and dentists are reported for adverse licensure, clinical privilege, and professional society actions.

Source: NPDB 2002 Annual Report, www.npdb-hipdb.com.

Table 6-4 Nurse Practitioners: Number of Medical Malpractice Payment Reports by Malpractice Reason (September 1, 1990–December 31, 2002)

Malpractice Reason	Nurse Practitioner
Anesthesia related	5
Diagnosis related	114
Equipment/product related	1
IV & blood products related	2
Medication related	31
Monitoring related	9
Obstetrics related	15
Surgery related	5
Treatment related	53
Miscellaneous	7
Total	**242**

This table includes only disclosable reports in the NPDB as of December 31, 2002. Medical malpractice payment reports that are missing data necessary to determine the malpractice reason are excluded.
Source: NPDB 2002 Annual Report, www.npdb-hipdb.com.

A hospital must report adverse clinical privileges actions against physicians and dentists lasting over 30 days and voluntary surrender of clinical privileges that occur while the practitioner is under investigation. Hospitals may report adverse clinical privileges actions taken against other health care practitioners. Professional societies must report adverse medical actions against physicians and dentists. Professional societies may report adverse medical actions taken against other health care practitioners.

Table 6-5 Physician Assistants: Mean and Median Medical Malpractice Payment Amounts by Malpractice Reason, 2002 and Cumulative (September 1, 1990–December 31, 2002)

Malpractice Reason	2002 Only			Cumulative Actual			Inflation Adjusted	
	Number of Payments	Mean Payment	Median Payment	Number of Payments	Mean Payment	Median Payment	Mean Payment	Median Payment
Anesthesia related	1	$ 415,000	$ 415,000	3	$ 140,963	$ 6,000	$ 141,219	$ 6,298
Diagnosis related	85	$ 187,909	$ 100,000	370	$ 154,759	$ 80,000	$ 166,072	$ 91,981
Medication related	8	$ 366,108	$ 79,930	53	$ 105,550	$ 25,000	$ 112,636	$ 29,593
Monitoring related	0	$ —	$ —	7	$ 129,627	$ 55,000	$ 145,194	$ 67,081
Obstetrics related	1	$ 125,000	$ 125,000	2	$ 437,500	$ 437,500	$ 477,415	$ 477,415
Surgery related	5	$ 21,100	$ 15,000	31	$ 60,176	$ 25,000	$ 69,716	$ 25,253
Treatment related	21	$ 54,393	$ 22,500	167	$ 81,156	$ 24,999	$ 89,597	$ 25,000
Miscellaneous	3	$ 126,667	$ 105,000	25	$ 60,140	$ 50,000	$ 63,419	$ 52,482
Total	**124**	**$169,910**	**$ 81,250**	**658**	**$124,593**	**$ 54,500**	**$134,530**	**$ 60,254**

This table includes only disclosable reports in the NPDM as of December 31, 2002. There have been no reports for physician assistants in the "Equipment/product related" and "IV & blood related" categories.

Source: NPDB 2002 Annual Report, www.npdb-hipdb.com.

Table 6-6 NPDB Summary Report

This data covers the period from September 1, 1990, through August 21, 2004.

Data Disclaimer: Adverse licensure actions against nonphysicians and nondentists are not report-able to the NPDM. Therefore, the numbers included in the "Licensure, Clinical Privileges, and Professional Society Membership Reports" column do not represent a complete picture nor do they represent a good sample of all adverse actions taken against nonphysicians and nondentists.

Profession	State	Medical Malpractice Reports	Licensure, Clinical Privileges, and Professional Society Membership Reports	Medicare/ Medicaid Exclusion Reports
Physician Assistant, Allopathic	AK	4	1	2
	AL	2	1	0
	AR	1	0	0
	AZ	38	2	6
	CA	57	1	49
	CO	24	0	2
	CT	5	0	0
	DC	1	1	0
	DE	1	0	0
	FL	92	2	9
	GA	37	1	7
	IA	13	0	1
	ID	4	0	1
	IL	4	0	3
	KS	10	1	2
	KY	4	2	1
	LA	7	1	0
	MA	12	0	2
	MD	11	0	7
	ME	10	2	0
	MI	62	2	17

(continued)

Profession	State	Medical Malpractice Reports	Licensure, Clinical Privileges, and Professional Society Membership Reports	Medicare/ Medicaid Exclusion Reports
	MN	8	0	1
	MO	4	1	1
	MS	1	0	2
	MT	9	0	2
	NC	44	2	9
	ND	4	0	0
	NE	6	1	2
	NH	4	3	0
	NJ	2	0	4
	NM	12	2	2
	NV	10	0	2
	NY	106	12	42
	OH	7	0	5
	OK	8	2	0
	OR	9	0	0
	PA	26	1	5
	SC	5	1	1
	SD	4	0	1
	TN	10	0	1
	TX	62	4	6
	UT	13	1	3
	VA	10	0	0
	VT	4	0	0
	WA	30	2	7
	WI	4	0	1
	WV	7	0	0
	WY	6	1	0
	UNLISTED	1	0	0
	TOTAL	**815**	**50**	**206**

Profession	State	Medical Malpractice Reports	Licensure, Clinical Privileges, and Professional Society Membership Reports	Medicare/ Medicaid Exclusion Reports
Physician Assistant, Osteopathic	AL	1	0	0
	AZ	2	0	0
	CA	2	1	0
	CO	1	0	0
	FL	4	1	0
	GA	1	0	0
	IA	1	0	0
	IL	1	0	0
	MA	1	0	0
	MI	4	0	0
	MN	1	0	0
	MO	2	0	0
	MT	2	0	0
	NC	1	0	0
	NE	1	0	0
	NM	1	0	0
	NY	2	0	0
	SC	1	0	0
	TX	2	0	0
	VA	1	0	0
	WA	1	0	0
	WV	1	0	0
	WY	1	0	0
	TOTAL	**35**	**2**	**0**

Source: NPDB Summary Report, www.npdb-hipdb.com.

Table 6-7   HIPDB Reports Submitted by State Agencies and Health Plans

This report summarizes the number of adverse action reports (including licensure actions, any other negative actions or findings, and other adjudicated actions) and civil judgment or criminal conviction reports submitted for each professional category including the number of state agencies and health plans that have submitted reports under each category. This data is current as of August 21, 2004.

Data Disclaimer: Not all state agencies and health plans have submitted reports, and some have submitted reports that were rejected and therefore not included here. Furthermore, the reporting entity may not have taken reportable actions since August 21, 1996, and, consequently does not have reportable actions to submit to the HIPDB.

Profession	State	Adverse Action Reports	Judgment or Conviction Reports
Physician Assistant, Allopathic	AK	23	0
	AL	11	0
	AR	4	0
	AZ	31	0
	CA	76	0
	CO	20	0
	CT	5	0
	DE	1	0
	FL	17	0
	GA	31	0
	IA	6	0
	ID	1	0
	IL	6	0
	IN	1	0
	KS	3	0
	KY	5	0
	LA	1	0
	MA	5	0
	MD	13	0
	ME	20	0
	MI	48	0
	MN	8	0
	MO	11	0
	MS	1	0
	MT	8	0

Profession	State	Adverse Action Reports	Judgment or Conviction Reports
	NC	34	0
	ND	5	0
	NE	3	0
	NH	7	0
	NJ	5	0
	NM	5	0
	NV	7	0
	NY	73	2
	OH	33	0
	OK	26	0
	OR	19	0
	PA	45	0
	SC	4	0
	TN	15	0
	TX	14	0
	UT	12	0
	VA	11	0
	WA	54	1
	WI	3	0
	WV	6	0
	TOTAL	**737**	**3**
Physician Assistant, Osteopathic	AK	2	0
	DE	1	0
	FL	2	0
	IA	4	0
	MA	2	0
	MI	2	0
	MO	1	0
	OH	2	0
	PA	3	0
	WA	1	0
	TOTAL	**20**	**0**

Source: HIPDB Reports Submitted by State Agencies and Health Plans, www.npdb-hipdb.com.

Table 6-8   HIPDB Reports Submitted by Federal Agencies

This report summarizes the number of adverse action reports (including licensure actions, any other negative actions or findings, and other adjudicated actions) and civil judgment or criminal conviction reports submitted for each professional category including the number of federal agencies that have submitted reports under each category. This data is current as of August 21, 2004.

Data Disclaimer: Not all federal agencies have submitted reports, and some have submitted reports that were rejected and therefore not included here. Furthermore, the reporting entity may not have taken reportable actions since August 21, 1996, and, consequently does not have reportable actions to submit to the HIPDB.

Profession	Federal Agency	State	Adverse Action Reports	Judgment or Conviction Reports
Physician Assistant, Allopathic	AFMSA SGOC	FL	1	1
	Drug Enforcement Administration	NJ	1	0
	Executive Office for US Attorneys	DC	1	0
	HHS Office of Inspector General	GA	0	1
		AK	2	0
		AZ	6	0
		CA	49	0
		CO	2	0
		FL	9	0
		GA	7	0
		IA	1	0
		ID	1	0
		IL	3	0
		KS	2	0
		KY	1	0
		MA	2	0
		MD	7	0
		MI	17	0
		MN	1	0
		MO	1	0

Profession	Federal Agency	State	Adverse Action Reports	Judgment or Conviction Reports
		MS	2	0
		MT	2	0
		NC	9	0
		NE	2	0
		NJ	4	0
		NM	2	0
		NV	2	0
		NY	42	0
		OH	5	0
		PA	5	0
		SC	1	0
		SD	1	0
		TN	1	0
		TX	6	0
		UT	3	0
		WA	7	0
		WI	1	0
	VA Medical Center	IA	1	0
		TOTAL	**210**	**2**
Physician Assistant, Osteopathic		**TOTAL**	**0**	**0**

Source: HIPDB Reports Submitted by Federal Agencies, www.npdb-hipdb.com.

HEALTHCARE INTEGRITY AND PROTECTION DATA BANK (HIPDB)

The Healthcare Integrity and Protection Data Bank (HIPDB) was established through the Health Insurance Portability and Accountability Act of 1996, Section 221(a), Public Law 104-191. HIPDB is a national data-collection program for the reporting and disclosure of certain final adverse actions taken against health care practitioners, providers, and suppliers. Information regarding licensure, exclusions from state and federal health programs and criminal convictions and civil judgments related to health care are contained in HIPDB. To alleviate the need to report to both entities, a combined system was developed allowing only one report to be filed. The system will automatically send the pertinent information to the correct data bank. Similarly both systems can be queried at the same time. (See Tables 6-7 and 6-8.)

It is estimated that over half of all adverse events resulting from medical errors could have been prevented. The most common malpractice actions brought against PAs are in the areas of diagnosis, with a mean payment of $187,909; treatment related with a mean payment of $54,393; and medication related, with a mean payment of $366,108.[11] The best defense to a malpractice claim is a complete and timely medical record graphed in flow sheets in a predictable place in the chart. Once a practitioner has one or two claims filed against him or her, even if the practitioner prevails, it becomes very difficult to obtain affordable malpractice insurance. Developing patient relationships is very important. Patients are less likely to sue a practitioner whom they like and who takes the time to answer their questions. Health care practitioners need to make the patients responsible for their actions and their care and document appropriately. Ultimately, documentation will be the deciding factor in a malpractice action.

REFERENCES

1. Starr, D. S. (2003, July/August). Medicolegal briefs. *Clinical Advisor.* July/August 2003:14.

2. Institute of Medicine Web site. To Eerr Is Human: Building a Safer Health System (IOM Report 2000). Available at http://www.iom.edu. Accessed March 2005.

3. Institute of Medicine Web site. Crossing the Quality Chasm, A New Health System for the 21st Century (IOM Report 2001). Available at http://www.iom.edu. Accessed March 2005.

4. Institute of Medicine Web site. Patient Management. Available at http://www.iom.edu. Accessed October 2004.

5. Bodenheimer, T. S., & Grumbach, K. (2002). The quality of health care. In *Understanding Health Policy: A Clinical Approach* (3rd ed.). New York: McGraw Hill (p. 39).

6. McCammon, G. (2004, September). Malpractice insurance: Change for the sake of change? Not really. *AAPA News.*

7. American Academy of Physician Assistants Web site. Insurance Information. Available at http://www.aapa.org. Accessed October 2004.

8. Health Integrity and Protection Data Bank (HIPDB) Reports Web site. Available at http://www.npdb-hipdb.com. Accessed September 2004.

9. National Practitioners Data Bank Information Web site. Available at http://www.npdb-hipdb.com. Accessed September 2004.

10. National Practitioners Data Bank 2002 Annual Report Web site. Available at http://www.npdb-hipdb.com. Accessed September 2004.

11. National Practitioners Data Bank Information Web site. Available at http://www.npdb-hipdb.com. Accessed September 2004.

CHAPTER 7

Risk Management

Documentation • Purposes of the Clinical Record • The Medical Record as a Legal Document • What Attorneys Look For • Alterations of the Medical Record • What to Include in the Medical Record • Documentation Guidelines • Things to Avoid When Documenting • Defenses to Malpractice • Avoiding Malpractice • Systems for Tracking Follow-Up • Patient Responsibility

DOCUMENTATION

The final decision whether to file a malpractice claim is based on the patient's record. The patient's record is the only document available 3–5 years after the suit is filed and the case is scheduled for trial. The patient's record should be legible, neat, objective, and consistent. The two most important factors in malpractice prevention are communication with your patients and proper documentation. Prior to filing a malpractice action the plaintiff's attorney will have a medical expert review the record to determine if the standard of care was met. Detailed documentation, which provides explanations as to why a certain treatment plan was followed, will discourage good medical experts from questioning a provider's care. If patient records are sloppy, the plaintiff's attorney will imply that a provider who has sloppy charting practices provides sloppy care to his or her patients. This approach has been successful in the past and a jury awarded a $1.8 million verdict to the plaintiff based on the fact that the provider's medical charting was sloppy.

Detailed documentation helps to prevent complications, increases patient compliance, helps providers obtain more informed consent, helps patients have a clear understanding of instructions, and aligns patient–provider expectations. Detailed documentation makes a difference in the courtroom as well; jurors have come to expect important facts will be documented. It is the only way a provider will receive acknowledgment for competent care. A jury looks for neatness, organization, and completeness of notes. The plaintiff's attorney will use technology to enlarge a provider's notes for everyone to view in the courtroom. This will magnify errors and inconsistencies. The plaintiff's attorney will look for inconsistencies between providers, nurses, and times and point these out to the jury.

The best defense against medical malpractice is prudent medical management, effective communication skills, and a well-documented medical record. It is important that a provider gets to know his or her patients and develops a relationship with them. Emergency department providers are sued at a higher rate than primary care practitioners because the patients do not have a relationship with the emergency room provider and it is easier to sue someone that you do not have a personal relationship with.

Of all malpractice claims, 35% to 40% are indefensible because of documentation problems. Adequate documentation can prevent a malpractice claim from being initiated and is invaluable in a successful malpractice defense. Clinical records should reflect that you acted reasonably and according to accepted standards of care, regardless of patient outcomes; a poor patient outcome does not mean that malpractice has occurred. Often patients choose to pursue a malpractice action because they are angry with their provider for some reason. They feel that their provider did not spend enough time with them, did not explain to them the alternate options of care, or ignored their questions.

Deficient medical records make it impossible to determine whether the care provided met or fell below the acceptable standards of care, make good care look bad, make bad care look worse, and make bad care result from what might have been good care. Deficient medical records are illegible, incomplete, do not show the provider's thought process as to why a certain course of action was taken or why a certain treatment plan was instituted, and do not document patient outcomes.

PURPOSES OF THE CLINICAL RECORD

The clinical record provides communication between the primary care provider, physicians, and other members of the health care team. It is the basis for evaluating the adequacy of care and it provides data to substantiate reimbursement. The patient's record protects the legal interests of the patient, the care provider, and facility. The clinical record is also used to provide clinical data for research and education.

THE MEDICAL RECORD AS A LEGAL DOCUMENT

The medical record as a legal document is used to construct the continuum of care. It is the only evidence that can be relied upon years later, and it is considered to be an accurate reflection of the care provided to the patient. It will be scrutinized by attorneys for both the plaintiff and the defense. The document should paint a factual word picture of past events. The plaintiff's attorney looks at the alleged injury and goes back and constructs a timeline of events.

The medical record is the most important source of evidence in a malpractice action. Human memory is fallible and has diminished credibility. If you did not document the care given to the patient in the patient's record, the jury will assume that you did not provide the care in question.

It is important to follow organizational and department policies regarding documentation. Daily progress notes should be written on inpatients and additional notes should be completed each time the person is seen. Notes should always include the time and date. The documentation of time can be very important in a malpractice action. Notes should be written or dictated as soon after the event as possible; timely entries are more believable, enhance communication, and improve the quality of care.

WHAT ATTORNEYS LOOK FOR

Attorneys look for evidence in the patient's record that the patient's care was appropriate, timely, and met the standard of care. An attorney will examine the medical record to see if it contains clinically pertinent information, if it includes the rationale for decisions that the clinician made, and if it includes patient outcomes. The majority of medical records do not provide a rationale for the decisions that the provider made or contain information regarding patient outcomes. Complete medical records must reflect why a practitioner made each decision; reflect that the patient made informed consent decisions; and contain discharge instructions, follow-up plans, clinically pertinent telephone calls, missed appointments, and attempted follow-up.

Attorneys will also look for patient complaints and practitioner responses to the patient's complaints. It is in a provider's best interest to respond to patient complaints and to document the responses. A provider should not ignore an unhappy patient. Unhappy patients are more likely to file malpractice actions against their providers. If a patient must be terminated from the practice, be sure to follow the appropriate steps. Otherwise a provider may be sued for abandonment of the patient.

ALTERATIONS OF THE MEDICAL RECORD

Attorneys will also look for alterations of the medical record. Experts are available to determine if the medical record has been altered. Experts will utilize X-rays and chemicals to determine if a medical record has been altered. A medical record should never be altered by writing in the margin, writing over an entry, or changing a date. If you need to make a correction to the medical record never obliterate, alter, or destroy an original note and do not use correction fluid or tape. When making a correction to original notes, adhere to your organization's policies regarding corrections of patient's records or use the SLIDE rule:

- Single
- Line
- Initial

- Date
- Error

This reminds you to put a single line through the mistake, initial the correction, date the change, and write the time and error next to the line.

A patient who is contemplating filing a malpractice action or the plaintiff's attorney often request the patient's clinical records prior to filing a malpractice action to evaluate the records. The office staff makes a copy of the original clinical records and sends the records to the party who made the request without ever notifying the practitioner responsible for the patient's care. The practitioner then receives notice that a malpractice claim has been filed. In certain instances a practitioner reviews the original clinical records and alters them improperly. The patient's attorney files a malpractice action. The practitioner sends a copy of the improperly altered records to the defense attorney and they are introduced at trial. Not only will the practitioner in this instance lose the malpractice action, the practitioner will be subject to disciplinary action by the licensing boards which may include loss of licensure, fines, and possible criminal prosecution depending upon state laws.

Alterations of the medical record can be made if done properly. Any alteration of the medical record should be made as contemporaneously to the actual event as possible, dated, and signed by the person making the alteration. A new entry should be made and should include a statement as to why the additional entry is being made. Changes, corrections, and additional information must be clearly identified as a subsequent entry by date and time. Supplemental information may be added if it is done within a reasonable time and clearly identifies the information as a subsequent entry by date and time. The person who renders care or treatment should be the individual documenting the information in the medical records.

Intentionally altering or destroying a patient's chart is considered unprofessional conduct. Most states will consider a practitioner who alters or destroys a patient's chart to have violated the applicable licensing statute and will sanction or suspend the practitioner's license to practice medicine. Health care providers should report any suspected alteration or destruction of a patient's medical record to the appropriate licensing board.

WHAT TO INCLUDE IN THE MEDICAL RECORD

A provider should document patient assessment, interventions, and patient outcomes. Providers often fail to document patient outcomes. History and physical exams should include positive and negative findings, complete treatment and medication orders, interventions based on findings, outcomes and patient responses, patient's refusal to cooperate or follow a recommended plan of care, precautionary measures, conversations with the patient and the family, discharge and follow-up instructions, follow-up on tests, referrals, and missed appointments. It is extremely important that practitioners document patient noncompliance including a patient's refusal to follow medical advice and the patient's decision to follow a treatment plan that the provider does not endorse—for example, a patient who decides not to follow up with oncology for a diagnosed cancer because the patient has decided to try herbal medications instead. Careful documentation of this type of a situation will help to prevent a malpractice action resulting from a poor patient outcome.

Patients should also be made aware of the consequences of not following a recommended treatment plan. The consequences should be documented in the patient's chart along with a statement that the patient understands and accepts these consequences. The patient should be asked to sign or initial this entry in his or her chart. Good medical practice and informed consent require practitioners to make patients aware of all the accepted treatment options for their medical conditions and allow the patient to choose the option that he or she feels is best personally. Documenting that the patient was given these options and chose a specific treatment option after a discussion of the risks and benefits of each option will help place the responsibility of the patient's choice back upon the patient.

To minimize documentation claims, record clinical findings clearly, comprehensively, consistently, and completely. The SOAP format should be followed for all office charting (unless the patient is being seen for a complete history and physical) and for progress notes on inpatients.

The SOAP format includes subjective and objective information and the assessment and plan in the following order:

- Subjective—Patient comments and complaints, nursing comments, appropriate review of systems, past medical history, family history, and social history
- Objective—Vitals: blood pressure, pulse, respirations, temperature, weight, height, oxygen saturation
  - Ins/outs—Intravenous fluids, oral intake (PO), emesis, urine, stool, drains
  - Exams—Objective physical findings
  - Medications—Pertinent routine and new medications
  - Labs—New laboratory or procedural results
- Assessment—Based on the subjective and objective findings in the order of importance
- Plan—Medication changes, laboratory tests and procedures and consults that are being ordered, etc.

For patients admitted to the hospital, practitioners should have a history and physical exam on the patient's chart within 24 hours of admission. The document must be labeled as a history and physical. A history and physical dictated between 8 and 30 days of admission is usually acceptable if the practitioner who recorded the original report or a practitioner within the same group updates the history and physical to reflect any changes in the original history and physical since the original history and physical was performed. Histories recorded within seven days of admission will usually be considered to reflect the current patient condition unless updated or noted in a progress note. Be sure to follow your facility's guidelines. The minimum required content for a history and physical includes:

- Patient identification
- Chief complaint
- History of present illness
- Past history
- Allergies
- Current medications
- Pertinent psychosocial and family history (e.g., alcoholism, drug abuse, elderly patient who lives alone)
- Appropriate review of systems

The physical examination must include:

- Vital signs
- Pulmonary assessment
- Cardiovascular assessment
- Details of other systems pertinent to the patient
- Assessment
- Plan

The history and physical exam should always include pertinent positive and negative findings.

For surgical emergencies a history and physical should be completed as soon as possible.

Consultation notes should be dictated within 24 hours of the request and should include the reason for the request. The consultation report must document evidence of review of the patient's record by the consultant, pertinent findings on examination, and the consultant's opinion and recommendations.

Operative reports should be dictated immediately following surgery.

Operative reports must include the following:

- Date of the surgical procedure
- Name of the primary surgeon and assistant(s)
- Preoperative diagnosis
- Postoperative diagnosis
- Procedures performed
- Detailed account of the findings during surgery
- Details of the surgical technique
- Immediate postoperative condition of the patient

- Specimens removed
- Estimated blood loss

All stays in the hospital over 48 hours must have a complete discharge summary except for normal obstetrical deliveries and normal newborns. No symbols or abbreviations should be used in the final diagnosis or the description of medical or surgical procedures.

The discharge summary should include the following:

- Admission and discharge dates
- Admission and final diagnosis
- Service name, attending and residents
- Referring physician
- Consults—Physicians, services, and dates
- Significant findings or complications
- Procedures preformed—Dates of surgeries, lumbar puncture, angiograms, etc.
- Treatment rendered and services provided
- Medications—Discharge medications with dosages, administration, and refills
- Condition at discharge
- Disposition—Discharged to home, nursing home, etc.
- Instructions—Activity restrictions, diet, dressing and/or cast care, symptoms that would require the patient to seek additional treatment
- Follow-up care—Follow-up appointment

A death summary is required for all deaths that occur in the hospital unless they occur in the emergency department.

Patients have a right to look at their records and the right to request that you as their provider make additions or corrections. If you do not agree with the change or requested additional information, the patient does have a right to submit an addendum to his or her record, which will become part of the record.

DOCUMENTATION GUIDELINES

Documentation should be legible, accurate, clear, concise, objective, chronological, and complete. There should not be any blank spaces in the record. A practitioner should be sure to use proper spelling and grammar. A patient's record should not be charted in advance of seeing the patient.

Prior to providing and documenting care a practitioner should read previous clinical record notations and verify that he or she has the correct patient's chart. Use objective and factual statements, quoting the patient whenever appropriate.

Ask yourself if your charting is timely; accurately reflects patient assessment. interventions, and outcomes; includes both positive and negative objective findings; is written legibly, with correctly spelled words and grammar; and consists of notes that are concise and clearly understandable by others.

THINGS TO AVOID WHEN DOCUMENTING

- Do not sign dictations without first reading and making corrections to the documents. Never stamp *dictated but not read* on a record.
- Do not use unapproved abbreviations or symbols when documenting in a patient's chart.
- Do not make notations that other health care workers were negligent or blame the hospital for inadequate equipment or staff.
- Do not make comments that suggest disapproval, annoyance, or frustration with difficult patients.
- Do not make comments that implicate your care as careless or that you are to blame for the patient's outcome.
- Do not make rationalizations about care provided to your patients.
- Do not make notations emphasizing differences of opinion between health care providers.
- Do not use words that may call into question the care provided to patients such as *unintentionally, inadvertently, somehow, unexplainable, unfortunately, appears to be, seems to be,* or *apparently.*
- Do not make subjective remarks in a patient's record.
- Avoid documentation problems that include illegible, messy records; entries that are not timed; insufficient documentation of the facts surrounding adverse events; inconsistencies; and gaps in time.

Your record should be as professional as the care you provide. Always be sure to read your dictations before signing them. The following are samples of actual dictations in medical records:

"The left leg became numb at times and she walked it off."

"Patient has chest pain if she lies on her left side for over a year."

"Father died in 90s of female trouble in his prostate and kidneys."

"Both the patient and the nurse herself reported passing flatus."

"Skin: somewhat pale but present"

"On the second day the knee was better, and on the third day it had completely disappeared."

"The pelvic examination will be done later on the floor."

"By the time she was admitted to the hospital her rapid heart had stopped and she was feeling much better."

DEFENSES TO MALPRACTICE

If you become involved in a malpractice action, your defense will be based on your compliance with the standard of care. The plaintiff's attorney will obtain an expert witness who will take the position that you failed to meet the standard of care, resulting in injury to the plaintiff. The expert that your defense lawyer retained will take the position that the care you provided met the standard of care and that the patient had a poor outcome but it was not a result of malpractice. (Unless there are documentation problems and the expert suggests trying to reach a settlement.) If the case does not settle before it goes to trial, the jury will be left to decide based on the facts of the case and the expert testimony whether the standard of care was met or if malpractice occurred.

Another defense that may be used in a malpractice case is comparative negligence. Comparative negligence comes into play when it is contended that two or more parties failed to perform at the standard of the "ordinary reasonable person." For example, suppose one person was driving too fast on a snow-covered road on the highway and hit a car—but the car that was hit did not have its lights on as it should have. In a situation where each party has some degree of negligence in causing an accident, the responsibility to the other person(s) is reduced by the other's degree of negligence. For example, suppose a jury decides that the driver going too fast on the snow-covered highway was 70% responsible for the accident, while the driver without vehicle lights on is 30% responsible. If the driver who didn't have his lights on would have recovered $10,000, his recovery would be reduced to $7000 because of his 30% contributory negligence. Whether the speeding driver would recover anything will depend on state law—in some states the driver who bears over 50% of the responsibility would recover nothing.

Comparative negligence is often used in malpractice cases when multiple providers and hospitals are involved in the care of a patient and can be used in cases where the patient can be shown to be negligent for not following medical advice. This pattern of noncompliance on the patient's part should be clearly documented in the patient's chart along with the risks and consequences of not following the treatment plan.

AVOIDING MALPRACTICE

Diagnostic errors account for the majority of malpractice actions against primary care providers. There are complaints with a statistically high probability for lawsuits in primary care. These are considered "red flag" complaints. "Red flag" complaints include abdominal pain, back pain with neurological symptoms, breast mass, chest pain, and pregnancy. It is important to be on alert when dealing with a patient who has a "red flag" complaint. The provider should approach each patient complaint by ruling out "the worst thing first," keeping in mind that certain patient complaints put the provider at an increased risk of being sued. Example: A 40-year-old attorney presented with chest pain, which began at work. He was seen in his primary care provider's office that day and was diagnosed with musculoskeletal spasm and was prescribed a muscle relaxant. Eight hours later he went to the emergency department with chest pain. A chest X-ray was ordered and the patient was again diagnosed with musculoskeletal spasm and discharged. The next day the patient returned and an electrocardiogram was performed, indicating that the patient had a myocardial infarction. The patient sued the first two providers for failure to diagnose and treat the myocardial infarction.[1]

When a patient or parent is insistent on having a test done, be sure to give the request adequate consideration before deciding whether to deny the request. Example: A 36-year-old pregnant female requested an amniocentesis and was told by two practitioners that it was unnecessary. The patient gave birth to a child with Down's syndrome and sued the two providers who told her that the test was unnecessary.[2]

Be sure to give adequate attention to ongoing problems. A practitioner should keep a log on the front of the patient's chart with a problem list. Each time the patient comes to the office the practitioner can review the problem list with the patient and address ongoing problems. This will prevent ongoing problems from being overlooked on subsequent visits. Example: A patient presented with a breast rash; the practitioner diagnosed mastitis and prescribed antibiotics. The patient was instructed to follow up with a dermatologist in 3 weeks if the rash did not resolve. The patient returned to the practitioner and did not complain about the breast rash. The practitioner did not question the patient regarding the rash to see if it resolved. The patient never followed up with the dermatologist. The patient died one year later of Paget's disease of the breast. The patient's family sued the practitioner.

Be sure to do a pregnancy test on all female patients of childbearing age prior to instituting a medical plan that might result in fetal harm. Do not rely on the patient to give you accurate information regarding her last menstrual period or her sexual activity.

Before giving a patient a diagnosis that may have a significant impact on his or her life, such as the diagnosis of a sexually transmitted disease, be sure to perform the appropriate diagnostic testing.

Do not overlook a diagnosis in a patient who has a significant mental health history or who has been given a diagnosis of hypochondriasis. Always perform a thorough review of systems and an appropriate exam to rule out a physical reason for the patient's complaint; do not assume that the complaint is the result of a psychological problem.[3]

Never request a patient to call you for lab or test results. You are responsible to call patients with their results. The majority of practitioners will schedule a follow-up appointment with patients in order to go over the results of labs and tests, especially if the results are sensitive in nature. Patients should not be required to wait unreasonably long periods of time to be seen by their practitioner if they are waiting for the results of labs or tests. Unreasonably long waiting periods will increase patients' anxiety and may anger them. A practitioner should not leave himself or herself open to a delay-of-treatment claim because of overly long patient waiting times.

Document telephone calls in the chart and do not give advice over the phone without having the patient's chart in front of you.

Dispense instructions sheets about medications, treatments, exercise, diets, and patient instructions. Document in the patient's chart that the instruction sheets were given to the patient, discussed with the patient, and that the patient understood the instructions and was given an opportunity to ask questions. Videotapes are also being used to provide patient education. If a video is used, documentation should be made in the same fashion as instruction sheets. To go one step further, it is wise to have patients initial the chart that they received the instructional material, that all their questions were addressed, and that they understood the instructions and the risks and consequences of not following the treatment plan.

When referring a patient to the emergency department, provide patients with a written description of the reason for the referral. If at all possible, call the ED and speak with the receiving provider in the ED to report on the patient's condition and reasons for sending the patient to the ED. If you cannot speak directly with the receiving provider, the ED staff should confirm the reason for referral of patients sent from another provider.

Develop a rapport with your patients. Patients are less likely to sue a practitioner that they have a relationship with. Involve your patients in their treatment. Discuss treatment options with them, including the risks and benefits of each treatment, and allow the patient to decide which treatment is best for him or her. Document the alternatives discussed with the patient as well as the risks and benefits and document which treatment option the patient decided to pursue and the reasons the patient chose this option.

Document a patient's refusal of treatment, tests, and laboratory procedures. Document a patient's failure to comply with medical advice and compliance with medications and that you have explained to the patient the risks involved with the patient's continual noncompliance.

Preprinted forms can cut down on the time spent charting. Often-used phrases do not have to be written repeatedly and the forms will help prevent practitioners from missing parts of the exam.

Checklist documentation of telephone calls is another means to cut down on the risk of becoming involved in a malpractice action. Telephone checklists should always become part of the patient's chart and not part of telephone logs. A patient's chart will be subpoenaed in a malpractice action; a telephone log will not.

A system for logging referrals should also be developed and checked on a monthly basis. Following up on referrals and abnormal lab results will help to prevent a malpractice action based on delay of treatment.

Be sure that everyone is using the same clock to time documentation made in a patient's record. A few minutes' difference can make a big difference when dealing with an obstetrics case.

SYSTEMS FOR TRACKING FOLLOW-UP

On the front of each patient's chart keep a problem list and a medication flow sheet, which lists refills, herbal medications, and known allergies. This sheet should be updated at each visit, when refills are ordered, and referred to when there is a telephone communication with the patient.

The office should develop a log system to track diagnostic tests on a daily basis. The system should track diagnostic tests performed, evaluated, reviewed by the practitioner, and results communicated to the patient. The system should also track the follow-up of abnormal test results and track tests to be sure that they are repeated at the rates recommended by the current standards.

There should also be a backup system in place so lab results are followed up on when a practitioner is out of the office.

PATIENT RESPONSIBILITY

One of the most common complaints of the public is that they are not involved with their own health care. Practitioners should document that they educated patients regarding their medical conditions and make patients more responsible for their own care. Have patients initial and date a document check-off sheet that lists all the care the patient received along with all the education materials given and viewed by the patient.

When patients come to your office have them fill out a history form for you. The history form should emphasize, "The following information is very important to your health. Please take the time to fill it out completely." At the end of the form include verifying language in order to make the patient responsible for the information that they have provided, such as "The above knowledge is true and complete to the best of my knowledge," and have the patient sign the form. If the patient refuses to sign the form, that should be documented on the form and placed in the patient's chart.

Develop a personal health plan for your patients in which the patient and the practitioner collaborate in the patient's health care. This can be done in a letter with bulleted points that highlight the patient's responsibility for his or her health care. This is a very successful risk management tool.

Practitioners taking care of obstetrics patients can provide the patients with an OB journal. The journal should contain all the initial information you give to new patients including contraindications, phone numbers, drugs to stay away from, frequently asked questions, and Web sites where patients can obtain additional information. The patients should be instructed to bring the journal to each visit so that the patient's weight and blood pressure can be documented. The patient can write down questions that she would like to ask at the visit as well. The journal is considered to enhance patient education and care and should cut down on phone calls to the office as well.

Developing an "at risk" file for patients who put you at risk as a practitioner is another way to increase patient responsibility. Patients who miss follow-up appointments and are noncompliant should become part of the "at risk" file. These patients should receive letters outlining how their behaviors put them at risk and what they should be doing to improve their health. These letters should become part of the patient's chart.

REFERENCES

1. Bupert, C. (2000). Systems for avoiding malpractice. In: *The primary care provider's guide to compensation and quality: How to get paid and not get sued.* (pp. 133–134). Gaithersburg, MD: Aspen.

2. Bupert, C. (2000). Systems for avoiding malpractice. In: *The primary care provider's guide to compensation and quality: How to get paid and not get sued.* (pp. 135–139). Gaithersburg, MD: Aspen.

3. Bupert, C. (2000). Systems for avoiding malpractice. In: *The primary care provider's guide to compensation and quality: How to get paid and not get sued.* (p. 134). Gaithersburg, MD: Aspen.

CHAPTER 8

The Health Insurance Portability and Accountability Act of 1996

Standards for Privacy of Individually Identifiable Health Information • Uses and Disclosures • Consent • Consent vs. Authorization • Business Associate Agreements • Individual Rights • "Minimum Necessary" Provision • Privacy Program • Oral Communications • PHI Communicated over the Telephone • Communications by Fax • Parents and Minors • Department of Health and Human Services Office of Civil Rights • Responsibilities of the HIPAA Privacy Officer upon Receipt of a Patient Complaint • Violation of Privacy Policies or Procedures • Duty to Report • The Privacy Policy • Mandatory Reporting • Specially Protected PHI • Disclosures to Prevent Harm • Disclosures to Nonmedical Persons Involved in a Patient's Care • Uses and Disclosures of Genetic Information • Disclosure of HIV/AIDS Information • Accounting of Disclosures of a Patient's Protected Health Information • **Appendix 8-A** Sample Listing of Mandatory Reporting Requirements • **Appendix 8-B** Sample Privacy Policy

Health care providers have an ethical and a legal obligation to safeguard their patients' privacy. The Health Insurance Portability and Accountability Act of 1996 (HIPAA) is part of the Federal Health Care Reform Policy, and mandates that all health care providers and entities adopt federal patient privacy protection rules. HIPAA requires all medical practices to develop and implement a written privacy policy, which must be made available to all practice patients. HIPAA (P.L. 101–104) is a large and complex law. The Privacy Rules (45 CFR Parts 160 and 164) are the portion of the regulations that relate to health information.

STANDARDS FOR PRIVACY OF INDIVIDUALLY IDENTIFIABLE HEALTH INFORMATION

The Privacy Rule prevents individually identifiable health information from being released without patient consent or authorization. The law was created to stop abuses such as mortgage companies and employers obtaining health information on individuals and denying mortgages and employment based on health reasons. The Privacy Rule affects over 600,000 entities, every American, and will cost over $17 billion in the next 10 years.

The Privacy Rule became effective on April 14, 2002. The final compliance date was April 14, 2004. The Privacy Rule creates national standards to protect individuals' health information. The federal Privacy Rule applies as a set of minimum standards. More stringent state laws continue to apply.

Protected health information (PHI) is defined as information that relates to the past, present, or future physical or mental health or condition of an individual; the provision of health care to an individual; or the past, present, or future payment for the provision of health care to an individual; and identifies or could reasonably be used to identify the individual. This information may be electronic, paper, oral, media, or any other form (45 CFR sec. 160.103).

Individually identifiable health information is health information that includes patient identifiers such as name, social security number, patient identification number, address, demographic data, or any other information that would allow or could reasonably allow a person to be identified from that record.

Deidentified health information means health information without any of the following identifiers:

- Names
- Account numbers
- Medical record numbers
- Social security number
- All elements of dates (except years) for dates directly related to an individual, including birth date, admission date, discharge date, date of death, and all ages over 89
- Telephone numbers
- Fax numbers
- All geographic subdivisions smaller than a state including street address, city, county, precinct, and zip code (except for the initial three digits if the population exceeds 20,000)
- Health plan beneficiary numbers
- E-mail addresses
- Internet protocol address numbers (IP addresses)
- Web uniform resource locators (URLs)
- Device identifiers and serial numbers
- Certificate/license numbers
- Vehicle identification numbers and serial numbers
- Full-face photographic images and any comparable images
- Biometric identifiers such as finger and voice prints
- Any other unique identifying number, characteristic, or code

Limited data set means health information that contains only a limited number of identifiers that combined carry little risk of allowing identification of the individual. A limited data set should include only the following specific identifiers:

- Zip code
- Age

- Admission date
- Discharge date

Sensitive protected health information (sensitive PHI) means protected health information that pertains to an individual's HIV status, treatment of an individual for an HIV-related illness or AIDS, an individual's substance abuse condition, the treatment of an individual for a substance abuse disorder, an individual's mental health condition, or treatment of an individual for mental illness.

USES AND DISCLOSURES

The term *use* is defined as an application or manipulation of information by the covered entity *internally*. Disclosure involves sharing PHI with another person for *external* application of the information or data (45 CFR sec. 160.103). A covered entity may use or disclose PHI to the patient, for purposes of treatment, payment, or for health care operations for itself, to another covered entity, or to its agents. Additionally, a covered entity may disclose PHI as required by law (see Appendix 8-A) or with a patient's authorization (45 CFR sec. 164.502).

Treatment covers a wide array of patient-related activities including providing health care, coordinating health care services, referring patients, and consulting among health care providers (45 CFR sec. 164.501).

The term *payment* is defined as including activities relating to the financial aspects of health care. PHI can be released to obtain reimbursement, billing, utilization review, and claim processing (45 CFR sec. 164.501).

Health care operations include a wide range of administrative and management activities, in which covered entities engage (Table 8-1) (45 CFR sec. 164.501).

Table 8-1 Health Care Operations

Health care operations include the following:
<ul><li>Quality assessments and outcomes development</li><li>Guidelines and protocol development</li><li>Case management and patient care</li><li>Reviewing qualifications of professionals and credentialing</li><li>Training students</li><li>Risk management</li><li>Legal services (auditing, advice, business planning)</li></ul>

CONSENT

Patient consent must be obtained prior to providing patient care services on the first visit. Consent only needs to be obtained once. The consent is valid until the patient revokes the consent. The consent form is a short document referring to patient notification of the practice's (or covered entity's) privacy policies. The patient does not have to be given the entire policy. The policy must be written, and the patient must have the opportunity to read the entire policy prior to signing the consent. The patient's signature is required on the consent. New consent must be obtained if the patient revokes the initial consent in writing. If a patient revokes the consent, the consent can still be relied upon for payment for services prior to the revocation of the consent.

Consent is not needed in emergency situations, but a practitioner should obtain consent as soon as possible.

Joint consent can be used for integrated entities and is sufficient for group practices. Practitioners can consult with other providers without the consultant having first obtained patient consent.

New consents should be obtained, with pertinent references to compliance with the privacy rules and the privacy practices of the office, for patients established with a practice prior to the April 2004 HIPAA compliance date.

Patient consents should be maintained for six years from the date they were last effective.

CONSENT VS. AUTHORIZATION

Consents cover uses and disclosures for treatment, payment, and health care operations. Prior to disclosing PHI for any other reason the practitioner must obtain a valid authorization from the patient, unless the disclosure is mandatory or required by law. A practitioner can condition treatment on consent, but not on authorization for any reason.

Authorizations must be very specific, detail what PHI will be disclosed, to whom it will be disclosed, and contain an expiration date (Table 8-2). Authorizations are required prior to releasing information to life insurance providers and a patient's legal counsel.

Individual authorizations must be obtained before patients can be sent any type of marketing materials. Covered entities cannot give or sell names of individuals for marketing purposes (e.g., giving pregnant women's names to formula companies).

Table 8-2 Authorizations

A valid authorization must contain the following information:
• A specific description of the PHI to be disclosed
• Who will use or disclose the PHI
• To whom the PHI will be disclosed
• Expiration date
• Right to revoke in writing (valid forward, but not retroactively)
• Risks of unprotected redisclosure
• Signature of the individual whose PHI is to be released (or his or her personal representative)

BUSINESS ASSOCIATE AGREEMENTS

The privacy rules only apply to covered entities. Business associates are entities or persons that perform a function for the covered entity such as dictation, billing, legal services, or accounting and are not subject to the Privacy Rule. When PHI is disclosed to business associates it must be pursuant to a business associate agreement. The business associate must assure the covered entity that the PHI will not be disclosed except as provided in the contract, and that the business associate will not violate any federal or state privacy laws. The business associate agrees to report a breach of the agreement, to destroy all PHI at the end of the contract, and to implement any necessary further security measures, such as encrypted communications (45 CFR sec. 164.504e). A covered entity will be held liable for any breach of the Privacy Rule by a business associate.

INDIVIDUAL RIGHTS

The Privacy Rule creates certain privacy rights for individuals, including the following:

- Individuals must receive written notification from a covered entity describing the privacy policies of the entity (45 CFR sec. 164.520).
- Patients have a right to access and copy their medical records (45 CFR sec. 164.524).
- Patients have the right to request an amendment or correction of the protected health information if it is inaccurate or incomplete, and may submit a written supplement to be included in their record. A covered entity may decline to make the amendment, but it must allow the individual to submit a correction to be placed in the record. The covered entity may also include its own rebuttal (45 CFR sec. 164.528).
- Patients have a right to an accounting of all the disclosures of their record. Covered entities must track all PHI disclosures, to whom they are made, when they are made, and for what purpose. Covered entities must provide an accounting to patients upon their request. A business associate who receives PHI on individuals must help the covered entity track the disclosures (45 CFR sec. 164.528).

A covered entity may limit patient access to his or her PHI to a 'designated record set.' The designated record set does not have to include, and the patient may not be granted access to, the following:

- Psychotherapy notes about the patient
- Personal notes and observations about the patient created by a health care provider (provided such notes and observations are not included in the patient's medical record)

- PHI that is compiled in reasonable anticipation of, or for use in, a civil, criminal, or administrative action or proceeding. A provider does not have to make available information accumulated in contemplation of litigation; however, the underlying medical record must be made available (65 FR 82554).

The term *psychotherapy notes* may be defined as notes recorded in any medium (e.g., on paper, electronically, etc.) by a mental health care provider who is documenting or analyzing the contents of a conversation during a private counseling session or a group, joint, or family counseling session and that are kept separate from the rest of the patient's medical record.

Psychotherapy notes **exclude the following:**

- Medications, prescriptions, and monitoring
- Counseling session start and stop times
- Modalities and frequencies of treatment furnished
- Results of clinical tests
- Any summary of the patient's diagnosis, functional status, treatment plan, symptoms, prognosis, and progress to date

Personal notes are defined as the practitioner's speculations, impressions (other than tentative or actual diagnosis), observations, and reminders, if they are maintained by a practitioner outside the patient's actual medical record.

Psychotherapy and/or personal notes should not be documented or included in the patient's medical record. If psychotherapy and/or personal notes are documented or included in the patient's medical record, they will be considered part of the patient's medical record and must be disclosed to the patient who requests access to or a copy of his or her medical record.

A covered entity does not have to provide a patient with access to, the opportunity to inspect, or a copy of any PHI created by a provider or entity outside of the covered entity. The covered entity can require the patient to come to the covered entity's place of business during normal business hours to access or inspect his or her PHI and has the right to have a records custodian or other employee physically present during the access or inspection.

A covered entity should develop specific request forms including the following:

- Request for an amendment to health information.
- Request for an accounting of disclosures.
- Request for restrictions on uses and disclosures of health information. A patient should be required to fill out the appropriate form to exercise his or her rights

"MINIMUM NECESSARY" PROVISION

The Privacy Rule contains a *minimum necessary* provision that limits the use or disclosure of, and requests for, protected health information to the minimum necessary to accomplish the intended purpose. The practitioner will be held to a "reasonableness standard" that requires the practitioner to use professional judgment to determine how much PHI should be released. If a request is made by another health care provider to obtain PHI necessary to treat the patient, the *minimum necessary* provision *does not* apply.

PRIVACY PROGRAM

To comply with the Privacy Rule, covered entities must develop a privacy program. Each entity must designate a Privacy Official and develop a privacy policy (see Table 8-3 and Appendix 8-B: Sample Privacy Policy). A mechanism for making complaints must be developed, as well as sanctions defined for violations of the privacy policy by workforce members or business associates. Safeguards must be implemented to protect individuals' PHI. Passwords and encrypted e-mail must be used to prevent access to PHI by unauthorized individuals. Employees must be trained during orientation and annually in privacy practices. The Privacy Official should maintain documentation of training sessions and refresher courses.

Table 8-3 Components of a Privacy Policy

The privacy policy should cover the following:
• Identify the Privacy Officer and define his or her duties
• Describe employee training regarding patient privacy protection
• Describe who has access to medical records
• Detail how records are to be shared, and with whom
• Note that the practice restricts releasing information for nonmedical purposes
• Describe the patients' rights
• Discuss enforcement of the privacy rules

Source: Adapted with permission from Gossman, J. (2003). Putting the PA in HIPAA: Privacy policy can be simple. *ADVANCE for Physician Assistants,* 11(3):11.

ORAL COMMUNICATIONS

Reasonable safeguards should be practiced relating to oral communications involving patients' PHI. Patient information should not be discussed in the elevator. Sign-in sheets can be used in the office and patients' names can be called in the waiting area. Postcards for appointment reminders or leaving appointment reminders on answering machines should be avoided.

PHI COMMUNICATED OVER THE TELEPHONE

If a caller states that he or she is a patient and that he or she is requesting PHI about himself or herself, a provider employee should *not* provide the PHI unless reasonable efforts have been made to confirm that the caller is the patient. The provider employee should, prior to disclosing PHI, ask specific questions that could only be answered by the patient, for example, the patient's date of birth, address, father's name, or mother's name. The provider employee may choose to place a return call to the patient using the telephone number documented in the patient's file rather than immediately disclosing the patient's PHI to the caller initiating the telephone conversation.

If the caller states he or she is an immediate family member (e.g., father, mother, child, sibling) of the patient, an employee should notify the health care provider who will, by asking specific questions, approve or disapprove the disclosure of PHI to the caller.

If the caller states he or she is a friend, relative, or acquaintance of the patient, or if the caller is unrelated to the patient (e.g., the patient's employer, a disinterested third party, a policeman, a reporter, etc.), the employee should *not* disclose PHI without the patient's authorization or should provide only directory information about the patient.

The term *directory information* is defined as the following:

- The patient's name
- The patient's location
- The patient's condition—described in general terms that do not communicate specific PHI about the patient (e.g., *good, stable, critical*, etc.)

If the patient or his or her personal representative has requested confidential status (i.e., that no information is to be provided), the employee should respond, "I can neither confirm nor deny that (patient name) is a patient."

COMMUNICATIONS BY FAX

The confidentiality of protected health information (PHI) must be maintained when transmitting or receiving it by facsimile (fax). Fax machines provide a useful mechanism for rapidly and cost-effectively conveying information and documents both within an organization and to outside entities. The transmission of PHI by fax poses significant privacy risks associated with misdirected faxes and the delivery to or receipt of faxes in unsecured locations. Employees should only transmit PHI by fax when the transmission is time sensitive and delivery by regular mail will not meet the reasonable needs of the sender or recipient. Providers and their employees should take reasonable steps to ensure that a fax transmission is sent to and received by the intended recipient (Table 8-4).

Table 8-4   Fax Transmissions Including PHI: Reasonable Steps for Protection of PHI

- Employees will confirm with the intended recipient that the receiving fax machine is located in a secure area or that the intended recipient is waiting by the fax machine to receive the transmission.
- Fax machines will be preprogrammed with the fax numbers of those recipients to whom PHI is frequently sent to avoid errors associated with misdialing. Preprogrammed fax numbers will be tested frequently to confirm they are still valid.
- When a fax number is entered manually (because it is not one of the preprogrammed numbers) the employee entering the number will visually check the recipient's fax number on the fax machine prior to starting the transmission.
- Employees will use a standard fax cover sheet that contains the following PHI statement:

  This facsimile is intended only for the use of the named addressee and may contain information that is confidential or privileged. If you are not the intended recipient, or you are not the employee responsible for delivering the facsimile to the intended recipient, you are hereby notified that any dissemination, distribution or copying of this facsimile is strictly prohibited. If you have received this facsimile in error, please notify the sender immediately.

- The name, business affiliation, telephone number, and fax number of the intended recipient, as well as the number of pages contained in the transmission will also appear on the cover sheet.
- Fax confirmation sheets will be checked immediately, or as soon as possible after the fax has been transmitted, to confirm the material was faxed to the intended fax number. If the intended recipient notifies the sender that the fax was not received, the sender will use his or her best efforts to determine whether the fax was inadvertently transmitted to another fax number by checking the fax confirmation sheet and/or the fax machine's internal logging system.
- If an employee becomes aware that a fax was sent to the wrong fax number, the employee will immediately attempt to contact the recipient by fax or telephone and request that the faxed documents, and any copies of them, be immediately returned or destroyed. The employee's supervisor or the HIPAA Privacy Officer will also be notified of the misdirected fax.
- Those recipients who regularly receive PHI via fax will be periodically reminded to notify the covered entity of any change to the recipient's fax number.
- Fax confirmation sheets will be attached to and maintained with all faxed materials.
- Sensitive PHI (such as HIV/AIDS results, status, or substance abuse and mental health treatment records) should never be sent by fax.
- When faxing PHI, employees will comply with all other privacy policies.

Providers and their employees who are the intended recipients of faxes that contain PHI should take reasonable steps to minimize the possibility that faxes are viewed or received by someone else. Fax machines that receive faxes that include PHI should be located in a secure area. If a provider or his or her employee receives a fax containing PHI on a fax machine that is not in a secure area, the recipient of the fax will promptly advise the sender that the receiving fax machine should not be used for the transmission of such information. Fax machines will be checked on a regular basis to minimize the amount of time incoming faxes that contain PHI are left on the machines. Employees who monitor the fax machines, or an employee who sees such a fax on the machine, will promptly remove incoming faxes and deliver them to the proper person. If an employee receives a fax addressed to someone other than the employee, the employee will promptly notify the individual to whom the fax was addressed and deliver or make arrangements to deliver the misdirected fax as directed by the intended recipient.

PARENTS AND MINORS

A minor is an individual who is under 18 years of age and who is neither married nor the parent of a child.

A *minor's personal representative* is the minor's parent, legal guardian, or another with documentation proving he or she has legal custody of the minor (e.g., a stepparent who presents valid custody papers).

Because a parent is considered the personal representative of a minor, the minor's PHI can be given to the parent except in instances when an adolescent can consent to treatment. If an adolescent can consent to treatment (e.g., in the case of a pregnant adolescent) no information can be given to the parent without the minor's authorization. If a court appoints a representative for a minor other than a parent, or if a parent agrees to a confidential relationship between the minor and the provider, or if the provider suspects the parent of abuse or neglect, no PHI should be released to the parent without the minor's authorization.

Minor's Right to Consent to Certain Treatment

In most instances, a minor who is over the age of 12 may seek and receive the following types of health care services independently (parental consent is *not* required) from his or her personal representative:

- HIV/AIDS testing and treatment
- Testing and treatment for venereal and sexually transmitted diseases
- Pregnancy and prenatal care
- Abortion
- Chemical dependency services
- Mental health outpatient services

The minor's personal representative does not have the right to the minor's PHI if the minor alone consented to the treatment, unless the minor authorizes its release.

Abuse

If a health care provider reasonably believes a minor has been or is subject to domestic violence, abuse, and/or neglect by the minor's personal representative, and that keeping the minor's PHI related to the abuse confidential is in the best interests of the minor, the health care provider may refuse to release or provide access to the minor's abuse-related PHI to the minor's personal representative.

DEPARTMENT OF HEALTH AND HUMAN SERVICES OFFICE OF CIVIL RIGHTS

The Department of Health and Human Services Office of Civil Rights is responsible for enforcing privacy protections and protecting the rights of consumers. Individuals can file complaints with the Office of Civil Rights and it will investigate the complaint. If a patient wants to file a complaint with the Secretary of HHS, he or she should be directed to follow the steps provided on the Office for Civil Rights Web site (www.hhs.gov/ocr/hipaa). There are both civil and criminal sanctions for the improper disclosure of PHI. If PHI is used for commercial benefit, sanctions can include fines as high as $250,000 and 10 years in prison.

RESPONSIBILITIES OF THE HIPAA PRIVACY OFFICER UPON RECEIPT OF A PATIENT COMPLAINT

The HIPAA Privacy Officer should document each privacy complaint received, including in the documentation a brief description of and the basis for the complaint. The HIPAA Privacy Officer should conduct an investigation to determine the following:

- What, if any, PHI was misused or improperly disclosed
- If PHI was misused or improperly disclosed, whether such misuse or improper disclosure violates privacy policies and procedures
- What, if any, privacy practices or forms require modification
- Whether additional training is required to avoid a repeat violation

If the HIPAA Privacy Officer determines a violation has occurred, designated officials should determine what sanctions, if any, will be imposed against the individual who committed the violation. The HIPAA Privacy Officer should include documentation of the investigation and any actions taken in response to the complaint.

The HIPAA Privacy Officer should notify the patient submitting the complaint of the results of the investigation in writing. All documentation relating to the patient's complaint should be maintained for a minimum of six years.

A covered entity cannot intimidate, threaten, coerce, discriminate, penalize, or take other retaliatory action against a patient who exercises his or her rights under HIPAA or who files a complaint with the Secretary of Health and Human Services.

VIOLATION OF PRIVACY POLICIES OR PROCEDURES

Failure to comply with privacy policies or procedures should result in disciplinary action against the individual committing the violation. Privacy policies, procedures, and sanctions must be enforced consistently throughout an organization.

The following types of conduct on the part of a member of the workforce should result in disciplinary action against the individual engaging in the conduct:

- Accessing a medical record for any purpose outside of treatment, payment, or health care operations
- Discussing a patient's PHI in a public area
- Failing to log off or leaving a computer monitor on and unsecured
- Using a patient's PHI for personal reasons rather than for legitimate and authorized business reasons
- Copying or compiling PHI with the intent to sell or use the PHI for personal or financial gain

Disciplinary Action

The disciplinary sanction imposed should be determined on a case-by-case basis, taking into consideration the specific circumstances and severity of the violation, and may result in termination of employment or of the business relationship, if appropriate.

Other sanctions that may be imposed include the following:

- A letter to the employee's personnel file
- Administrative leave without pay
- Attendance at and successful completion of additional training
- Reimbursement of expenses incurred by the entity to resolve the matter

DUTY TO REPORT

Any provider employee who observes, becomes aware of, or suspects a wrongful use or disclosure of PHI is required to report his or her suspicion, the wrongful use, or disclosure as soon as possible to his or her supervisor or the HIPAA Privacy Officer.

A provider employee who makes a report of a suspected or actual improper use or disclosure in good faith cannot be retaliated against for making the report.

A provider employee who fails to report either a suspected or actual violation should be considered to have violated the entity's privacy policy and may be subject to disciplinary action, up to and including termination.

THE PRIVACY POLICY

A privacy policy should alert patients that an office will use, disclose, or release a patient's protected health information (PHI) as required by, and in accordance with, city, state, and federal law, even if the patient has not provided written authorization. The privacy policy should make patients aware of how the health care organization will use and disclose a patient's PHI, the patient's rights and responsibilities with respect to his or her PHI, and the covered entity's duties with respect to a patient's PHI. The patient's chart should contain documentation of receipt and acknowledgment of the covered entity's privacy policy.

Patients should be made aware that all PHI, including any PHI maintained electronically, is confidential and is not normally used, disclosed, or released without the patient's written authorization. However, there are times when practitioners are required by law to report or provide PHI to state or federal agencies or other authorities, or when they must respond to judicial or administrative requests for PHI.

MANDATORY REPORTING

A patient's authorization is not required for mandatory reporting to certain authorities and agencies. A patient's request to restrict the reporting of his or her PHI cannot be granted if the request interferes with a mandatory reporting obligation. (See Appendix 8-A for a sample list of mandated reporting requirements.)

When providing PHI in response to a mandatory reporting requirement, a provider should document the name, title, and contact information of the individual to whom the PHI was provided, the agency name and address (if known), the date the PHI was provided, and a brief summary of the PHI provided (e.g., demographic information about the patient, copy of face sheet showing diagnosis, etc.) for each patient whose PHI is reported or released.

The person providing PHI to an individual, agency, or authority in response to a mandatory reporting requirement must take reasonable steps to confirm and verify the identity and authority of the individual, agency, or authority prior to providing the PHI. Reasonable steps should include the following:

- Obtaining the contact name, title, and telephone number of the individual making the request
- Recognizing the requester's voice if the request or report is made over the telephone
- Recognizing the requester's telephone number, fax number, or address if the report is made by fax or delivery

Documentation of disclosures of PHI that is required as part of a mandatory report can be maintained in each individual patient's file or on a log. If documentation is included in the patient's file, the entry should *not* be considered part of the patient's designated record set.

A list of the mandatory reporting disclosures for each patient should be provided to the HIPAA Privacy Officer.

Responding to Law Enforcement Inquiries

Protected health information provided to a federal official or law enforcement official without first obtaining the patient's written authorization must be in accordance to both federal and state law. If the law enforcement official requests PHI via a court order, subpoena, warrant, summons, or other similar document, the PHI requested should be relevant and material to the law enforcement inquiry as well as specific and limited in scope to the extent reasonably practicable. Deidentified PHI should be used if at all possible, and the court order, subpoena, warrant, summons, or other similar document must comply with state law, which in some cases may require patient authorization to release the PHI.

If you are presented with a court order, subpoena, warrant, summons, or other similar document, immediately notify your supervising physician and the HIPAA Privacy Officer to discuss and evaluate the document and determine whether and how the disclosure of PHI will be made. No PHI should be disclosed in response to a court order, subpoena, warrant, summons, or other similar document prior to discussing the document with an attorney or the HIPAA Privacy Officer.

SPECIALLY PROTECTED PHI

An employee who receives a request from a federal, state, local, national security, or law enforcement official for PHI that includes HIV/AIDS information, mental health information, or substance abuse and treatment records must immediately contact his or her supervisor and the HIPAA Privacy Officer. Under no circumstances should PHI that includes HIV/AIDS information, mental health information, or substance abuse and treatment records be released to the requesting official unless the disclosure is approved by the HIPAA Privacy Officer.

DISCLOSURES TO PREVENT HARM

A patient's PHI may be disclosed without the patient's authorization if there is a reasonable and good faith belief that disclosure is necessary to prevent or reduce a serious and imminent threat to the health or safety of the public. The disclosure should be made only to a person or persons reasonably able to prevent or reduce the threat. The disclosure may be made to the target of the threat.

Disclosure may be made to law enforcement authorities, as necessary, to identify or apprehend an individual if the patient admits participation in a violent crime that caused or may have caused serious physical harm to a victim, or if it appears from all circumstances that the patient escaped from a correctional institution or from lawful custody. Disclosure of a patient's PHI should not occur if the admission was made during the course of counseling or therapy treating the patient for his or her propensity to commit the criminal conduct.

If a disclosure of the patient's PHI is made to prevent a serious threat to health or safety, the PHI disclosed should be limited to the following:

- Patient's statement in which he or she admitted participating in a crime
- Patient's name and address
- Patient's date and place of birth
- Patient's social security number
- Patient's ABO blood type and Rh factor, if known
- Type of injury
- Date and time of the patient's treatment
- Date and time of death, if applicable
- Description of any distinguishing physical characteristics including height, weight, sex, race, hair and eye color, presence or absence of facial hair (i.e., beard or moustache), scars, and tattoos

Specially protected PHI, such as genetic or HIV/AIDS information should not be disclosed.

DISCLOSURES TO NONMEDICAL PERSONS INVOLVED IN A PATIENT'S CARE

Practitioners must be committed to protecting patient privacy and to disclosing patient PHI in accordance with the patient's desires. However, when the patient's desires are not known or have not been expressed, it may be necessary to disclose a patient's PHI to a member of the patient's family, a friend of the patient, or someone else who is directly involved in the patient's care. It may also be necessary to disclose a limited amount of the patient's PHI to locate the patient (for example, in case the patient elopes) or to locate or notify a member of the patient's family or a friend of the patient.

When the Patient Is Physically Present

An individual who is physically present with the patient can generally be assumed to be an individual who is directly involved in the patient's care unless the patient specifically states otherwise. Before disclosing a patient's PHI to an individual who is physically present with the patient, the patient should be asked whether he or she agrees to the disclosure and should be given an opportunity to object. If the patient does not object to the disclosure, disclosures can be made to the individual at that time or any time in the future, or until such time as the patient revokes his or her consent. If the patient fails to respond, a health care professional treating the patient should use his or her professional judgment and experience to decide whether disclosing the PHI to the person physically present with the patient is in the patient's best interest. If the patient objects to the disclosure, the practitioner should provide the patient with a copy of the institution's Request for Restrictions on Uses and Disclosures of Health Information form (or a similar document) and ask the patient to complete it and forward it to the HIPAA Privacy Officer.

Copies of a patient's PHI should only be released to a patient's family member, a friend of the patient, or someone directly involved in the patient's care if the individual requesting the PHI presents a valid authorization (signed by the patient) that has not been revoked.

Questions regarding whether an authorization is valid or whether release of a patient's PHI to a particular individual is appropriate should be directed to the HIPAA Privacy Officer.

When the Patient Is Unable to Communicate

The health care professional may disclose a patient's PHI to an individual who is physically present with a patient who is unable to communicate when, based on the health care professional's judgment, the health care professional is reasonably sure under the circumstances that the patient would not object.

When the Patient Is Not Present

If the individual requesting the PHI is physically present but the patient is not, the PHI should be released only if the individual meets one of the following criteria:

- Is known to be a family member or personal friend of the patient
- Is someone who the patient has previously identified as someone involved in the patient's care
- Is someone whose direct involvement in the patient's care is obvious

The PHI that is released must be released as follows:

- Disclosed orally (not provided in writing)
- Limited to the minimum amount of information necessary to allow the individual to help the patient
- Directly relevant to the individual's involvement in the patient's care
- Necessary to help the patient with health care or with payment for health care

Locating a Patient

A practitioner may need to disclose a patient's PHI to the patient's family members, the patient's friends, or other individuals for purposes of locating the patient (if the patient has eloped or otherwise disappeared). Disclosure of a patient's PHI may be necessary—to the patient's family members, the patient's friends, or other individuals responsible for the patient's care—to notify them of the patient's location, general condition, or death.

USES AND DISCLOSURES OF GENETIC INFORMATION

The use and disclosure of genetic information should be done in accordance with its extremely confidential nature, but also as required by city, state, and federal laws and regulations, including the Health Insurance Portability and Accountability Act of 1996 (HIPAA). Genetic information is protected health information (PHI) and, as such, is protected by city, state, and federal laws and regulations. However, because of its extremely sensitive nature, if genetic information is improperly used or released, the patient's privacy, health care, or other interests may be irreparably damaged.

The term *genetic information* means any written or recorded individually identifiable health information resulting from genetic testing or medical evaluation to determine any of the following:

- The presence or absence of variations or mutations, including carrier status, in a patient's genetic material
- The presence or absence of genes that are scientifically or medically believed to cause a disease, disorder, or syndrome
- The presence or absence of genes that are associated with a statistically increased risk of developing a disease, disorder, or syndrome that is asymptomatic at the time of testing
- The findings or results of a genetic test
- The documentation of counseling sessions to convey the genetic information to the subject individual

The terms *genetic testing* or *genetic test* mean a test used to diagnose a presymptomatic genetic factor, including analysis of human DNA or RNA, mitochondrial DNA, chromosomes, proteins, or metabolites.

A patient's genetic information should not be disclosed without obtaining a written authorization from the patient unless required by law (Table 8-5).

Table 8-5 Genetic Testing That May Be Required by Law

- To establish parentage
- To determine the presence of metabolic disorders in a newborn by testing conducted pursuant to newborn screening and protocols
- To furnish genetic information relating to a decedent to the blood relatives of the decedent for the purpose of medical diagnosis
- In connection with a criminal investigation or prosecution
- Under a specific order of a state or federal court
- For identification of the individual
- For the identification of human remains

DISCLOSURE OF HIV/AIDS INFORMATION

A patient's HIV/AIDS information should not be disclosed except to the following individuals in the following instances:

- To the patient himself or herself or, when the patient lacks the capacity to consent, a person legally authorized to consent to health care for the patient
- Any person pursuant to a valid, written authorization signed by the patient
- Another health care provider or facility when knowledge of the HIV/AIDS information is necessary to provide appropriate care or treatment to the patient, a child of the patient, a contact of the patient, or a person authorized to consent to health care for a contact of the patient
- A health care facility or health care provider in relation to the procurement, processing, distribution, or use of a human body or body part for use in medical education, research, therapy, or transplantation
- A medical staff committee, accreditation, or oversight review organization—provided the recipient of the HIV/AIDS information will not further disclose the confidential information except as required by law
- A federal, state, county, or local health officer when such disclosure is required by federal or state law
- An authorized foster care or adoption agency, provided, however, that such an agency agrees not to further disclose the information except as required by law
- Pursuant to a court order
- An employee or agent of the Parole Division, Probation and Correctional Alternatives Division, the Commission of Correction, or a Medical Director of a local correctional facility
- A legal guardian appointed by a court to represent a minor with respect to the minor's HIV information

Any disclosure of a patient's HIV/AIDS information should be documented in the patient's medical record and maintained for six years.

ACCOUNTING OF DISCLOSURES OF A PATIENT'S PROTECTED HEALTH INFORMATION

One of the rights granted to patients under the Health Insurance Portability and Accountability Act of 1996 (HIPAA) is the right of the patient to request and receive an accounting of the disclosures made of the patient's PHI. Practitioners must respond appropriately to requests from patients for an accounting of disclosures, which is a listing of disclosures made of the patients' protected health information (PHI) by the covered entity. Although most of the disclosures of a patient's PHI are subject to an accounting, there are some disclosures that are *not* required to be included in an accounting of disclosures provided to the patient (see Table 8-6).

Table 8-6 Disclosures of a Patient's PHI That Do Not Need to Be Documented

- Those made prior to April 14, 2003
- Those made to carry out treatment, payment, or health care operations
- Those made to the patient
- Those made pursuant to a valid and effective authorization (one that complies with the requirements of state law as well as with the HIPAA Privacy Regulations) signed by the patient
- Those made to persons involved in the patient's care or in other notification and location purposes
- Those made to federal officials for national security or intelligence purposes
- Those made to a correctional institution or law enforcement official that has custody of a patient
- Those made to a health oversight or law enforcement official or agency provided the official or agency notifies the covered entity in writing that providing an accounting of disclosures to a specific patient would be reasonably likely to impede the official's or agency's activities

Like some other rights, this right requires action on the part of the patient (making the required request in writing) before the covered entity can respond.

Responsibility to Document Disclosures

Individuals who disclose a patient's PHI should document those disclosures that must be included in an accounting of disclosures (see Tables 8-7 and 8-8).

Table 8-7 Disclosures That Are to Be Documented

- Those to a business associate of the covered entity—unless the disclosure to the business associate is made for purposes of the business associate providing treatment, payment, or health care operations activities on behalf of the covered entity
- Those required by law, including mandatory reporting to local, state, and federal agencies and authorities
- Those for purposes of public health activities (e.g., for preventing or controlling disease, injury, or disability; for reporting of disease, injury, birth, or death; and for conducting public surveillance, public health investigations, and public health interventions)
- Those about victims of abuse, neglect, or domestic violence
- Those for health oversight activities
- Those for judicial and administrative proceedings
- Those for law enforcement purposes pursuant to process and for identification and location purposes
- Those to coroners, medical examiners, and funeral directors
- Those for cadaveric organ, eye, or tissue donation purposes

(continued)

Table 8-7 (continued)

- Those for research purposes
- Those to avert a serious threat to health or safety
- Those for specialized government functions including military and veterans activities, national security and intelligence activities, protective services for the President of the United States and other public officials, correctional institutions and other law enforcement custodial situations
- Those for workers' compensation

Table 8-8   The Information to Be Documented for Each Disclosure

- The date of the disclosure
- The name of the entity or person who received the PHI and, if known, his or her address and contact information
- A brief description of the PHI disclosed (e.g., records for visit on June 7, 2003, all radiology reports related to broken wrist, etc.)
- A brief statement of the purpose of the disclosure that reasonably informs the patient of the basis for the disclosure

Documentation should be maintained so it can be retrieved quickly upon a request from the HIPAA Privacy Officer, who is responsible for compiling the disclosures and providing the accounting of disclosures to the patient. Questions about what types of disclosures must be documented should be directed to the employee's supervisor or the HIPAA Privacy Officer. If a patient requests an accounting of disclosures, the individual receiving the request must ask the patient to complete and forward a Request for an Accounting of Disclosures form to the HIPAA Privacy Officer. The individual receiving the patient's request should provide a blank Request for an Accounting of Disclosures form to the patient.

All completed requests for Accounting of Disclosures forms should be maintained for a minimum of six years.

Disclosures of a patient's PHI to the patient or pursuant to the patient's authorization need not be documented.

Documentation of any disclosures of PHI made should be maintained for a minimum of six years and may be stored in the patient's file or on a disclosures log. If the documentation of disclosures made is stored in the patient's file, it should not be considered part of the patient's file and would *not* be provided as part of the patient's medical record.

Sample Listing of Mandatory Reporting Requirements

Agencies and authorities that must be reported to and the types of personal health information (PHI) that must be reported include the following.

(Mandatory reporting requirements vary by state, so be sure you are in compliance with both state and federal privacy laws prior to making any disclosure.)

Agency/Authority Receiving	Subject/Category of Required Report
City, county, or district health official	Suspected or confirmed cases of communicable diseases
Local health official	Exposure to animal suspected of having rabies
Local health official	Patients infected with tuberculosis who vacate an apartment or premises by death or are removed from the premises
Local health official	Pregnant women who test positive for Hepatitis B
Local health official	Syphilis tests on pregnant women
National Practitioner Data Bank	Specified information regarding malpractice payments and adverse actions
City Department of Health	All immunizations administered to any child age 7 and under
City Department of Health	Cases, carriers, and persons who at their time of death were affected by any communicable diseases
City Department of Health	Deaths from natural causes
City Department of Health	HIV, HIV-related illnesses, and AIDS
City Department of Health	Deaths not a result of natural causes
City Department of Health	Tuberculosis
City Department of Health	Births

Agency/Authority Receiving	Subject/Category of Required Report
State Board of Medicine	Specified information regarding malpractice payments and adverse actions
State Department of Child Welfare	Suspected child abuse or maltreatment or failure to immunize infants for Hepatitis B if the mother is Hepatitis B positive
State Department of Health	Alzheimer's disease upon diagnosis or confirmation of presence of illness
State Department of Health	Cardiac reporting
State Department of Health	Cases of communicable diseases diagnosed after death
State Department of Health	Habitual narcotics users
State Department of Health	Hepatitis B test results for all women with newborn children
State Department of Health	HIV, HIV-related illnesses, and AIDS
State Department of Health	Increased incidence of nosocomial infections or nosocomially acquired communicable diseases
State Department of Health	Radioactive cadavers
State Department of Health	Sexually transmitted diseases (STDs)
State Department of Health	Blood sample from every newborn to be tested for certain diseases
Occupational Safety and Health Administration (OSHA) area office	Death of an employee or multiple employee injuries
Police	Violent injury—bullet wound, gunshot wound, powder burn, other injury caused by a gun or firearm. All injuries that are likely to or do result in death and appear to be caused by a knife, ice pick, etc.
U.S. Department of Health and Human Services, Centers for Medicaid and Medical Services (CMS)	Deaths—caused by restraint or seclusion
U.S. Department of Labor	Death of an employee or multiple employee injuries

Sample Privacy Policy

BEST IN TOWN INC. PRIVACY POLICY

The Best in Town (BIT) medical group's mission is to provide quality, affordable, personalized health care.

Best in Town is committed to patient confidentiality and will adhere to the requirements of the Health Insurance Portability and Accountability Act (HIPAA).

Privacy Officer

John Smith, physician assistant-certified (PA-C), will monitor regulations changes, oversee staff training, and enforce policy.

Training

Upon employment and annually thereafter, all employees will receive a copy of BIT's privacy policy. An in-service training will be conducted that will cover the need for a federal privacy policy, the requirements for disclosures of medical information and patients' rights, and emergency exceptions. Annually, the Privacy Officer will review federal regulations to assure BIT is in compliance with them.

Access to Health Records

Health care providers (physicians and physician assistants) and the Privacy Officer are the only individuals who will review and study medical records at BIT.

Support staff [licensed practical nurses (LPNs) and medical assistants] will access medical records for "need to know" information for the purposes of scheduling tests, refilling medications, and so on. The secretarial staff will only scan a chart to assure completeness (such as the provider's signature). The Privacy Officer and the billing staff will review charts at compliance meetings for the purpose of assuring billing compliance with insurance guidelines.

No staff member will read a medical record. Charts will not leave the premises.

Release of Medical Information

Medical records will be sent only with a written authorization at the request of the patient. Only the minimum amount of information necessary to satisfy a patient's needs will be sent. In the event of referring physicians, information will be exchanged with the specific verbal consent of the patient.

The Privacy Officer will decide what information will be released. Information will not be released for non-health-related purposes such as employment, financial, political, or marketing purposes. Pharmaceutical manufacturers will not have access to patient names or addresses. Emergency situations and public safety concerns are exceptions to the usual authorization process.

Patients' Rights

Patients have the right to request a copy of their records for personal perusal. If there is an area of dispute, the patient and the provider will discuss the entry, and amendments will be determined mutually.

BIT's patient brochure has a section that specifically informs patients of their rights and about the privacy policy of this practice.

Personal and Professional Conduct Rules

Medical care is very personal and intimate. We have an ethical and legal obligation to never betray a person's trust. We have access to information about patients that could be damaging, not only to the patient's privacy, but also to the person's reputation and social relationships.

Our responsibility to maintain professional patient confidentiality continues into our personal and community lives. In fact, it is outside of work where the most damage can occur. Our shared 8:00 to 5:00 experiences need to be kept as privileged information and not be detailed to others. "How was your day?" kind of questions should be answered in generalities.

No BIT staff member will reveal the identities of patients, their visits to the office, their medical conditions, or their financial obligations to BIT.

Enforcement

Failure to adhere to the privacy policy or breach of confidentiality is grounds for termination.

Each employee must sign and date the privacy policy. Include language such as, "This is to certify that I have received a copy of Best in Town Inc.'s privacy policy. I have read and understand the policy and will adhere to the policy."

A copy of the HIPAA rules can be obtained from the Health and Human Services (HHS) Web site at www.hhs.gov/ocr/hipaa.

With your practice in mind, analyze the rules for risk areas and current office systems that could lead to privacy breaches before writing your policy.

Source: Adapted with permission from Gossman, J. (2003). Putting the PA in HIPAA: Privacy policy can be simple. *ADVANCE for Physician Assistants, 11*(3): 11.

CHAPTER 9

Evaluation and Management Coding

Documentation Requirements • Key Components • Final Determination of CPT Code

Author: Mark Kauffman, DO, PA

Proper visit documentation allows for appropriate coding and reimbursement. Missing key components in the documentation can be costly to the practice both financially and in lost time. Denied or reduced reimbursements can result in a large loss of manpower hours spent in chart review and resubmission, and not infrequently result in *writing off* the collections.

Many times core components of services that need to be documented are performed but not documented. This is often a result of a lack of time for each patient encounter, and the chart is sacrificed in lieu of time spent with the patient. To the payer of the claim, this can result in the use of the adage, "If it wasn't documented, it wasn't done," and hence, reimbursement can be reduced. Practitioners who are cognizant of the components of evaluation and management (EM) coding can use these skills to obtain higher reimbursements for their services, thus justifying the salaries they command.

The centers for Medicare and Medicaid services have developed guidelines for EM coding. Either the 1995 or 1997 guidelines may be used. These guidelines incorporate the American Medical Association's Current Procedural Terminology (CPT) codes.

Accurate coding can be a complex task. It is first broken down into categories based on whether the patient is new to the provider or previously established, whether the patient is seen in consultation, and the location of the encounter—such as outpatient, hospital, extended care facility, or home visit. Each category is then assigned a CPT code based on the level of services provided with regard to three key components: history, physical examination, and medical decision making, along with the contributing factors of counseling, coordination of care, nature of the problem, and time spent with the patient. These aspects will each be revisited in detail.

Further requirements include documentation of medical necessity and appropriateness, accurate reporting of the service provided, and a complete and legible medical record that includes the reason for the encounter. This documentation is typically presented as the chief complaint, the history, physical examination, and test results. In addition, the complete record will include an assessment, impression, or diagnosis with an associated plan of care and indication of complexity. Finally, a date and legible identity of the health care provider must be noted. Financial loss is easily encountered merely because of illegible documentation. Electronic medical records, if and when implemented, have alleviated much of this concern.

DOCUMENTATION REQUIREMENTS

EM coding is first broken down into categories. For each patient encounter, the site of service must be identified. See Table 9-1.

Table 9-1 Encounter Sites

Categories	Required Number of Key Components
New patient visits: outpatient	3 of 3
Established patient visits: outpatient	2 of 3
Consultations	3 of 3
Initial hospital visits	3 of 3
Subsequent hospital visits	2 of 3
Hospital observation care	3 of 3
Emergency department visits	3 of 3
New and annual nursing facility care	3 of 3
Established nursing facility care	2 of 3
New domiciliary: rest home, custodial care	3 of 3
Established domiciliary care	2 of 3
New house calls	3 of 3
Established house calls	2 of 3

There are three key components that constitute the encounter. They are history, physical examination, and medical decision making. This is further detailed later in this chapter.

A *new patient* by definition is a patient who has not been seen by the provider, or another provider within the same group, for the last three years. The three key components, "3 of 3," must be completed to code at this category. This means that any encounter that is coded as a new patient must have (1) a documented history, (2) a physical examination, and (3) medical decision making easily identifiable in the record.

An *established patient* by definition is a patient who has been seen by the provider, or another provider within the same group, within the last three years. In this case, only two of the three key components, "2 of 3," must be completed to code at this category.

Consultations are defined to include both new and established patients. Again, all three key components must be completed. A consultation must be requested by another provider who documents the need for the consultation and the specific problem to be addressed. If the consultation is performed as an outpatient service, the provider must document the visit in a written report. A consultation on an inpatient can be documented as a note on the patient's chart. Consultants may initiate diagnostic or therapeutic strategies. If a consultant is assuming all care for the patient, such as in a "transfer to the service of Dr. John Smith," the encounter should not be coded as a consultation, but rather, as a new or established visit.

Initial hospital visits by definition require "3 of 3" key components. These codes are used for the first inpatient encounter by the admitting physician. If a patient is seen as an outpatient or in an emergency room and subsequently admitted, the services should be combined and billed at the higher EM level.

Subsequent hospital visits are defined as requiring "2 of 3" key components. Each note requires a chief complaint, interval history, and billed diagnoses that may change from day to day as new diagnoses are made.

Hospital discharge services are coded based on time. Different CPT codes are applied based on the time spent on preparing the discharge, one for 30 minutes or less, the other if greater than 30 minutes is spent. The actual time must be documented. Discharge services cannot be billed if the patient was admitted for observation only.

In general, encounters with new patients require "3 of 3" key components, whereas visits with established patients require just "2 of 3" key components.

KEY COMPONENTS

The following are the three key components involved in selecting a level of EM service:

1. History
2. Physical examination
3. Medical decision making

There are also the following contributory factors:

1. Counseling
2. Coordination of care
3. Nature of presenting problem
4. Time spent face to face with the patient

History

History, the first key component, contains four criteria, the chief complaint (CC), a history of the present illness (HPI), a review of systems (ROS), and the grouped past medical history, family history, and social history (PFSH).

The Chief Complaint

The chief complaint is required on all encounters and is usually stated in the patient's own words. This concise statement should describe the symptoms, diagnosis, "provider recommended return," or other reasons for the encounter. The following are two examples:

- CC: "I have a pain in my chest" x 6 hours
- CC: For 3-month follow-up for diabetes mellitus

History of Present Illness

The HPI is defined as *brief* or *extended*, based on the number of key components. See Table 9-2. A *brief* encounter will have from one to three components. An *extended* encounter will have four or more components or the status of three chronic conditions.

Table 9-2   History of Present Illness

Components	
Location	Where symptom is located
Quality	Description of symptom
Severity	Intensity
Timing	Onset and chronology
Duration	Time since onset
Context	Circumstances causing the problem
Modifying factors	Aggravating or alleviating factors
Associated signs or symptoms	Concurrent findings

Review of Systems

The ROS is an inventory of symptoms related to the body systems. See Table 9-3.

Table 9-3 Review of Systems

Constitution	Fever, chills, weight changes, night sweats, fatigue
Eyes	Change in vision, double vision, eye pain, redness
Ears, nose, mouth, and throat	Ear pain, epistaxis, discharge, dysphagia, tinnitus
Cardiovascular	Palpitations, chest pain, peripheral edema, claudication
Respiratory	Shortness of breath, orthopnea, dyspnea on exertion, coughing, wheezing
Gastrointestinal	Dyspepsia, nausea, vomiting, diarrhea, constipation
Genitourinary	Dysuria, hematuria, urgency, hesitancy, frequency
Musculoskeletal	Arthralgia, myalgia, cramping, fractures, joint swelling
Integumentary/breast	Rashes, lesions, hair loss, nail changes, dimpling
Neurologic	Memory loss, paresthesias, weakness, slurred speech
Psychiatric	Depression, anxiety, thoughts of hurting self or others
Endocrine	Polyuria, polyphagia, polydipsia, heat or cold intolerances, excessive sweating
Hematologic/lymphatic	Easy bruising or bleeding, anemia, transfusion history
Allergic/immunologic	Allergies, eczema, recurrent infections

Encounter documentation for the ROS is based on the number of systems addressed. A *problem pertinent* ROS is a review of only one system that is directly related to the problem.

An *extended* ROS includes both the system directly related to the problem and the addition of two to nine other systems.

A *complete* ROS documents at least a 10-system review. It is acceptable to note both positive and pertinent negative responses followed by the summary statement "all other systems negative."

Past Medical, Family, and Social History

In the PFSH, past medical history includes any prior diagnosis of medical conditions, operations, illnesses, medications, and allergies.

The *family history* may vary on depth of detail, but includes current medical conditions, health status, and causes of death of parents, siblings, and other first- and second-degree relatives whose heath history may impact the patient. For example, a family history of early onset coronary artery disease in uncles and cousins would be pertinent.

The *social history* includes past and present use of tobacco, alcohol, and drugs. This section may also include marital status and living arrangements, employment and occupational exposures, level of education, recent travel, and household pets.

A *pertinent* PFSH reviews the history directly related to the HPI and documents at least one item from either the past medical history, family history, or social history areas. For example, in a patient presenting with a cough, the social history for tobacco use would be pertinent.

A *complete* PFSH documents at least one specific item from at least two of the three areas. For example, in a patient presenting with chest pain, the three history areas could easily include a past medical history of hyperlipidemia, a family history of early onset coronary artery disease, and a social history of tobacco use, all of which increase the patient's risk of coronary artery disease.

Determining Level of History

Combining the four criteria defines the level of service. See Table 9-4.

Table 9-4 Level of Service Criteria

HPI	ROS	PFSH	Level of History
Brief 1 to 3 components	None	None	Problem Focused
Brief	Problem pertinent	None	Expanded Problem focused
Extended 4 or more components or the status of 3 chronic conditions	Extended System related, plus 2 to 9 other systems	Pertinent At least 1 item from past medical, family, or social history	Detailed
Extended	Complete Review of at least 10 systems	Complete At least 1 item from 2 areas	Comprehensive

The highest level obtained is determined by the least complete assessment. For example, if the HPI and ROS is *extended*, but no PFSH was *none*, the level of history could not exceed *expanded problem focused*. If, however, a *complete* PFSH was done, the level of history would be *detailed*, limited by the *extended* ROS. To obtain a *comprehensive* level of history, the ROS would have to be expanded to include at least 10 systems.

Physical Examination Component

Physical examination is the second key component. Two documentation guidelines exist, the 1995 and 1997 Documentation Guidelines for Evaluation and Management Services, and either may be implemented. The 1995 guideline breaks down the physical examination into body areas and systems, whereas the 1997 guideline uses a general multisystem examination with bulleted components. Level of service is determined by the number of body areas or systems (or bullets) documented. See Table 9-5.

Table 9-5 1995 and 1997 Physical Examination Guidelines

1995 Body Areas (bolded) and *Systems* (unbolded)	1997 General Multisystem Examination Bullets
Constitutional: vitals, general appearance	• Measurement of 3 of 7 vital signs: pulse, respirations, temperature, height, weight, supine blood pressure, or standing/seated blood pressure • General appearance
Head (including face)	
Eyes	• Inspection of conjunctiva and lids • Examination of pupils and irises • Ophthalmoscopic exam
Ears, nose, throat, and mouth	• External inspection of ears and nose • Otoscopic examination • Auditory acuity • Inspection of internal nasal structures • Inspection of lips, teeth, and gums • Examination of oropharynx
Neck	• Examination of neck • Examination of thyroid
Respiratory	• Assessment of respiratory effort • Palpation of the chest • Percussion of chest • Auscultation of lungs
Cardiovascular	• Palpation of heart • Auscultation of the heart with notation of abnormal sounds or murmurs • Examination of carotids, aorta, femoral, and pedal pulses, edema and/or varicosities

(continued)

Table 9-5 *(continued)*

1995 Body Areas (bolded) and *Systems* *(unbolded)*	1997 General Multisystem Examination Bullets
Chest (including breast and axillae)	• Inspection of the breasts • Palpation of the breasts and axillae
Back (including spine)	
Gastrointestinal/**abdomen**	• Inspection and palpation of the abdomen with notation of masses or tenderness • Examination of the liver and spleen • Examination for presence or absence of hernia • Examination of anus, perineum, and rectum • Stool sample for occult blood
Genitalia, groin, buttocks	
Male genitourinary	• Examination of scrotal contents • Examination of the penis • Digital rectal examination of the prostate gland
Female genitourinary	Pelvic examination including: • External genitalia and vagina • Urethra • Bladder • Cervix • Uterus • Adnexa/parametria
Hematologic/lymphatic/ immune	• Palpation of lymph nodes in 2 or more areas: neck, axillae, or groin
Extremities	
Musculoskeletal	• Examination of gait and station • Inspection or palpation of digit or nails • Examination of joints, bones, or muscles of 1 or more of the following areas: (1) head and neck, (2) spine, ribs, and pelvis, (3) right upper extremity, (4) left upper extremity, (5) right lower extremity, or (6) left lower extremity. • Inspection/palpation with notation of misalignment, asymmetry, crepitation, defects, tenderness, masses, or effusions • Range of motion noting pain, crepitation, or contracture • Assessment of stability noting dislocation, subluxation, or laxity • Assessment of strength and tone noting atrophy or abnormal movements

(continued)

1995 Body Areas (bolded) and *Systems* (unbolded)	1997 General Multisystem Examination Bullets	
Skin	• Inspection of skin and subcutaneous tissue • Palpation of skin and subcutaneous tissue	
Neurologic	• Testing of cranial nerves noting deficits • Examination of deep tendon reflexes noting pathological reflexes • Examination of sensation	
Psychiatric	• Description of patient's judgment and insight Brief assessment of mental status including: • Orientation to time and place • Recent and remote memory • Mood and affect	
1 body area or system	**Problem focused**	1 to 5 bullets
Up to 7 body areas or systems	**Expanded problem focused**	At least 6 bullets
Up to 7 body areas or systems	**Detailed**	At least 2 bullets from each of 6 body systems/areas or at least 12 bullets from 2 or more systems/areas
8 or more body areas or systems	**Comprehensive**	At least 2 bullets from each of 9 systems/areas

Source: Adapted from www.cms.hhs.gov/medlearn/master/.pdf.

Medical Decision Making

The third and final key component is medical decision making and is composed of three areas: (1) number of diagnoses or treatment options, (2) amount or complexity of the data reviewed, and (3) risk of complications and/or morbidity or mortality. These three areas combined determine the overall complexity of the medical decision making.

The number of diagnoses or treatment options is based on the problem status. Each problem or diagnosis should be classified as stable or controlled, improved or resolving, worsening, uncontrolled, or failing to improve. Each problem is then categorized as self-limited or minor, as an established problem, or as a new problem.

The amount and/or complexity of the data reviewed require documentation of each area reviewed by the provider. These data include the reviewing or ordering of clinical laboratory tests, imaging, testing, discussing test results with the performing physician, obtaining the history from others or others' records, reviewing and summarizing of old records, discussing the case with another provider, and visualizing images, tracing, or specimens oneself as opposed to being interpreted by another provider.

Assigning a level of risk to the risk of complications and/or morbidity or mortality is more complex. There are four levels of such risk: minimal, low, moderate, and high.

A *minimal* level of risk reflects one self-limited or minor problem, with minimal diagnostic workup such as laboratory analysis, ECG, or basic imaging, and recommendations for supportive care that would not include medications.

A *low* level of risk includes two self-limited or minor problems, one stable chronic problem, or one new uncomplicated illness or injury. This level includes more advanced, nonemergent, diagnostic testing such as pulmonary function tests, noncardiovascular contrasted imaging, superficial needle and skin biopsies, or laboratory tests requiring arterial puncture. Management recommendations may include over-the-counter medications, occupational or physical therapy, and minor surgery. Nonadditive intravenous fluids are also included in this level.

A *moderate* level of risk includes chronic illnesses with mild exacerbation, two or more stable chronic conditions, a new problem with an uncertain prognosis, or an acute systemic or complicated illness or injury. The diagnostic workup is more advanced and includes stress tests, endoscopies or cardiac imaging with no identified risk factors, deep needle or incisional biopsies, and any procedure where fluid is obtained from a body cavity. Management at this level includes minor surgery where risk factors are identified, major elective surgery, prescription drug management, therapeutic nuclear medicine, intravenous fluids with additives, and closed treatment of fractures or dislocations.

Finally, a *high* level of risk includes chronic problems with severe exacerbations, abrupt changes in mental status, or any acute illness or injury that threatens life or bodily function. This level includes endoscopies or cardiovascular imaging when risk factors are identified, for example, cardiac catheterization with troponin elevation, cardiac electrophysiology, and discography. This level has the highest degree of management including elective major surgery with identified risk factors, emergency major surgery, dispensing of controlled substances or those requiring monitoring for toxicity, and a decision to withhold resuscitation or decrease the level of care due to a poor prognosis.

These examples are not all-inclusive, but demonstrate the escalating level of care provided as the level of risk rises.

Time

Finally, the contributory factor of *time* may be determined. If more than 50% of the encounter was spent face to face with the patient for counseling or coordination of care, either in an office or hospital setting, none of the above calculations are necessary, and the EM service can be based on time alone. The encounter documentation must delineate the exact time spent with the patient, reflecting that more than 50 percent of the time was spent on counseling or coordination of care. This may include differential diagnosis, prognosis, treatment options, risks and benefits, education, instructions, compliance, or discussions with other providers.

FINAL DETERMINATION OF CPT CODE

Each category is then broken down into levels. Each level increase reflects an increase in the complexity of the case determined by merging the three key components. Based on the number of required key components, coding must reflect the highest completed level of service.

Case Study

Review the following progress note and determine its proper level of CPT coding. The patient is seen in the outpatient clinic.

Case presentation:

Date/Time   CC: Chest pain x several months

Subjective:

Mr. B is a 42-year-old well-known patient who presents complaining of chest pain. He states the pain began several months ago. He describes the pain as a burning in the epigastric and retrosternal areas. Originally he experienced the pain on a weekly basis but now relates an increase in frequency to nearly daily occurrences, especially after eating, and lasting for several hours at a time. He admits occasional radiation of the pain into the left side of his neck. He scales the pain as a 4 or 5 out of 10. Eating prior to going to bed makes it worse, as do spicy foods. Taking Mylanta helps for about an hour.

He admits some associated nausea (but denies diaphoresis), abdominal or back pain, vomiting, diarrhea, constipation, bloody or dark-colored stools, coughing, and wheezing.

Past medical history: childhood asthma, no hx of PUD, hyperlipidemia, or
   hypertension
Family history: no history of early cardiovascular disease
Social history: lifetime nonsmoker, admits two to three beers twice a week

Objective:

Vitals: pulse 72, bp 150/88, respirations 16, ht 6'2", wt 232, temperature 97.2 F
ENT and mouth: teeth without erosions
Lungs: clear to auscultation without wheezes, crackles, or rubs
Heart: regular rhythm without murmur, rub, or gallop
Abdomen: obese, normoactive bowel sounds, tenderness to palpation in the
   epigastrium. No masses or organomegaly
Neurologic: clear phonation

(continued)

(continued)

EKG: sinus rhythm

Impression/plan:

1) Chest pain—suspect Gastroesophageal Reflux Disease (GERD)

   Trial of ranitidine 150 mg PO q hs, #30, refill 2

   Pt education to avoid spicy foods, alcohol, and eating prior to bedtime

   Pt to call in 2 weeks if no improvement

   Doubt cardiovascular disease with normal ECG; however, repeat cholesterol to assess risk as the last panel was 2 years ago

2) Elevated systolic blood pressure without prior diagnosis of hypertension

   First documented visit with systolic elevation

   Pt has blood pressure cuff at home. Will take bp daily x 2 weeks and will have nurses call to obtain results

   Pt education for reducing sodium in diet and beginning daily exercise routine

3) Increased body mass index

   Patient education for low-fat, high-fiber diet with daily exercise as above

_____

Provider signature

Coding for this encounter begins with categorizing the visit. This is an established patient seen in an outpatient setting. Reference the CPT coding manuals available from the American Medical Association.

As an established patient, two of the three key components are necessary. A chief complaint is identified. The HPI is *extended,* completing four or more of the components such as location, quality, severity, timing, context, modifying factors, and associated signs and symptoms.

The ROS is included in the subjective area and is *extended,* an evaluation of from two to nine systems, including constitutional (diaphoresis), cardiovascular (chest pain), gastrointestinal (nausea, vomiting, constipation, diarrhea), and respiratory (cough and wheezing).

The PFSH is *complete* including all three areas of pertinent past medical history, family, and social history. The level of history must then be *detailed,* limited by an *extended* ROS. Had the ROS included 10 systems, the history component would have had a *comprehensive* level.

The second key component is physical examination. Six body areas or systems were examined including constitution, ENT/mouth, respiratory, cardiovascular, abdominal, and neurologic. This reflects an *expanded problem focused* or *detailed* examination according to the 1995 documentation guidelines.

HPI	ROS	PFSH	Level of History
Brief 1 to 3 components	None	None	Problem focused
Brief	Problem pertinent	None	Expanded Problem focused
Extended 4 or more components or the status of 3 chronic conditions	Extended System related plus 2 to 9 other systems	Pertinent At least 1 item from past medical, family, or social history	Detailed
Extended	Complete Review of at least 10 systems	Complete At least 1 item from 2 areas	Comprehensive

If following the 1997 guidelines, there are seven bullets, or an *expanded problem focused* examination. Thus far, we have a *detailed* history and an *expanded problem focused* or *detailed* examination.

The final key component is medical decision making. There are three diagnoses in this examination. The patient presented with the complaint of chest pain, which after complete evaluation was diagnosed as GERD. This is a new diagnosis as is the second, elevated systolic blood pressure without diagnosis of hypertension. Both require additional workup. The third diagnosis of increased body mass index is not new, with the patient having similar weights on prior examinations. His weight has not increased so the problem can be considered stable, not worsening. "Possible" or "rule out" diagnoses will be rejected. For example, a problem should be documented as "chest pain," not "rule out myocardial infarction (MI)."

The second component in medical decision making is type of data. A clinical laboratory test, the cholesterol panel, was ordered. An ECG was performed and interpreted.

The final component of medical decision making is risk. The fact that prescription drug management incurred places the risk at *moderate*, for an overall *moderate complexity* in medical decision making.

Now we bring the three key components together for the final determination of the CPT code. Again, this was an established patient seen in an outpatient setting. The history was *detailed*, the examination *expanded problem focused* or *detailed*, and medical decision making was *moderate*. This visit would then be assigned a CPT code of 99214. See Table 9-6.

Table 9-6 Office or Other Outpatient Services—Established Patient

History	Examination	Medical Decision Making	Time (minutes)	Level 2 of 3
Minimal visit, not requiring the presence of a physician, PA, or NP				99211
Problem focused	Problem focused	Straightforward	10	99212
Expanded problem focused	Exp problem focused	Low complexity	15	99213
Detailed	Detailed	Moderate complexity	25	99214
Comprehensive	Comprehensive	High complexity	40	99215

As is evident, proper coding can be a complex task; however, the provider fluent in proper documentation of the clinical encounter assures maximum reimbursements appropriate to the level of service provided.

CHAPTER 10

Reimbursement for PA Services

Methods of Reimbursement • Government-Sponsored Insurance • Private Insurance • Compliance

Author: Holly Jodon, MPAS, PA-C

The goal of every physician assistant (PA) should be to serve patients in the most competent and cost-efficient manner. The escalating costs of both health care and health care insurance in the United States have moved these issues to the forefront of our national agenda. Rising costs have made medical insurance unaffordable for some, a financial strain for those who wish to maintain it, and a challenge for employers and the government to continue to finance the coverage they now offer. Patients who are uninsured are responsible for all costs they incur and these are paid out-of-pocket directly to the health care provider. Patients who present with health insurance may also be responsible for a portion of their medical expenses, which can add up very quickly. To secure health care coverage, a monthly premium must be paid to a health plan either by the individual and/or his or her employer, or by the government. The insured patient may also be responsible for a yearly deductible, which is the first out-of-pocket expense that must be paid by the insured before the insurance coverage takes effect. The policy may also have a limit on the amount that will be covered, usually 80%, leaving the insured responsible for the remaining amount, or *coinsurance*. Some plans also require a *copayment*, which is the out-of-pocket expense the insured pays at the time of service or for prescription drugs or both. Most insured patients must have the ability to pay for at least a portion of their care even when utilizing their health care plan. Another stipulation for the health plan to pay for coverage is that the insured must be seen by a provider who is enrolled or participates in that health plan. Insurance companies will credential providers before accepting them into the health plan. This credentialing process is to verify that the provider meets the professional standards of training, certification, and licensure, as well as to review any background history regarding privileges, malpractice, violations, or limitations. For all of these reasons, it is challenging for PAs to maintain competency as providers and to practice medicine efficiently, which will result in helping control costs for patients and ultimately provide them with the highest quality care.

METHODS OF REIMBURSEMENT

Quality patient care must remain the first priority of every PA. Once the patient has been appropriately assessed and a plan implemented, the medical record should reflect the severity of illness, the level of care, and the service that has been rendered. Based on this documentation, a PA can assign a diagnosis code using the *International Classification of Diseases*, 9th edition, *Clinical Modification (ICD-9-CM)* manual.[1] A code appropriate for the encounter is also assigned using the *Physicians Current Procedural Terminology* (CPT) manual for the level of service provided, such as an evaluation and management (E/M) code (as described in Chapter 9) or a procedure code.[2] These codes will be used to establish a fee that is billed to the insured patient's health plan. This contracted health plan will then reimburse the provider for services rendered to the insured. In most instances, payment for PA services is made directly to the employing physician or practice. The method of payment can be administered in one of the following four ways:

1. Fee-for-service—Payment is made based on the E/M or procedure code, plus every other service or supply is individually itemized on the bill. The insured patient may belong to a Preferred Provider Organization (PPO) that allows him or her to self-refer to a limited number of providers within the organization, usually at a discounted fee-for-service rate.
2. Episode of illness—A *global* surgical fee is a single payment to the provider for the procedure, preoperative, and postoperative care. In a similar manner, a global obstetrical fee is just one payment to the provider for the delivery, prenatal, and postnatal care. Hospital reimbursement is based on diagnosis-related groups (DRGs), in which payment is based on the patient's diagnosis (such as congestive heart failure), regardless of the patient's length of stay in the hospital.
3. Capitation—This is the reimbursement method used in managed care organizations (MCOs) such as a health maintenance organization (HMO). The HMO requires the insured member to select a primary care physician (PCP) from a group of contracted providers. One monthly or annual payment is made to the selected provider for the prospective medical treatment of that HMO member. The total reimbursement is based on the number of HMO members or *heads* enrolled with that provider. This amount is prepaid, usually per member per month, regardless of whether or not the HMO member utilizes the provider.
4. Salary—Providers employed full time by hospitals, by MCOs, or by the government are reimbursed in one lump sum for all care provided over a specific duration of time, whether a month or a year.[3]

Because the health plan is the third party in the patient–provider relationship and is responsible for reimbursement payments, it is called a *third-party payer*. When a provider submits a bill for reimbursement there are a number of possible third-party payers a patient may be insured with:

1. Government-sponsored
   - Medicare (MC)
   - Medicaid (MA)
   - State Children's Health Insurance Program (SCHIP)
   - TRICARE
   - Federal Employees Health Benefit Program (FEHBP)
2. Private insurance
   - Traditional (fee-for-service)
   - Managed care organizations (MCOs)

The U.S. Census Bureau, reporting the principal source of health insurance coverage for the population in 2003, stated that 60.4% of the population was covered by employment-based private insurance, 26.6% was covered through government financing, and an estimated 15.6% of the population was uninsured.[4]

GOVERNMENT-SPONSORED INSURANCE

Medicare

The federal government created Medicare in 1965 to provide health care coverage for the elderly. Medicare Part A provides partial hospitalization coverage including subsequent care in a skilled nursing facility, some skilled home health care, and hospice care for a doctor-certified terminal illness. Anyone who pays into Social Security for 10 years is automatically enrolled in Medicare Part A, as well as his or her eligible spouse, upon the age of 65 years. Medicare also covers persons (who qualify) younger than 65 years old with a disability or chronic kidney disease requiring dialysis or a transplant. Medicare Part B provides the elderly with insurance coverage for medical expenses such as a physician's services, skilled therapy, diagnostic tests, and medical equipment. To qualify for Part B, individuals must be eligible for Part A and pay a monthly premium.[5]

Historically, Medicare has utilized a fee-for-service method of reimbursement. Medicare sets the physician reimbursement fee schedule on a resource-based, relative-value scale (RBRVS). Each medical and surgical service is assigned a value based on the time and intensity of work involved. Time is broken down into preservice work, intraservice work, and postservice work. Intensity is broken down into mental effort and judgment, technical skill, physical effort, and psychological stress.[6] The RBRVS is then multiplied by a conversion factor to arrive at the actual amount of Medicare's reimbursement. Fee reimbursements also vary geographically to account for differences in costs associated with practice expenses and professional liability. Each year the Center for Medicare and Medicaid Services (CMS) proposes revisions and changes to the policy for payment. Medicare's payment rate increased by 1.5% in 2005, but reimbursement is scheduled to decrease in 2006 unless Congress takes legislative action.[7, 8]

The federal government began reimbursing physicians for services provided by their PAs under Medicare Part B with the Rural Health Clinic Services Act in 1977. Incrementally and at varying reimbursement rates, coverage grew to include hospitals, nursing homes, Rural Health Professional Shortage Areas, and surgical first assisting. The Balanced Budget Act (BBA) of 1997 increased and standardized the reimbursement rate Medicare paid for services provided by a PA. It also gave PAs greater latitude in providing care to Medicare patients by expanding coverage to all practice settings. With the physician supervising in accordance with state law, Medicare currently reimburses PA employers 85% of the physician's fee schedule for services provided by their PA when it is billed under the PA's provider identification number (PIN). This is the same for inpatient and outpatient practice settings including office, clinic, hospital, skilled nursing facility, and home visits. Some differences do arise, such as the care provided at a Federally Qualified Health Center (FQHC) or Rural Health Clinic (RHC), which are cost-based reimbursement sites. Also, the fee for a surgeon to first assist is 16% of the primary surgeon's fee; therefore, PA reimbursement for first assisting in surgery is 85% of 16%, which is a net amount of 13.6% of the primary surgeon's fee.[9].

Fee-for-service reimbursement requires contributions from patients in the form of yearly deductibles, coinsurance, and the entire cost of medications. These costs can sometimes be prohibitive for those on a fixed income, especially in the wake of a hospitalization. For this reason, many Medicare patients purchase a supplemental or secondary insurance, called Medigap, or qualify for Medicaid as a secondary insurance to cover the cost of deductibles and coinsurance. Once Medicare has reimbursed the provider at the allowable rate, the secondary insurance is also billed. To try and offset the additional expense of secondary insurance, or the costs associated with the lack thereof, Medicare began allowing beneficiaries to enroll in MCO options in 1985. Later the BBA expanded plan options under Medicare to include Medicare HMOs called Medicare Part C or Medicare + Choice. These MCO plans offer some prescription drug benefits, preventive care, and eliminate deductibles and coinsurance. Beneficiaries enrolled in HMOs typically are restricted to receiving their medical care from within the network and are required to obtain referrals from their PCP to be seen by a specialist. Medicare HMOs may offer a *point-of-service* (POS) option. The point-of-service plan allows the insured to be seen outside of the group of HMO contracted providers or to self-refer, but at a cost in the form of higher deductibles, coinsurance, and copayments. Market forces, such as increasing expenses and limits on MC payment increases, have made it difficult for some MC plans to offer extra benefits.[10]

The Medicare Prescription Drug, Improvement, and Modernization Act (MMA) was enacted on December 8, 2003, to give Medicare beneficiaries more options and better benefits. This broadens the Medicare MCO options to include PPOs, which are the most popular health plan choices for non-Medicare beneficiaries. Medicare + Choice was renamed Medicare Advantage. The MMA also implemented the Medicare Prescription Drug Benefit, which will take effect January 1, 2006, and provides for medication, limited preventive services such as an initial "Welcome to Medicare" physical examination and screening tests for diabetes and coronary artery disease.[11]

Medicare Enrollment

All physician assistants who treat Medicare patients, either under fee-for-service or through an MCO, must have a PIN. To qualify for enrollment, the PA must fulfill the following requirements:

1. Have graduated from a physician assistant educational program that is accredited by the Accreditation Review Commission of Education for the Physician Assistant (ARC-PA) or a predecessor agency
2. Have passed the national certification examination that is administered by the National Commission on Certification of Physician Assistants (NCCPA)
3. Be licensed by the state to practice as a physician assistant[12]

Physician assistants should enroll through the Center for Medicare and Medicaid Services (CMS) Web site where applicants are directed to contact their local MC carrier, who is accessible by a link on the Web site.[13] The local MC carrier, typically a Blue Cross/Blue Shield (BC/BS) provider, is contracted by the government to administer the MC program in that local area, including processing medical claims and enrollment applications. These local contractors enroll PAs in the MC program through a credentialing process to verify the PA meets professional standards. The American Academy of Physician Assistants (AAPA) reimbursement staff recently reported the only form PAs are required to submit is the CMS 855I for Individual Health Care Practitioners enrollment form.[14] The certification statement must be signed, dated, and mailed to the local Medicare contractor. At the present time, upon enrollment the PA will receive a Medicare PIN for each practice site and a *unique* provider identification number (UPIN). The PIN will change by employer, but the UPIN is permanent. Most applications are processed within 60 days and the PIN remains valid for 12 months. The PA must submit claims to Medicare, as allowed by state law, under this provider number for the PIN to be maintained.

Physician assistants should be aware of changes in this enrollment process that are currently under way. The Health Insurance Portability and Accountability Act of 1996 (HIPAA) established Administrative Simplification provisions. These mandate the Department of Health and Human Services (HHS) adopt a standard unique health identifier for health care providers. Regulations issued by HHS on January 23, 2004, established the national provider identifier (NPI). This is a 10-digit identifier that all health care providers, including PAs, are required to obtain and use for reimbursement of medical claims. When the NPI is implemented, all standard transactions will require the use of only the NPI to identify health care providers. Previous identification numbers, such as the UPIN, those from Medicaid, from TRICARE, or from private plans will not be permitted. Health care providers may apply for NPIs beginning May 23, 2005, and once assigned, NPIs will not expire. The compliance date for full implementation is May 23, 2007, with the exception of small health plans which must comply by May 23, 2008.[15]

Once a PA is credentialed by Medicare he or she becomes an *approved provider*. The PA becomes a *participating provider* upon entering into an agreement with the Department of Health and Human Services (HHS) based on the following stated conditions:

> To accept payment based on the reasonable cost of the items and services furnished, not to charge the beneficiary or any other person for covered items and services, except deductibles and coinsurance amounts, and to return any money incorrectly collected.[16]

Under the fee-for-service payment method, MC is billed at the full 100% reimbursement rate, then as a participating provider the PA's provider number will automatically generate the 15% reduction to 85% of the physician fee schedule.

Covered Services

Services rendered by a PA may be covered under Medicare Part B if all of the following requirements are met:

1. The services are those typically rendered by a physician.
2. The provider meets all the qualifications set forth for a PA.
3. State law authorizes the PA to provide such services.
4. The physician supervises those services, as defined by state law.
5. Those services have not been previously excluded from coverage.[17]

Examples of covered services include physical examinations, minor surgery, casting of simple fractures, X-ray interpretation, and independent patient assessment and treatment. As state law allows, PAs are authorized to perform a physical examination to determine the need and to order the certificate of medical necessity for durable medical equipment (DME)[18] and to order outpatient physical therapy after establishing a rehabilitation treatment plan.

Physician assistants may bill using Current Procedural Terminology E/M codes for all levels of service and diagnostic tests if the PA is authorized within the scope of practice for his or her state license, and if the services are furnished under the general supervision of a physician. [19, 20]

Surgeons are reimbursed from Medicare under one global surgical fee. This includes the preoperative history and physical examination performed within 24 hours prior to surgery, intraoperative care rendered by the surgeon and PA, and any postoperative care, usually for 90 days after major procedures, and for 10 days after minor procedures. Medicare does cover surgical PA first assist services for procedures that commonly require an assistant surgeon. Procedures provided by a PA are distinguished by a modifier code attached to the procedure code. When submitting for PA first assist services, the modifier most commonly used by MC is AS (assist services); however, it is important to clarify with the local MC carrier which modifier code it requires. This will generate the 13.6% PA reimbursement.

Some restrictions apply to reimbursement for surgical PA first assisting. Medicare has a list of 1800 CPT codes that are not eligible for PA services. This list can be accessed at the AAPA Web site.[21] Restrictions also apply to surgical PA first assisting in teaching hospitals. Medicare requires surgeons to use a resident if an approved, accredited residency program exists in the surgical specialty. Medicare will reimburse for PA first assist services if the following exceptions exist:

1. The surgeon has an across-the-board policy of never involving residents in the care of patients.
2. A resident is not available because of a regularly scheduled training conference or involvement in a concurrent surgical case.[22]

Incident To

Physician assistant services are eligible for reimbursement at 100% of the physician's fee schedule if those services are furnished *incident to* the services of an MD or DO and billed under the physician's name and provider number. To qualify under this provision, specific criteria must be met. Only those services provided in an office or clinic setting are eligible. The PA must be an employee, leased employee, or independent contractor of the physician, or of the entity that employs or contracts with the physician. As a provider, the PA must be licensed and working within his or her scope of practice under state law. The services rendered by the PA must also meet the definition of *incident to* as set forth in the Medicare Carriers Manual. Those services must be provided according to the following guidelines:

1. "Furnished as an integral, although incidental, part of a physician's professional services in the course of diagnosis or treatment of an injury or illness"
2. Commonly rendered in an office or clinic setting and commonly included in the physician's charges
3. Performed under the direct supervision of the physician[23]

For the services provided by a PA to be covered as incident to the services of a physician and reimbursed at 100% of the physician's fee schedule, those services "must be performed under the direct supervision of the physician as an integral part of the physician's personal in-office service."[24] The Medicare Carriers Manual gives a further explanation with the following qualifications:

1. Direct supervision does not imply the physician must actually perform the service or be present in the room. The physician must, however, be present in the office suite and available for immediate assistance if it is required. Access by telephone or elsewhere within the institution does not qualify for direct supervision. In these instances the PA should bill under his or her own provider number and receive 85% of the physician reimbursement fee schedule.

2. The physician must provide direct, personal service to initiate the course of treatment furnished by the PA. This means the physician must personally diagnose the medical condition and treat a new patient on his or her initial visit and must make the diagnosis of a new medical condition in established patients who present for follow-up. The PA may provide subsequent care of a previously diagnosed condition.

3. The physician must continue to follow the patient at a frequency that establishes continued participation and management of the patient's medical condition. The frequency of physician visits may be governed by state law.[25]

These are the rules as set forth by Medicare for incident to billing. If there is any doubt as to whether an encounter is eligible, or if documentation does not substantiate an incident to encounter, it is best to bill under the PA's provider number rather than risk an ineligible claim.

Shared Hospital Visit

As of October 25, 2002, CMS approved *shared visits*. This allows hospital inpatient, hospital outpatient, or emergency department visits provided by a PA and a physician on the same day to be combined. Both providers must work for the same group practice for the shared visit to be billed under the physician's provider number for 100% reimbursement. The physician is required to see the patient face to face when providing any portion of the evaluation and management encounter and to document this in the medical record. This applies to new and/or established hospital to emergency department visits, but does not include procedures.[26]

Medicaid

The enactment of Medicare in 1965 also included the creation of Medicaid (MA), which provided health insurance coverage for low-income individuals, persons young and old who are disabled with chronic illnesses, and institutionalized individuals. Medicare is a federal program, whereas Medicaid, though funded through federal and state taxes, is a state-run program. The federal government mandates certain services be covered, such as hospitalization, physician's fees, laboratory work, X-rays, preventive, prenatal, nursing facility, and home health care. The states regulate eligibility and reimbursement and policies vary from state to state. Currently all 50 states reimburse employers for services rendered by their practicing PAs. Enrollment through the CMS Web site directs providers to contact their state MA programs.[27] For enrollment and reimbursement information, the AAPA reimbursement staff has collated a state-by-state guide of MA programs (in the "members only" section) on the AAPA Website. This provides each state's program information as to whether PAs are credentialed, issued provider numbers, considered covered providers, and if so, at what reimbursement rates. It distinguishes if PAs should submit bills under their own PIN, with modifiers, or under the physician's PIN. It also lists physician supervision requirements, the types of plans offered, and provider contact information.[28]

Historically, MA utilized a fee-for-service method of reimbursement with payment for PA services the same or slightly lower than physicians and made directly to the PA employer. Unfortunately, overall poor reimbursement discouraged many providers from participating. Recently, states are changing to MCOs because of the increasing number of MA beneficiaries and increased costs associated with their care.

The federal government has also created the State Children's Health Insurance Program (SCHIP). This provides coverage for uninsured children whose family income is up to 200% of the federal poverty level, but above the income requirements for MA (i.e., they are ineligible for MA, yet unable to afford insurance). In SCHIP, physician assistants may be considered covered providers and are typically reimbursed for PA services at 100% of the physician fee schedule with general physician supervision.[29] However, this should be clarified with each individual state program.[30]

Military-Related Coverage

TRICARE, formerly known as CHAMPUS (Civilian Health and Medical Program of the Uniformed Services), insures active duty or retired service members and their families, as well as qualified reservists and their families. This includes members from any of the seven uniformed services: Army, Air Force, Navy, Marine Corps, Coast Guard, Public Health Service, and the National Oceanic and Atmospheric Administration.[31] TRICARE will cover all necessary medical services provided by a PA if his or her physician supervises the PA according to state law, is an authorized TRICARE provider, and bills for the services of the PA. The fee-for-service reimbursement for PA services is 85% of the physician's allowable fee and first assisting in surgery is 65% of the physician's allowable fee. TRICARE has two managed care plans that recognize PAs as eligible providers. TRICARE *Prime* operates much like an HMO, and TRICARE *Extra* operates much like a PPO.[32]

Federal Employees Health Benefit Program (FEHBP)

The Federal Employees Health Benefit Program (FEHBP) provides the widest selection of health plans in the country to federal employees, retirees, and their survivors. These beneficiaries include federal civilian employees, Federal Deposit Insurance Corporation (FDIC) employees, and United States Postal Service (USPS) employees, including the American Postal Workers Union (APWU), the National Association of Letter Carriers (NALC), the National Rural Letter Carriers Association (NRLCA), and the Government Employees Health Association (GEHA).

The list of possible plans includes private insurance, both traditional and MCO, as well as government or group-sponsored insurance. Beneficiaries may choose from a variety of plans including fee-for-service, fee-for-service with PPO, HMO, or HMO + POS. Some programs are nationwide and open to all enrollees. Some plans may limit enrollment to the location the plan is offered, to certain employee groups, or to membership-paying organizations that sponsor the plan.[33] These FEHBP programs typically do not credential PAs, but choose instead to reimburse PA services under the supervising physician's provider number. Physician assistants should contact the plans offered in their area and utilized by the patients in their practice for information regarding PA provider status and reimbursement policies.

PRIVATE INSURANCE

Traditional

Nonprofit and commercial insurance carriers offer service plans that can be purchased by employers who provide employment-based coverage, or by individuals who are self-employed or are uninsured. The insured person and/or his or her employer pays a premium to the insurers, who are known as the *third-party payers*. The insurance carrier is then responsible for reimbursing the provider for services rendered to the insured. The method of payment is usually fee-for-service with the insured responsible for a yearly deductible and additional coinsurance. Another form of insurance, known as *indemnity*, requires the insured to pay the provider directly and then seek reimbursement from the insurance carrier.

Private health insurance companies are not mandated to follow Medicare's policies. They are entitled to formulate their own policies and procedures regarding PAs. Many consider the PA a covered provider whose services can be billed under the physician's PIN for 100% reimbursement if the PA is supervised according to the private insurance company's policy, which may be state law. Some companies do require the PA to bill under his or her own PIN, and sometimes a modifier may be required. Some insurance companies reimburse PA employers for services provided by PAs in medically understaffed areas with only indirect physician supervision. There has been a recent increase in the number of insurance companies reimbursing for surgical PA first assist services.

Currently, there is a wide array of differences between private insurance companies, as well as differences in patient policies and provider contracts within the same company. The AAPA has profiled the reimbursement data for the top private insurance companies, collated it state by state, and made it available to members on their Web site. The site provides information as to whether the PA is a covered provider, credentialed, or has been given a PIN number. It lists supervision requirements, covered services, specific billing and reimbursement instructions, as well as company contact information.[34] It is strongly recommended that each insurance company be contacted individually to clarify its specific policies regarding PAs.

Managed Care Organizations (MCOs)

Managed care has emerged as an attempt to control rising medical costs and as a way to ensure the quality of medical care. Managed care organizations contract with selected providers to form a *network* for the plan. Included in this network are providers for outpatient services, inpatient services, and prescription coverage. Insured members must stay within the network of the managed care plan they select, except in emergent situations or with specific authorization; otherwise, they are responsible for paying for all out-of-network care.

Managed care plans may be in the form of a PPO that is offered to persons with traditional private insurance. This allows the member to self-refer to providers in the network at discounted fee-for-service rates. Members agree to utilization review, which requires mandatory second opinions and precertification for elective surgeries or procedures, and case management of their hospitalization care.

HMO-managed care plans prepay for comprehensive health care services by contracting with providers in a designated geographic area. There are different types of HMOs. *Group* practice plans contract with groups of physicians who practice at medical centers. *Individual* practice plans contract with physicians or groups of physicians who practice within their own offices. *Mixed models* combine group practice and individual practice plans. Insured members choose their primary care physician from one of these plans. The PCP also serves as the patient's "gatekeeper" by making appropriate referrals within the network and ensuring patients receive the most appropriate level of care when it is needed. PCPs are reimbursed on a capitated basis, whereas specialists within the network are usually reimbursed using a fee-for-service method.[35]

Medicare MCOs follow MC reimbursement guidelines; however, as with other private insurance carriers, private MCOs develop their own PA policies and procedures. As a nonphysician provider (NPP), the PA is responsible for treating MCO patients utilizing services within the network. Some MCOs prefer the NPP to bill under the physician's PIN and others assign PAs provider numbers. Some plans offer incentive programs where additional reimbursement is provided to augment capitation for selected preventive services. It is important for the PA to review the MCO contracts within his or her supervising physician's practice and follow the guidelines stipulated in those contracts.

COMPLIANCE

It is imperative that PAs stay abreast of the ongoing changes in the field of insurance reimbursement to maximize their earning potential and to remain compliant. Physician assistants need to learn the governmental and major private insurance carriers in their practice and be aware of updates to their policies and regulations. A participating provider agreement with Medicare designates you as a government contractor with all the responsibilities implicit in that agreement. Typical third-party payer medical claim forms include a statement verifying the provider understands the rules and regulations and intends to follow them. Pleading ignorance does not excuse providers from being held accountable. Failure to meet those requirements could lead to a penalty and/or prosecution. Medicare, Medicaid, and private insurance companies (such as BC/BS) have initiated task forces to review for fraudulent billing.

Medicare defines fraud as "an intentional representation that an individual knows to be false or does not believe to be true and makes, knowing that the representation could result in some unauthorized benefit to himself/herself or some other person."[36] The most common forms of fraud in MC include the following:

1. Billing for unfurnished services
2. Justifying payment with a misrepresentation of a diagnosis
3. Being involved in kickback schemes
4. Separately billing for services that should be bundled
5. Justifying payment by falsifying medical records, treatment plans, or certificates of medical necessity
6. Upcoding a service to a higher level than was rendered[37]

The complex nature of insurance regulations makes the task of understanding all aspects of billing almost insurmountable. Reviewers are interested in seeing a good-faith effort to try to comply on the part of providers. This can be accomplished with a voluntary compliance plan to identify, correct, and prevent coding and/or billing not consistent with the regulations. The Office of the Inspector General (OIG) has published Federal Register notices addressing compliance program guidance for a number of providers, including one for individual and small group physician practices.[38] The OIG recommends a step-by-step approach to implementing the following seven components of a voluntary compliance plan:

1. Internally audit patient charts and billing practices.
2. Publish and utilize practice compliance standards.

3. Designate a compliance officer
4. Educate providers and office staff.
5. Rectify errors.
6. Communicate inconsistencies.
7. Establish and publicize consequences for failure to comply.[39]

As a first step, the OIG recommends the physician's office begin by adopting components that will address their known areas of billing and compliance problems. One of the most important aspects of a successful compliance plan is to take corrective action when a problem is identified.

Areas that a physician assistant should be astutely aware of include the following:

1. Medical documentation for evaluation and management coding must be done properly and accurately. The chief complaint must be present in every medical record. Medical records must reflect the level of service billed. If the documentation does not substantiate the severity of illness or the level of intensity required for a high-level visit, the service is considered not billable at that level.
2. All the requirements of *incident to* billing in the office must be met; otherwise, the service is to be billed under the PA's PIN.
3. The requirements for a shared visit in the hospital must be met; otherwise, the service is to be billed under the PA's PIN.
4. Restrictive physician supervision requirements must be understood and followed for licensure purposes and for appropriate billing practices.[40]

It is important for PAs to know the regulations that pertain to their clinical situation. Along with the right to provide services under a PA license goes the responsibility to maintain its precepts and convey them to coworkers. It is not recommended to rely solely on the supervising physician, office manager, or coding specialists. The AAPA stays abreast of the implementation and interpretation of reimbursement issues affecting PAs. One that will be of interest to all PAs is the implementation of the NPI. The requirement for an insurance company to assign PAs a provider number will be eliminated, as the NPI will be the only one allowed to do so by law. The impact this will have on the provider status of PAs within the insurance industry is yet to be seen.

The following resources are available to PAs and serve to enhance understanding of the constantly changing and complex guidelines for reimbursement:

1. Attendance at the Reimbursement, Billing, and Coding Seminar at the AAPA's Annual Physician Assistant Conference
2. AAPA Web site for reimbursement information at www.aapa.org. keyword: reimbursement
3. *Physician Assistant Third-Party Coverage* available from the AAPA's online store at www.aapa.org/aapastore/index.html

4. Medicare Part B newsletter and Nonphysician Practitioner newsletter
5. Centers for Medicare and Medicaid Services. Reference Guide for Medicare Physicians and Supplier Billers Part B. Available at: www.cms.hhs.gov/medlearn/billingguideB/referencej.pdf. Accessed November 28, 2004.

BIBLIOGRAPHY

1. Igenix, Inc. (2005). *Physician ICD-9, International classification of diseases, 9th revision, clinical modification* (6th ed). Salt Lake City, UT: Author.

2. American Medical Association. (2003). *Physicians current procedural terminology: CPT 2004* (4th ed). Chicago: Author.

3. Bodenheimer TS, Grumbach K. (2005). *Understanding health policy: a clinical approach* (4th ed). New York: McGraw-Hill.

4. U.S. Census Bureau. Health insurance coverage: 2003. Available at http://www.census.gov/hhhes/hlthins/hlthin03/hlth03asc.html. Accessed November 28, 2004.

5. Centers for Medicare and Medicaid Services. Medicare plan choices. Available at http://www.medicare.gov. Accessed November 28, 2004.

6. Centers for Medicare and Medicaid Services. Physician fee schedule: work relative value units—chapter 1. Available at http://www.cms.hhs.gov/physicians/pfs/wrvu-ch1.asp. Accessed November 28, 2004.

7. Power M. (2004, September 10). Medicare issues proposed 2005 regulatory changes. *American Academy of Physician Assistants Reimbursement Watch.* Alexandria, VA: Department of Government and Professional Affairs.

8. Centers for Medicare and Medicaid Services. Medicare program: revisions to payment policies under the physician fee schedule for calendar year 2005. Available at http://www.cms.hhs.gov/regulations/pfs/2005/1429p.asp. Accessed November 28, 2004.

9. American Academy of Physician Assistants. Professional issues: reimbursement. Available at http://www.aapa.org/gandp/3rdparty.html#PAcoverage. Accessed November 28, 2004.

10. Centers for Medicare and Medicaid Services. Facts about the Centers for Medicare and Medicaid Services. Available at http://www.cms.hhs.gov/researchers/projects/APR/2003/facts.pdf. Accessed November 28, 2004.

11. Centers for Medicare and Medicaid Services. Medicare modernization act. Available at http://www.cms.hhs.gov/medicarereform/. Accessed November 28, 2004.

12. Department of Health and Human Services. (2002, March 12). *Medicare carriers manual: physician assistant services.* Baltimore, MD: Centers for Medicare and Medicaid Services. Transmittal 1744, section 2156.

13. Centers for Medicare and Medicaid Services. Medicare fee-for-service provider/supplier enrollment. Available at http://www.cms.hhs.gov/providers/enrollment/forms/. Accessed November 28, 2004.

14. Reimbursement question and answer. (2004, November 30). *American Academy of Physician Assistant News*:3.

15. Centers for Medicare and Medicaid Services. Overview of the national provider identifier. Available at http://www.cms.hhs.gov/hipaa/hipaa2/regulations/identifiers/default.asp. Accessed November 26, 2004.

16. Centers for Medicare and Medicaid Services. Provider reimbursement manual part 1: chapter 24 payment to providers. Available at http://www.cms.hhs.gov/manuals/pub151/PUB_15_1.asp. Accessed November 29, 2004.

17. Department of Health and Human Services. (2002, March 12). *Medicare carriers manual: Physician assistant services.* Baltimore, MD: Centers for Medicare and Medicaid Services. Transmittal 1744, section 2156.

18. Powe, M. (2004, September 10). *Medicare issues proposed 2005 regulatory changes.* American Academy of Physician Assistants Reimbursement Watch. Alexandria, VA: Department of Government and Professional Affairs.

19. Department of Health and Human Services. (2002, March 12). *Medicare carrier manual: Physician assistant services*. Baltimore, MD: Centers for Medicare and Medicaid Services. Transmittal 1744, section 2156

20. Department of Health and Human Services. (2001, March 19). *Medicare program memorandum carriers*. Baltimore, MD: Centers for Medicare and Medicaid Services. Transmittal B-01-28.

21. American Academy of Physician Assistants. Medicare first assisting in surgery: 2003 surgical denial list. Available at http://www.aapa.org/gandp/mcsurglist.html. Accessed November 28, 2004.

22. Department of Health and Human Services. (2002, November). *Medicare carriers manual: Supervising physicians in teaching settings*. Baltimore, MD: Centers for Medicare and Medicaid Services. Section 15016.

23. Department of Health and Human Services. (2002, August 28). *Medicare carriers manual: Incident to physician's professional services*. Baltimore, MD: Centers for Medicare and Medicaid Services. Transmittal 1764, section 2050.1-2.

24. Department of Health and Human Services. (2002, August 28). *Medicare carriers manual: Incident to physician's professional services*. Baltimore, MD: Centers for Medicare and Medicaid Services. Transmittal 1764, section 2050.1-2.

25. Department of Health and Human Services. (2002, August 28). *Medicare carriers manual: Incident to physician's professional services*. Baltimore, MD: Centers for Medicare and Medicaid Services. Transmittal 1764, section 2050.1-2.

26. Department of Health and Human Services. (2002, October 25). *Medicare carriers manual: Evaluation and management service codes: examples of shared visits*. Baltimore, MD: Centers for Medicare and Medicaid Services. Transmittal 1776, section 15501.

27. Centers for Medicare and Medicaid Services. Medicaid provider relations. Available at http://www.cms.hhs.gov/Medicaid/stprovrel.pdf. Accessed November 28, 2004.

28. American Academy of Physician Assistants. State Medicaid surveys. Available at http://www.aapa.org/members/gandp/medicaidprofile.html. Accessed November 28, 2004.

29. American Academy of Physician Assistants. State children's health insurance program. Available at http://www.aapa.org/gandp/schip.html. Accessed November 28, 2004.

30. Centers for Medicare and Medicaid Services. State children's health insurance program. Available at http://www.cms.hhs.gov/schip/html. Accessed November 28, 2004.

31. Office of the Assistant Secretary of Defense. Military health system. Available at http://www.tricare.osd.mil/. Accessed November 28, 2004.

32. Office of the Assistant Secretary of Defense. Become a TRICARE certified provider. Available at http://www.tricare.osd.mil/provider/provider_cert.cfm. Accessed on November 30, 2004.

33. U.S. Department of Personnel Management. Federal employees health benefits program. Available at http://www.opm.gov/insure/health/index.asp. Accessed November 30, 2004.

34. American Academy of Physician Assistants. Private insurance company surveys. Available at http://www.aapa.org/members/gandp/privatepayer.html. Accessed November 28, 2004.

35. Kongstvedt, P.R. (2002). *Managed care: What it is and how it works* (2nd ed). Gaithersburg, MD: Aspen Publishers, Inc.

36. Centers for Medicare and Medicaid Services. Medicare definition of fraud. Available at http://www.cms.hhs.gov/providers/fraud/DEFINI2.ASP. Accessed November 30, 2004.

37. Centers for Medicare and Medicaid Services. Medicare definition of fraud. Available at http://www.cms.hhs.gov/providers/fraud/DEFINI2.ASP. Accessed November 30, 2004.

38. Office of Inspector General. Compliance Program for Individual and Small Group Physician Practices. Available at http://www.oig.hhs.gov/authorities/docs/physician.pdf. Accessed November 30, 2004.

38. Office of Inspector General. Compliance Program for Individual and Small Group Physician Practices. Available at http://www.oig.hhs.gov/authorities/docs/physician.pdf. Accessed November 30, 2004.

40. Scott, D. (2004, August 15). Knowing if your practice implements a compliance program is critical to your job. *American Academy of Physician Assistant News*, 6.

CHAPTER 11

Political and Legislative Action

"I Have No Interest in Politics" • A Few Definitions and Concepts • Liberty of Practice • The Need for an Agenda • Political Action Education • A Broader View • A Familiar Face • Model State Legislation

Author: William Duryea, PhD, PA-C

The professional life of the physician assistant in our current world involves more than clinical practice, educational updating through continuing medical education (CME), and "shop talk" at medical staff meetings. Today's practice climate is heavily influenced by the political activities of physicians and other allied health providers who may be working at odds with physician assistant political and legislative interests. In its relatively brief period of existence, the PA profession has learned that an active political agenda, pursued vigorously and persistently with legislators, translates into regulations and laws that improve the practice conditions for professionals who diligently work to achieve change. Physicians, nurses, nurse practitioners, physical therapists, and others have demonstrated that a strong base of political support is necessary for favorable legislative action.

Compared to other health professions, the number of PAs is still small, making it difficult for the profession to compete in the political and legislative arena. Nationally, about 60,000 PAs are in practice, and some states have incredibly small populations of PAs compared to other providers. However, small numbers can still be effective forces for political and legislative change if well organized and persistent about pressing their agenda. This chapter will present elements of political and legislative action and will provide a few blueprints for PAs to employ toward legislative change.

"I HAVE NO INTEREST IN POLITICS"

It is not unusual to hear an ordinary citizen say, "I'm too busy with my work and family, and I lack the time to be interested in politics." A person who lives in Pittsburgh, for example, might follow his or her favorite sports team, such as the Pirates, with passionate allegiance. That person might be familiar with all the players, their statistics, salaries and might be able to argue the wisdom of trading this or that player. But the same person may not know the name of the mayor of Pittsburgh and probably is less able to recall the names of any of the city council members.

This contrast is not unusual because sporting events are relatively simple, making it easy to focus on the immediate action. Politics, however, tend to be more complex, requiring more thought and insight into the often subtle, abstract, multidimensional conflicts of ideas, interests, and issues. "The irony is that athletic fans so often seem unaware that although sports may give them pleasure and touch their imagination, politics control their lives."[1]

A FEW DEFINITIONS AND CONCEPTS

- Legislative change—A new law (statute or act) or change in an existing law is enacted by a state or national legislative body. For example, legislation to enable PA practice in a particular state may be enacted as part of an existing medical practice act.
- Regulatory change—A rule-making activity that provides specific language for elements defined by the law. For example, if a PA practice law provides for prescribing authority, regulations (rules) must be written and published to specifically describe how prescribing shall be done by PAs.
- Registration—PAs may be required to register with a state medical board in order to obtain the right to practice in that state. The state board will maintain an official list (registry) of all PAs having the right to engage in clinical practice.
- Certification—PAs obtain certification by passing the Physician Assistant National Certification Exam (PANCE), after which they are entitled to use the professional title: PA-C. Physician assistants may be "certified" to practice in a particular state after having passed the PANCE. Recertification must be done every two years via CME and every six years via a recertification examination. Failure to recertify will result in the loss of practice privileges.
- Licensure—Signifies permission to practice upon the submission of appropriate qualifications (i.e., certification) and approval by the appropriate regulatory agency. Licensure is obtained independently of the PA's employment status and is renewable.
- Supervising physician—A licensed physician (MD or DO) authorized by the state regulatory agency to supervise physician assistants. Such a physician delegates certain clinical activities and services to PAs and accepts responsibility for the services provided by his or her PAs.
- Scope of practice—This is the breadth of a PA's responsibilities as delegated by a supervising physician.
- Locum tenens—The temporary provision of health care services by a substitute provider.

LIBERTY OF PRACTICE

Within the law, one could argue that PAs should enjoy the liberty to practice medicine and surgery consistent with their education and clinical experience. But it is abundantly clear that this liberty is, by varying degrees, constrained by laws and regulations that hamper the PA's ability to provide the best quality of care currently available. For example, a PA hired by an oncology practice to care for patients who suffer chronic pain should not be prohibited from prescribing appropriate pain medications for such patients, especially when it can be demonstrated that the PA has received appropriate training in the use of such medications.

Should liberty to practice continue for those elements of a PA's training that he or she may use very little? Shue argues, "Having a liberty can be valuable in itself, even if one does not actually exercise it...and the belief in the usability of the liberty must be correct and not subjected to standard, baseless threats."[2] If "the usability of the liberty [is] correct," laws and regulations governing PA practice must have some solidity and should not be altered without clear and defensible reasons. Such clear and defensible reasons should emanate principally from PAs, and not from those prone to "standard, baseless threats."

It would be a mistake to assume that PAs' liberty to practice is written in stone; such liberty must be protected by constant attention to the prevailing political climate and by diligent action to counter political efforts to undermine and limit PA practice.

THE NEED FOR AN AGENDA

Political action without an agenda is akin to a ship without a rudder. Any group seeking legislative or regulatory change must have a clear, well-conceived plan with realistic goals and objectives. The agenda must be specific, well-researched, and supported by the PA's constituency. The political action plan emanates from the agenda, but may have secondary objectives apart from the agenda, such as recruiting a lobbyist, fund-raising, and so forth. No agenda is stamped in stone, and each should be modified as circumstances and events dictate.

Who is in charge of the agenda? A group's decision to embark on a political action campaign commonly results in the establishment of a committee or task force made up of leaders who step forth to do the work of developing the agenda. Typically, the leadership sets the agenda with input from its constituents. Since agendas are often works in progress, it is the responsibility of the leadership to have periodic meetings to update the agenda and to move in new directions when necessary. Clearly, this is a dynamic process, requiring dedicated leaders and a committed constituency.

POLITICAL ACTION EDUCATION

It would be fair to speculate that most PAs are clinicians with little or no experience in the arena of political action. At one time or another, many PAs have probably given some thought to becoming politically involved over some practice issue that needs immediate attention; however, the thought seldom translates into action. Perhaps the lack of action is related to a sense of isolation and perceived lack of support from others with common interests. PAs with an interest in political and governmental affairs can readily find comrades within their state and national organizations. State PA societies and the American Academy of Physician Assistants (AAPA) welcome new members who have this interest. To foster political action at the national level, the AAPA sponsored a Constituent Chapters Officers Workshop (CCOW) in Washington, D.C. Delegates from state societies composed the CCOW participants. The CCOW generally consisted of several parts: a series of seminars devoted to educating participants about current, "hot" legislative issues of concern to PAs and sessions devoted to methods for effectively getting the PA message across to legislators. All of this activity culminated in opportunities for participants to visit their congressperson's offices to solicit his or her support for the key legislative issues outlined in the CCOW seminars. The success of the congressional visits was then evaluated at the end of CCOW. The CCOW provided excellent lessons in political action, particularly by demonstrating the effectiveness of face-to-face exchanges of views with legislators. The AAPA continues to encourage PAs and state societies to take part in legislative visits with their representatives.

A BROADER VIEW

The need for political action transcends PA self-interest in obtaining the best professional climate in which to practice and make money. The profession must subscribe to a wider view: that a better health care system benefits providers and patients together. The pathetic reality is still that millions of people in this country have no access to health care. Preventable diseases are on the increase. Reimbursement for health promotion and disease prevention services is grossly inadequate. Patient advocacy is desperately needed to alleviate the miserable situation that many of our poor and needy face in today's world. The need for political activism to address these issues has never been greater. There is no doubt that PAs can be an effective political force in seeking positive change.

Political activism resources are widely available on the Web, where everything from "anarchists" to "Zionists" can be found. An exceptionally comprehensive Web site to survey "all things political" is www.kimsoft.com/kimpol.htm. Political activists are persistent, relentless, and vocal. They know the issues they represent inside and out, and they know who to target with their information. Legislators are sensitive to public opinion, especially to the depth of opinion that translates into votes. When political activism takes on the appearance of a grass roots campaign with wide support, one can be certain that legislators will stand up and take notice. The adage "the squeaky wheel gets the grease" encapsulates the motivating force and persistent energy required to keep a hot issue cooking on the front burner until it gets proper attention. If issues are kept cooking long enough, political action is likely to convert into legislative action.

A FAMILIAR FACE

Legislative representatives at the state and national levels keep apprised of issues that are politically advantageous to them and their constituents. Issues that are close to home get the most attention, particularly when they are currently popular and politically charged. Legislators are hungry for information that will give them a competitive edge. Legislators employ aides who are specialists at gathering useful information from expert sources. PAs are excellent, reliable sources of information about many of the important issues surrounding health care in this country today. Legislators want to know what PAs know so they can convincingly argue for change (and also "feather their own nests" at election time). The PA who is a familiar face in a legislative office is an effective voice for such change. Many PAs are known on a first-name basis by some of the most prominent members of Congress and are respected as vital sources of information on the status of our current health care system. More familiar faces are needed.

MODEL STATE LEGISLATION

Every state in this country has enacted legislation to enable physician assistants to practice medicine under the supervision of a licensed physician. However, such legislation is not uniform from state to state, and regulations governing PA practice contain glaring deficiencies, inconsistencies, and contradictions in most states. Clearly there is a need for better laws and regulations governing PA practice so that patients are provided with the best care available in today's health care environment. To that end, the American Academy of Physician Assistants has proposed model state legislation for PAs that reflects two vital conditions: "that PAs should be licensed to practice medicine with physician supervision, and that PA scope of practice should be determined by supervising physicians."[3]

Many states still do not license PAs; they are instead "certified" or "registered" to practice.

The lack of licensure confers a "second-class citizenship" status on PAs, whereby the denial of certain rights and privileges conferred by licensure creates unfavorable practice conditions. For example, reimbursement clauses in provider contracts with third-party payers often contain the language, "medical services reimbursed only to licensed providers." It is vital that practices employing PAs be reimbursed for all covered services that PAs provide. PA licensure continues to be a political action issue that must stay on the front burner in those states lacking a licensure law.

REFERENCES

1. Moore, J. A., Jr., & Roberts, M. (1989). The pursuit of happiness. New York: Macmillan, 192.

2. Shue, H. Basic rights. Princeton, NJ: Princeton University Press, 68–69.

3. Web site of the American Academy of Physician Assistants. Model state legislation for physician assistants. http://www.aapa.org/gandp/modelaw.html. Accessed 2004.

CHAPTER 12

Ethics: Principles and Guidelines in Practice

Ethical Principles • Professional Code of Ethics • Ethical Decision Making • Mistakes in Medicine: What the Provider Should Know • The Provider's Obligation to Disclose Information Regarding Medical Mistakes • The Effects of Veracity on Medical Errors • Scenarios for Analysis • Conclusion

Author: Catherine Gillespie, DHSc, MPAS, PA-C

ETHICAL PRINCIPLES

"Ethics" are standards set forth to guide and maintain the definition of what constitutes correct conduct. The American Academy of Physician Assistants holds that ethical principles are based on the following four main tenets of autonomy, beneficence, nonmaleficence, and justice:

- Autonomy—Is allowing the patient freedom to choose his or her own direction, and respecting the wishes of the patient and the culture that he or she values
- Beneficence—Refers to the promotion of good towards the patient, acting in such a manner as to look out for the best interest of the patient
- Nonmaleficence—Is refraining from actions that may create or cause harm to the patient
- Justice or fairness—Equates to equal treatment for all, regardless of age, sex, race, ethnicity, disability, socioeconomic status, culture, religion, or sexual orientation[1]

These principles serve to guide the practice of health care in promoting the best interests of the patient. Further principles that add clarity to these tenets are informed consent, confidentiality, and veracity.

"Informed consent" is the act of providing the patient with information regarding a diagnosis that includes the nature and purpose of the diagnosis, proposed treatments, known risks, and consequences associated with the treatment or abstaining from treatment. The provider must present the necessary information in a manner the patient can understand. According to the American Medical Association the communication should include the following:

1. The patient's diagnosis, if known
2. The nature and purpose of a proposed treatment or procedure
3. The risks and benefits of a proposed treatment or procedure
4. Alternative treatments or procedures
5. The risks and benefits of the alternative treatment or procedures
6. The risks and benefits of not receiving treatment[2]

The patient must be provided with the appropriate information as listed previously and be competent in understanding the relevant consequences of his or her decision. The provider must not judge the patient's competence based on the patient's education level, nor is he or she to judge the patient on his or her decision when it is contrary to the provider's beliefs or the general norms of society. Respect for the patient's wishes must be maintained and the patient must also be free from coercion.

Misuse of the obligation to provide the patient with information is to utilize "therapeutic privilege." Therapeutic privilege is withholding information from the patient when the provider believes that the disclosure will have an adverse effect on the patient's condition or health. This is a specific form of strong paternalism, in that the provider is making the decision for a patient on the grounds of anticipated emotional difficulty.[3] This practice overlooks the patient's autonomy and dignity, leading to a relationship that will eventually be lacking in trust.

The obligation to obtain informed consent prior to treating a patient may be excluded in the case where there is the need for immediate treatment and the risk of life or serious impairment. If the patient is incapacitated, and there is no lawful surrogate to give consent, then the justification to omit informed consent is valid.

"Confidentiality" is the act of respecting patient communications and information in the strictest privacy. The patient–provider relationship is based on trust and the importance of confidentiality. Communication between the patient and the provider is privileged; to violate this entrusted information is harmful to the patient, the medical profession, and society. The provider must hold the patient's confidentiality in the highest regard.

The provider *does* have the right to consult other health care providers in an effort to provide his or her patient with the best health care. This consultation must be carried out in a professional manner, away from public access. The elevator, hallway, and a busy nursing station are not appropriate places for consultation regarding a patient's private information. By the same token, this right of consultation must not be misconstrued so as to allow providers to seek information simply to satisfy curiosity.

Exceptions to confidentiality may be enforced in situations where there is potential harm to the patient, to someone else, or in the case of minors. Providers are encouraged to know state and federal laws in reference to confidentiality and to be aware of the consequences of a breach in confidentiality.

"Veracity" reflects accuracy, honesty, and truthfulness. The principle of veracity binds the provider to honesty. These three aforementioned areas are the hallmark of or focus in the patient–provider relationship.

According to Hippocrates, the physician was to be the healer and authoritarian, and no one was to question this icon. This emphasis was maintained through the 1800s, as it was professed that giving the patient true information may actually prove harmful to the patient.[4] This is a strong example of the paternalism that was encouraged in medicine, where the physician was the strong father figure that made decisions for the patient despite the patient's wishes or consent. It was not until the 1970s that the attitude of telling the truth made an abrupt turnaround. The factors that have been credited in this change include advances in cancer treatment and the greater recognition of the patient as a person deserving dignity and autonomy. Clinicians have a duty to tell the truth and act beneficently toward the patient to preserve the patient's dignity.[5]

Forms of not telling the truth can be broadly defined as "concealment" or "deception." Concealment is intentionally avoiding the communication to another person of all relevant information. This can also be defined as "withholding" or "selective disclosure" of the information. Deception is the intentional causing of another person to adopt a false belief or to fail to reject a false belief. Forms of deception are lying, purposely misleading, and the use of placebo.[6]

Outright lying in medicine is less common; however, "misleading" may be the more common heading used for describing "nonlying" in terms of deception, wherein the provider means no harm. This is exemplified by the provider who may mislead by the use of euphemisms or by using vague descriptive terms rather than being specific with the diagnosis. For example, discussing cancerous growths with a patient but using the word lesions rather than cancer is an attempt not to overstimulate the patient with anxiousness and to soften the conversation. This is still deception, but as used in this example, it is not lying.

The practice of deception in medicine toes a very fine line. Who decides when a situation allows the provider to withhold the truth? This seems as though it may be creating a paternalistic pattern wherein the provider can then decide what is best to disclose to the patient. There is no doubt that there are circumstances in which clinicians may be tempted to withhold or modify information; however, the commitment to provide the truth is the clinician's ultimate responsibility and obligation. Providers who engage in routine deception are in time creating a personal risk of erosion of public trust along with negative views of his or her integrity, character, and professionalism.[7]

The American Medical Association holds that it is the physician's ethical responsibility to be truthful with patients at all times. Any deviation from the truth erodes the integrity of the patient–provider relationship. Physician assistants are bound to relationships that involve patients, physicians, and society. These relationships must be based on respect utilizing the described ethical principles.[8]

PROFESSIONAL CODE OF ETHICS

Professional "codes of ethics" are descriptive guides that offer direction in providing the highest level of service to the patient, the supervising physician, one's peers, and the community. The code of conduct outlines guidance in reference to issues of professionalism, collaboration with other health care professionals, the health care system, and society. See Figure 12-1 for the statement of values of the physician assistant profession.

Figure 12-1   Statement of Values of the Physician Assistant Profession

Physician assistants hold as their primary responsibility the health, safety, welfare, and dignity of all human beings.

Physician assistants uphold the tenets of patient autonomy, beneficence, nonmaleficence, and justice.

Physician assistants recognize and promote the value of diversity.

Physician assistants treat equally all persons who seek their care.

Physician assistants hold in confidence the information shared in the course of practicing medicine.

Physician assistants assess their personal capabilities and limitations, striving always to improve their practice of medicine.

Physician assistants actively seek to expand their knowledge and skills, keeping abreast of advances in medicine.

Physician assistants work with other members of the health care team to provide compassionate and effective care of patients.

Physician assistants use their knowledge and experience to contribute to an improved society.

Physician assistants respect their professional relationship with physicians.

Physician assistants share and expand knowledge within their profession.

Source: American Academy of Physician Assistants. (2003). From program to practice: A guide for PA practice. Alexandria, VA: AAPA.

The physician assistant is to be familiar with these guidelines and practice in a manner that upholds the basic principles essential to their profession. In times of ambiguity, the utilization of current knowledge, guidelines, and resources provided by the profession can assist the physician assistant in the direction of the best interests of all involved parties.

ETHICAL DECISION MAKING

Ethical decision making is often bound by ambiguity; dilemmas can be complex and involve gray areas. The provider must respond with tolerance and responsible practice. Faced with an issue, the provider who has a plan in place is more likely to have continued success in the patient–provider relationship. The following are guidelines that offer a therapeutic benefit or means toward a solution.

1. Recognize first, and then define the problem. Gather information and clarify if the problem is ethically, legally, or morally binding. Begin the process with appropriate documentation.
2. Develop solutions utilizing ethical guidelines and the support of colleagues. Review the code of conduct and consider the basic tenets of autonomy, beneficence, nonmaleficence, justice, informed consent, confidentiality, and veracity as they apply to the issue. Seek guidance from colleagues and professional organizations to assist with applicable laws and regulations.
3. Communicate with the patient to encourage him or her to become involved in the solution.
4. Determine the course of action, based on the best interests of the patient.
5. Be reflective; this is a powerful learning tool for future benefit.

These guidelines offer an outline of steps that will assist the PA in reaching a solution. The manner in which the provider takes the steps may not necessarily numerically follow the preceding presentation, which leaves the option to the provider to find the best fit of the guidelines to the situation.[9]

The foundations of ethical practice begin with the professional code of conduct as a guide. The provider must also take into consideration the need to employ critical thinking in a clear manner and without prejudice and to consider the basic tenets of ethics in the patient–provider relationship. The successful provider will base his or her actions on honesty, diligence of action and mind, and being sensitive to the needs of the patient.

MISTAKES IN MEDICINE: WHAT THE PROVIDER SHOULD KNOW

Errors are inevitable in medicine and may arise from medicine's inherent uncertainty. Mistakes may also arise as a result of oversights on the part of the individual provider. In each case the provider is faced with situations where he or she must address mistakes with the patient.[10]

How do mistakes occur? Most errors in medicine are not directly the result of gross negligence. A provider may make a mistake because of an incomplete knowledge base, an error in perception or judgment, or a lapse in attention. Making decisions on the basis of inaccurate or incomplete data may lead to a mistake. The environment in which a provider practices may also contribute to errors. Lack of sleep, pressures to see patients in short periods, and distractions may all impair an individual's ability to avoid mistakes.[11]

Errors that occur most often begin at the point of the administration of health care and prescribing. Insulin and anticoagulants are the drugs most likely to be involved in an error, with omission, improper dosing, and unauthorized drugs being the most frequently reported errors. Performance errors include failure to follow procedures or protocol and deficits in knowledge base because of distractions, excessive work loads, and inexperience. Many errors in health care go unreported as a result of the fact they have created little or no harm. These errors are usually not brought to the attention of the patient and are less likely to be reported.[12]

THE PROVIDER'S OBLIGATION TO DISCLOSE INFORMATION REGARDING MEDICAL MISTAKES

Providers have an obligation to be truthful with their patients. This duty includes situations where the patient suffers serious or nonserious consequences because of an error in medical management. The fiduciary nature of the relationship between a provider and patient requires that a provider deal honestly with the patient and act in his or her best interest.[13]

When a provider witnesses another health care provider making a major error, he or she is placed in an awkward and difficult position. The observing provider must maintain the same level of obligation as the acting provider to see that the truth is revealed to the patient. The observing provider should first approach the provider involved in the error and encourage disclosure. If that provider refuses to disclose the error, then the logical chain of command should be followed to fulfill the obligation of the observing physician.[14]

THE EFFECTS OF VERACITY ON MEDICAL ERRORS

The disclosure of medical errors should include the essential components of listening, empathy, respect, and apology. These move beyond the arena of blame and reinforce the relationship with the patient. When veracity is present and errors correctly disclosed, the level of trust in the patient–provider relationship is strengthened, which decreases the risk of subsequent malpractice suits. Forgiveness, trust, and confidence are often experienced when patients are treated with respect and given the truth.

Most patients desire some acknowledgment of even minor errors. Loss of trust will be far more serious when a patient feels something is being hidden from him or her. All that patients usually want is the truth. Patients are less likely to consider litigation when a physician has been honest with them about errors in medical management. Litigation is often used as a means of forcing an open and honest discussion that the patient feels he or she has not been granted. Furthermore, juries look more favorably on providers who have been honest from the beginning than those who give the appearance of having been dishonest.[15]

Veracity in medicine is not only an obligation of the provider, but an essential element in the patient–provider relationship. A relationship based on truth encourages a trusting relationship that often overpowers the desire to seek litigation in cases of error. If the patient is treated with respect and dignity, he or she may be more likely to respond to the apology with favor and respect.

Doing the right thing may prove difficult at times; however, our society expects a high level of ethical behavior. Health care providers must be able to deliver the best level of care in the most accountable way. Recognizing the trust placed in a provider, he or she should then offer the patient an earnest, straightforward, and complete conversation about the medical error. The patient should be given time to process the information. Excuses should be minimal and blaming absent. This honesty reflects the appropriate level of respect and professionalism warranted in the patient–provider relationship and leads to an easier transition from the problem to a successful conclusion.[16]

SCENARIOS FOR ANALYSIS

Consider the following scenarios as examples of ethical situations. Following each scenario there will be a discussion of the ethical concerns and standards that should be upheld. Evaluate the scenario on the basis of the standards of ethical care. What elements are absent, and what standards should have been in place to avoid the situation?

Scenario 1—Dr. Smith has treated Mrs. Preston and her family for many years. At the present time Mrs. Preston is suffering from end-stage renal disease and has a life expectancy of 6–12 months. During a recent appointment, Mrs. Preston points out to Dr. Smith a lesion on her right upper arm and her concern for the irregular appearance of the lesion. Dr. Smith observes the lesion and has concerns that the lesion is melanoma. He decides that because of her limited life expectancy there is no need to investigate this any further. Dr. Smith tells Mrs. Preston that it is nothing to worry about and could be a result of her current diagnosis of renal failure.

Discussion—Dr. Smith has certainly overstepped the situation by applying therapeutic privilege. The patient's autonomy and sense of justice have been violated. The fact that the patient has a terminal disease does not allow the physician to withhold information or care. Concurrent disease processes may have further implications for the patient and the patient's family.

Scenario 2—Dr. Sanson and PA Jones are discussing Mr. Olsen's case in the nurse's station. Mr. Olsen is a 75-year-old male who presented to the emergency room after a fall; he sustained a fracture to his right hip and now Dr. Sanson's orthopedic practice has been consulted in the case. PA Jones has completed an initial evaluation of the patient and during his evaluation of the patient found a chest X-ray result that notes a moderate-sized mass in the patient's right lobe. This is what he and Dr. Sanson are discussing. During their discussion, Betty James, a respiratory therapist overhears the conversation. Later in the day, Betty James approaches PA Jones with concerns about what she overheard. As it turns out, Mr. Olsen is her uncle, and after overhearing the conversation between Dr. Sanson and PA Jones she has great concern for the health of her uncle.

Discussion—This situation points out the importance of confidentiality. The nurse's station was not an appropriate place for PA Jones and Dr. Sanson to engage in consultation. This is further complicated by the patient's niece, another health care professional overhearing the conversation and creating a further ethical dilemma of confidentiality.

Scenario 3—Dr. Smith and PA White practice in a large internal medicine group; they are privately completing a small pilot study for personal use on two hypertensive medications to decide which one works best. Patients who present with new onset hypertension are randomly given either medication. The side effects of the medication are given in general terms, as the providers are concerned that the patient may be less likely to agree to the medication out of fear of the side effects. The patients are also not aware of the study the providers are conducting.

Discussion—Dr. Smith and PA White are not imparting informed consent and are also overstepping their therapeutic privilege. The veracity of the situation is also in question as the side effects of the medication and the study are not being completely disclosed to the patient.

Scenario 4—Family practice PA Wilson has had a busy afternoon with patients. The last patient of the day was a 5-year-old child presenting for a routine preschool physical examination and update of his immunization. PA Wilson completes the examination and orders the final series of immunizations for the child. Nurse Peters completes the task and while logging the immunizations in the patient's chart, realizes that one of the vaccines was slightly out of date. She discusses the issue with PA Wilson and they decide the outdated vaccine would most likely do no harm and that there is no need to take any further action.

Discussion—This presents the concern of nonmaleficence. Do both providers know for certain that this will do no harm to the patient? There are also potential concerns of the immunogenicity of the outdated vaccine. The final decision to not tell the patient is not truly in the hands of the PA and nurse. The PA must uphold the values of the supervising physician; he or she should also be apprised of the situation and take part in the decision making. Lastly, the obligation of truthfulness with the patient is foremost; disclosing information in reference to an error is best. This shows honesty, which is in the patient's best interest.

With any situation there is bound to be special circumstances and distinctions that unfold and complicate the situation. These scenarios are presented to encourage providers to learn by example and to practice ethical standards as the basis for their actions to avoid such situations in the future.

CONCLUSION

Ethics are means by which actions are deemed right or wrong. The principal tenets of ethics serve to provide a basis for practicing in the best interests of the patient, provider, and society. This responsibility is essential to the success of the entrusting patient–provider relationship.

The physician assistant profession has in place a professional code of ethics that serves to guide the provider toward the highest moral standards of professional behavior. The provider must be familiar with this code and readily embrace the substance of these values to be an effective practitioner. Ethical decision making is a difficult process; having a grounded sense of these standards and an action plan in place will lead to a more successful decision-making process and, ultimately, practice.

Dealing with medical errors in a lawful, truthful manner is in the best interest of the patient, as well as one's own. Being accountable, ethical, and earnest places PAs in a favored light with the patients, physicians, and community in which they serve.

REFERENCES

1. American Academy of Physician Assistants. (2003). *From program to practice: A guide for PA practice.* Alexandria, VA:Author.

2. American Medical Association. Informed consent. Available at http://www.ama-assn.org/ama/pub/category/4608.html. Accessed September 19, 2004.

3. Garrett, T., Baillie, H., & Garrett, R. (2001). *Health care ethics principles and problems.* Upper Saddle River, NJ: Prentice Hall.

4. Sugarman, J. (2000). *Ethics in Primary Care.* New York: McGraw-Hill.

5. Sugarman, J. (2000). *Ethics in Primary Care.* New York: McGraw-Hill.

6. Sugarman, J. (2000). *Ethics in Primary Care.* New York: McGraw-Hill.

7. Sugarman, J. (2000). *Ethics in Primary Care.* New York: McGraw-Hill.

8. American Medical Association. Informed consent. Available at http://www.ama-assn.org/ama/pub/category/4608.html. Accessed September 19, 2004.

9. American Academy of Physician Assistants. (2003). *From program to practice: A guide for PA practice.* Alexandria, VA:Author.

10. Diekema, D. Mistakes. University of Washington School of Medicine Ethics in Medicine. Available at http://eduserv.hscer.washington.edu/bioethics/topics/mistks.html Accessed November 2, 2002.

11. Diekema, D. Mistakes. University of Washington School of Medicine Ethics in Medicine. Available at http://eduserv.hscer.washington.edu/bioethics/topics/mistks.html Accessed November 2, 2002.

12. Kohn, L., Corrigan, J., and Donaldson, M. (Eds.) (2000). *To err is human: Building a safer health system.* Washington, DC: National Academy Press.

13. Diekema, D. Mistakes. University of Washington School of Medicine Ethics in Medicine. Available at http://eduserv.hscer.washington.edu/bioethics/topics/mistks.html Accessed November 2, 2002.

14. Diekema, D. Mistakes. University of Washington School of Medicine Ethics in Medicine. Available at http://eduserv.hscer.washington.edu/bioethics/topics/mistks.html Accessed November 2, 2002.

15. Diekema, D. Mistakes. University of Washington School of Medicine Ethics in Medicine. Available at http://eduserv.hscer.washington.edu/bioethics/topics/mistks.html Accessed November 2, 2002.

16. Sholas, M. Honesty is the best policy when discussing medical errors. Amednews.com. Available at http://www.ama-assn.org/amednews/2002/11/04/prca1104.htm. Accessed November 3, 2002.

Index